Research Methods in Pharmacy Practice

Methods and Applications Made Easy

Research Methods in Pharmacy Practice

Methods and Applications Made Easy

Zubin Austin BScPhm, MBA, MISc, PhD, FCAHS
Leslie Dan Faculty of Pharmacy
University of Toronto
Toronto, Canada

Jane Sutton BSc (Hons, Open), PhD, CPsychol, AFBPsS
Visiting Research Fellow
Department of Pharmacy & Pharmacology
University of Bath
Bath, UK

For additional online content visit StudentConsult.com

ELSEVIER

ELSEVIER

ISBN: 978-0-7020-7426-4

Content Strategist: Pauline Graham
Content Development Specialist: Trinity Hutton
Senior Project Manager: Kamatchi Madhavan
Designer: Patrick Ferguson
Illustration Buyer: Nichole Beard
Marketing Manager: Deborah Watkins
Cover Illustrator: Hannah Family

Printed in China

Last digit is the print number: 9 8 7 6 5 4 3 2 1

Working together to grow libraries in developing countries

www.elsevier.com • www.bookaid.org

CONTENTS

FINDING YOUR WAY AROUND THIS BOOK

PART I: INTRODUCTION

Chapter 1: Introduction to research: evidence-based practice; why research is important in health care and pharmacy. History of research methods; social sciences antecedents; inspiration to ensure rigorous research; duty to patients and health care staff; a taste of what is to come in the book. Introduction to our case study pharmacists.

Chapter 2: Planning research: which methodology and method to use including practical and ethical issues. This chapter also includes a section on how to conduct a literature review and introduces the concept of 'theoretical frameworks'. Examples are provided of some of the more commonly used frameworks, e.g. Theory of Planned Behaviour, and examples of how such frameworks may inform research design are given. The chapter ends with some advice on how to frame your research question.

Chapter 3: Levels of measurement from questionnaires to interviews; choosing the appropriate level of measurement; generalisability, when it is essential and how to achieve it.

PART II: QUANTITATIVE RESEARCH: DATA COLLECTION & ANALYSIS

Chapter 4: What is quantitative research and when would you use it?

Chapter 5: Reliability and validity: how do you know you are measuring what you think you are measuring?

Chapter 6: Planning a survey, designing your questionnaire and setting up a database.

Chapter 7: Choosing your participants: sampling issues.

Chapter 8: Experimental design and randomised controlled trials: deciding what treatment works.

Chapter 9: Analysing your results: a step-by-step guide to the principles underpinning how to choose the right statistics to use.

Chapter 10: Descriptive statistics: how many people said what and who were they?

Chapter 11: Inferential statistics: what might their answers mean? Interpreting and reporting your data.

PART III: QUALITATIVE RESEARCH: DATA COLLECTION & ANALYSIS

Chapter 12: Qualitative research; what it is; examples of where it might be used; reliability and trustworthiness.

Chapter 13: Interviewing participants: listening to your participants' voices. This section includes advice on how to design an interview schedule; developing the skills to conduct an interview, e.g. listening and prompting and how to deal with difficult interviews.

Chapter 14: Designing and conducting Focus Groups: including the impact of group dynamics. Interpreting and reporting data.

Chapter 15: Observational research: key principles and different types of observation. Explanation of some ethical issues. Doing case study research.

Chapter 16: Data analysis and coding: understanding how to make sense of qualitative data. Coding and theming explained.

Chapter 17: Data synthesis and presentation of qualitative findings: how to draw different strands together. How to write up qualitative research.

Chapter 18: Other qualitative methods: participant-observer research, action research, grounded theory as alternatives. More ethical issues explained.

PART IV: MIXED-METHODS RESEARCH

Chapter 19: Mixed-methods research; arguments for and against mixing methods including some of the key debates in this area of research; advice on how best to combine different methods in one research project. When to use mixed methods and how. Synthesising the data: drawing your findings together into a coherent whole.

PART V: CONCLUSIONS

Chapter 20: Discussion of different methods for disseminating the results of research (e.g. publications, abstracts, presentations, posters, etc.), along with tips for optimising success in competitive situations. Knowledge translation.

Chapter 21: Conclusions and the way forward leaving you equipped to become a researcher.

Dear reader

As a pharmacy practice researcher who has historically had to use a wide variety of sources to continually develop his expertise I have great pleasure in writing the forward for a book which brings together a wealth of knowledge on how to perform pharmacy practice research.

Representing a monumental amount of work by both authors it fully draws on both of their research experience and expertise. The additional incorporation of their knowledge of apocryphal research stories further helps the reader to both contextualise concepts and recognise their importance within the paradigm of health services research. The regular use of case studies throughout the chapters provides readers with the opportunity to apply their newly gained knowledge.

Aimed at both novice and experienced researchers the book contains a wealth of useful information which can be used to help write a research protocol from scratch, enhance a developing protocol, inform an ongoing research process or support the process of critical appraisal of published research.

Not only does it provide clear and concise guidance on how to undertake health services research from a pharmacy perspective using a wide variety of approaches, it also explains many of the key concepts for which understanding is frequently just assumed.

In recognising and discussing those difficult issues which are continually under review and development within health services research the book enables the reader to appreciate the complexity within the field and the fact that such research is not formulaic. Decisions regarding research design frequently have to be made in the knowledge that they are imperfect but are believed to be the best option when considering both the pros and cons of that chosen approach in comparison to the others.

Written in an accessible and engaging manner this book is suitable for use by undergraduate, postgraduate and independent pharmacy practice researchers and is an essential text for all pharmacy-practice-based academics.

I very much hope that you enjoy both reading this book for personal development purposes and using it to enhance the quality of any pharmacy practice research within which you are involved.

Yours faithfully

David Wright
Professor of Pharmacy Practice, University of East Anglia,
Norwich, England, UK
Professor of Clinical Pharmacy, University of Bergen,
Bergen, Norway

PREFACE

What is research?

a. A hoop to jump through as part of earning a degree in pharmacy
b. Something other, smarter people do
c. A lot of fuss and bother to simply restate what's obvious
d. None of the above

Practice-based research is one of the great underexplored areas of the pharmacy profession today. Practitioners and students – just like you – are increasingly finding ways to participate in and to lead important interesting research projects that are based on their day-to-day experiences and observations in their workplaces. Practice-based research is not a new innovation: our colleagues in medicine, nursing, rehabilitation sciences, social work and many other health and care professions have engaged in practice-based research for years. Their work has led to significant innovations in workplace redesign, patient-care management, administration and management of health care facilities, and clinical practice. Without the contribution of practitioner-researchers to the scientific literature and the evidence base, evolution and improvements in health care delivery for patients would be severely constrained.

With the growing importance of the pharmacy professions within the health care system, there is a greater need than ever for pharmacists, students and technicians to take the lead in practice-based research. As pharmacists become more involved in direct provision of primary patient care services, as students become better trained and more integral to professional practice, and as technicians assume new roles and responsibilities in health care delivery, the entire profession must come together to better understand what works, what doesn't work, what can be improved upon, and what opportunities for quality enhancements exist.

If you answered "a", "b" or "c" to the multiple choice question above – this book is for you. Many of us have misconceptions and biases about what research is and whether we are capable of actually performing it well. Unfortunately, for some, research is something that other people do, something that we merely consume rather than produce. For others, research has become a make-work project or an administrative requirement for degree completion. For practitioner-researchers, there is frequently intrinsic pride and joy in the act of studying day-to-day practice, particularly when there is an opportunity for quality improvement or process enhancement.

If you answered "d" to the multiple choice question above – good for you! You are well on your way to having the kind of open-minded curiosity that is at the heart of what practitioner-researchers do. Recognising that you have many of the raw materials needed to be a good researcher is the first step in the process: having curiosity, being able to observe the world and the practice around you, not being satisfied with the status quo, believing that improvements are possible…all of these are the important starting reagents for research.

What we hope this book gives you is the leg-up needed to take these reagents and use them in a careful, deliberate and strategic way to help you take charge of your own research. Through a series of case studies drawn from our own experiences, we hope we can illustrate why research is important to pharmacy professionals, and how these professionals can and should lead research themselves. We have divided this book into several broad categories corresponding to quantitative, qualitative and mixed methods traditions. Some of you may naturally gravitate to one method over another, but we hope that this book provides you with some inspiration to explore new areas and avenues for inquiry that may not come as easily or naturally to you.

The pharmacy profession is undergoing significant evolution, and with this evolution comes abundant opportunities. Members of the profession must seize their own destiny and lead their own future in an evidence-based, rigorous manner. If we as pharmacy professionals are unable or unwilling to study ourselves, our practices and our processes – who else will? If we are disinclined to look for opportunities for quality improvement and practice change – others will determine our future for us.

Research is a powerful tool for helping us and our profession through this turbulent period of change. Rigorous, well-executed research is the cornerstone of the modern health care system and the foundation of all professional practice. It is also one of the most exhilarating and professionally rewarding activities that pharmacists, students and technicians can do to stay engaged and involved in their own profession.

We hope the book inspires you to consider research opportunities in your own practice and that it provides you with the knowledge, skills and confidence to undertake disciplined and rigorous inquiry in your own practice. It was our honour to write this book and it will be an even greater honour for us if you put it to good use!

ACKNOWLEDGEMENTS

Students and staff at the Universities of Bath (MPharm program) and Toronto (Pharm D program), for their inspiration and interest in this work, and for being effective sounding boards for our thoughts and writing throughout the process.

To Hannah Family for her ongoing support and for her incredible artistry in designing the jacket cover of this book.

To Martha Bailes for getting us started on this exciting project and for helping us through the early days of writing and revising.

To my parents, Dina and Hosie, for their support and love and for sparking a lifelong interest in learning and research.
Zubin

To Ken for all his love and support throughout my career.
Jane

Introduction to Research in Pharmacy Practice

LEARNING OBJECTIVES

After reading this chapter you should be able to:
- describe what research is
- understand the importance of research theories and their origins
- understand the importance of learning about research

- explain evidence-based practice and the 'cycle' of research and practice
- understand the pharmacist's duty to patients and other health care staff
- describe how doing research 'fits' in learning and practice

1.1. INTRODUCTION TO RESEARCH IN PHARMACY PRACTICE

Why should pharmacists consider practice-based research as a valuable tool for addressing problems and opportunities in their daily work? Why do pharmacy students need to learn about research methods? Pharmacists have long been consumers and supporters of research, and work within health care systems that recognise the importance of research in supporting clinical decision-making. As an evidence-based, scientifically oriented profession, pharmacy has always placed a great premium on high-quality, rigorous, defensible research as the core of professional practice, and pharmacists recognise that the **scientific method**, as detailed in **Table 1.1**, is a crucial tool for separating fact from fiction and opinion from belief.

However, for many health care researchers, including pharmacists, and in many circumstances, such a method alone is not sufficient for them to understand all aspects of patient care. To explore some of the more subjective aspects of health care, such as how people feel about being diagnosed with a health condition, or why they behave in a certain way, researchers often turn to theories and methods drawn from the **social sciences**.

Choices about the most appropriate way to find answers to research questions are informed by the way we think about how we know what we know, or **epistemology**: is there one truth or set of truths that can be revealed by using

the scientific method (**positivism**)?; or are there a range of truths that can be revealed, often simultaneously, depending on which point of view you take (**constructivism**)? If you think that, for a particular research question, you can find one right answer (positivist), you may feel you are best served by methodologies and methods underpinned by the scientific method, such as **experimental research** (see Chapter 8) and **quantitative analysis** (see Chapters 4–11). If, on the other hand, you think that there may be many possible answers to a particular research question (constructivist), and that these cannot be reached by using the scientific method, you may turn to approaches underpinned by social science, such as qualitative research (see Chapters 12–18).

It's useful to remember that all kinds of health care research, including pharmacy practice research, are informed by such ideas about how we are to use this knowledge and about how research should be carried out, which in turn influences the methodology and methods employed (see Table 1.1 below). Although these might seem like abstract considerations, this understanding of the way we think about knowledge and how to acquire it is essential because it directly influences the decisions we make about our research, and as you read through this textbook you will see how these **epistemologies** relate to two main categories of research – quantitative and qualitative.

In this chapter we will set the scene for this textbook by drawing on research theory and relating this to pharmacy

TABLE 1.1 Types of Research

Experimental Research Methods	Opinion- or Attitude-based Research Methods	Observational Research Methods
Involves the manipulation of quantitative, independent variables that can be analysed using scientific measurements, e.g. interval or ratio-based. Generally known as 'the scientific research method' as the researcher is using the data to test hypotheses. Requires rigorous design and can be very expensive to conduct.	Used to access people's attitudes towards something. Information is usually collected by means of a questionnaire which asks people to give their preferences or feelings. Measurement is usually arbitrary, using ordinal or interval-type scales. Not as exact as the experimental research but gives an idea of the intensity of people's feelings.	Involves as little intervention as possible and is used to obtain information about how people and/or processes work in practice in their natural setting. Such methods are the opposite to the scientific method.

practice to answer the questions raised earlier. The chapter provides an introduction to research and why it is important in health care and pharmacy. It will give a brief background to where 'doing' research came from and some of the theories that have been drawn from the social sciences and applied in a health care research setting. Above all the authors hope that this textbook will inspire readers to learn about research and to understand how to implement it in practice. The case studies which run through this textbook are described in detail in this chapter so that we can prepare you for what is to come. All of the concepts that are introduced in this chapter are explained in greater detail in subsequent chapters of this book, and you will be signposted to these. Throughout the book we will also signpost you to topics that will help you design and conduct the research that you are doing during your studies. This might be as part of a research project or work carried out when on placement.

1.1.1. Professional Standards to Be Met by Pharmacists in the UK

The General Pharmaceutical Council (GPhC) is the statutory regulator for pharmacists and pharmacy technicians and is the accrediting body for pharmacy education in Great Britain. The GPhC is responsible for setting standards and approving the education and training courses which form part of the pathway towards registration for pharmacists. The UK qualification required as part of the pathway to registration as a pharmacist is a GPhC-accredited Master of Pharmacy degree course (MPharm). Please see 'Future pharmacists: Standards for the initial education and training of pharmacists' (2011) found at http://www.pharmacyregulation.org/sites/default/files/GPhC_Future_Pharmacists.pdf

All Higher Education Institutions providing education for pharmacists must conform to the 10 GPhC standards

in terms of what is taught in the Master of Pharmacy (MPharm) programme. The GPhC is also responsible for the premises in which pharmacy is practised (e.g. community pharmacies) and the way that pharmacists behave in their dealings with patients and the public. It is recommended that all pharmacy students familiarise themselves with the GPhC standards and that students practising in other countries familiarise themselves with any equivalent regulation. Please see (http://www.pharmacyregulation.org/standards/conduct-ethics-and-performance) for more information. Standard 10 of the document 'Standards for the initial education and training of pharmacists' sets out the outcome levels that must be achieved by students doing the MPharm course. A number of these outcomes refer to activities that relate to research, because in many cases knowledge of research that has been conducted in pharmacy-related subjects is essential for pharmacy activities. For example, outcome 10.2.1.h states that by the end of their degree students should be able to provide evidence-based medicines information.

The GPhC standards for conduct, ethics and performance 'set out the behaviours, attitudes and values expected of pharmacy professionals and explain the standards that all pharmacy professionals must comply with. They also inform patients and the public of the standards that they can expect of pharmacy professionals.' (http://www.pharmacyregulation.org/sites/default/files/standards_of_conduct_ethics_and_performance_july_2014.pdf).

All pharmacy professionals must behave in such a way that patients and the public are treated safely and effectively. It does not matter what sector of pharmacy you work in, or indeed whether your job involves interaction with patients (e.g. providing advice to other pharmacists) you must comply with the GPhC standards.

There are seven principles that pharmacists must work to; as a pharmacy professional you must:

1. make the patients your first concern
2. use your professional judgement in the interests of patients and the public
3. show respect for others
4. encourage patients and the public to participate in decisions about their care
5. develop your professional knowledge and competence
6. be honest and trustworthy
7. take responsibility for your working practices.

In order to meet these standards it is essential that you have sufficient knowledge and skills to do evidence-based practice. One of the primary tools you will need to do this is to be able to appraise the evidence for and against different treatments and practices. You have a duty to keep yourself up-to-date with research as this will help you identify gaps in knowledge and care. You must be discerning in your use of published research to ensure that research findings are appropriately applied – you can only do this if you understand how the research process works.

1.1.2. Research and the Undergraduate Programme

In the UK the MPharm programme is usually delivered at a university. In most cases this is through a School of Pharmacy and so the term 'School of Pharmacy' will be used throughout this book and refers to any department of an academic institution that has been accredited by the GPhC to deliver the MPharm programme. Most schools of pharmacy include in their programme a period of study specifically set aside to conduct activities relating to research. In some schools this is during the fourth year of study and can take the form of a research project conducted by a group of students under the guidance of a supervisor who is normally a member of staff. In other cases students who elect to go on an overseas placement will be expected to write a report of their experiences and engage in some data collection relating to their placement. Not all MPharm students do a pharmacy practice research project. Many do a laboratory-based project where they conduct a project relating to their supervisor's area of research, and in this case they often do not have a choice about the nature of their project. Students who are doing a pharmacy practice project are often given some choice in the topic and design of their project. For example, some pharmacy practice supervisors may allow their project groups to come up with their own research question and others may suggest some research questions for their group to choose from. Thus, not all students will have the opportunity to design their own research project from start to finish.

In this textbook we set out the research process from the research question to the reporting of results, while accepting that not all students will see the process through from beginning to end. Rather, we expect students to dip in and out of the chapters that they find most useful to them. However, they may find other chapters helpful once in practice if they are involved in research in their place of work.

Learning about research does not just happen in one block towards the end of the MPharm programme. You will generally begin to explore issues relating to evidence-based practice from year one, and so this textbook can be used throughout your MPharm degree course and beyond.

1.2. RESEARCH, PHARMACISTS AND EVIDENCE-BASED PRACTICE

As consumers of research, most pharmacists are comfortable with the principles of evidence-based medicine. Whether working in collaboration with patients and families or carers, physicians, nurses and other health care team members, or practicing in a more autonomous (e.g. **pharmacist independent prescribers**) fashion and assuming sole responsibility for clinical decisions, pharmacists apply principles of evidence-based decision-making on a regular basis. More recently, however, pharmacists have begun to recognise the potential value of becoming producers of research, rather than simply consumers. As the complexity of clinical practice increases and the explosion of information continues (paradoxically leading to greater uncertainty and ambiguity), pharmacists are assuming greater individual and collective responsibility for decisions and outcomes. Pharmacists (along with other health care professionals) are increasingly required to move beyond currently available literature, research and evidence. Instead they must gather and interpret data from their specific local context as a way of better meeting specific, local needs and requirements. As discussed later in this chapter (see Section 1.4) the health care professionals doing the work can often produce the best research.

The case studies which are described in detail later on in this chapter are examples from different areas of pharmacy practice where student pharmacists might consider doing some research. To do this they or their supervisors will all have identified an area of their practice where they would like to know more in order to better understand medicines' use and patients' responses to it. Our case studies have been carefully designed to represent what students and pharmacists would do in real life, to show how understanding of research can help inform practice at different stages in the education of student pharmacists, and pharmacists in practice.

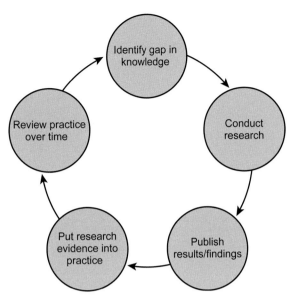

FIGURE 1.1 Cycle of research and practice.

The four case studies relate the experiences of two undergraduate students (Rosie and Serena), one postgraduate student (Dorothy) and one registered pharmacist (Sandy). Rosie is doing a research project in her final (fourth year) of studies and Serena (in the third year of her four year degree) wants to use what she has learned so far to help understand patient care in the pharmacy she works in at weekends. They will be working closely with their supervisors at university.

Dorothy and Sandy have been in practice for some time in very different areas of pharmacy practice. This means that they will be drawing upon the expert knowledge they obtained when in university, their experience of treating patients and their desire to continue their professional development and learn more to benefit their patients. Once they have conducted their research they will want to share their findings with other pharmacists, health care professional, patients, carers, researchers and other stakeholders. In this way a topic that was identified in practice becomes a piece of research and the findings are fed back into practice. Subsequently, another pharmacist or researcher or doctor or nurse may pick up this research and want to see if the findings apply in their own practice setting. We have called this process the 'Cycle of Research and Practice' and a diagram of this is given in Fig. 1.1.

1.2.1.   What Is Research?

Research can be described as a form of investigation into things that are happening in the world. In terms of the research described in this book pharmacists 'do' research to try to find out how things are done in a particular field of interest, why they are done and when, in order to be able to develop theories that might help them do things better in the future. This may seem like a very simplistic definition but doing research need not be a complicated process. In health care research we are ultimately trying to find better and more appropriate ways of treating patients so that they either recover completely or are able to live their lives with the help of medical interventions such as medication. It is also important to note that sometimes the best treatment option for certain patients may be no treatment. Research can help us to discover how to design treatment interventions that result in the maximum benefit to patients – either in large groups, e.g. patients with high blood pressure, or individual patients, e.g. one person's experience of being diagnosed with cancer of the bowel.

It is not necessary to be an academic researcher to do research. In some cases the people who do the most practical, applicable research are those who are working in the field of interest. Pharmacists are often the best people to identify needs in the populations they work with, e.g. identifying gaps in services or helping practices that find it difficult to conform to treatment, but with this comes the responsibility of creating guidelines to help assess if and how those needs might be better met. To be a researcher all you have to do is identify the needs, identify how those needs might be met and understand enough about research to be able to do some investigating for yourself – either alone or in collaboration with others.

Pharmacists are experts in medication, but research in pharmacy includes not only investigating how patients respond, say, to different medication options (or none) but also how pharmacists and their staff themselves do their jobs. During your training as a pharmacist you will learn (or will have learnt) about the anatomy and physiology of the human body and how drugs are developed to act on particular systems of the body. You will have been taught by people who are 'research active' – in other words people who are doing research into pharmacy and the pharmaceutical sciences as part of their job. The content of their teaching will likely be based on research that they or others have done, and so they are imparting to you the most up-to-date ways of doing things.

1.2.2.   The History of Research in Health Care and Pharmacy Practice

In 2005 the UK Department of Health defined health care research as 'research concerned with the protection and promotion of public health, research undertaken in or by the Department of Health, its non-Departmental Public Bodies and the NHS, and research undertaken by or within social care agencies' (https://www.gov.uk/government/uploads/system/uploads/attachment_data/file/139565/dh_4122427.pdf [Accessed 17_05_2015).

Health services research has a broad scope encompassing research conducted across all health and social care professions, but research into how to treat patients better has been done for a very long time. In fact the famous nurse, Florence Nightingale, conducted a significant amount of research into the prevention of infection and how best to treat wounds. Her work was conducted in the nineteenth century and was based on her understanding of what care was required by her patients. This put her in an excellent position to study innovations in health care. The research process is such that as work is carried out and shared with others, more research is done and thus our understanding of health care improves as time passes.

Pharmacy practice research as with other health care research may be best conceptualised as a continuum or a relay race, one in which individuals and groups build upon each other's work sequentially and in this way collectively advance understanding and knowledge within an area. This relay race may eventually lead to the design and testing of an intervention using gold-standard methods, or it may not. In either case, findings are still relevant and meaningful.

Of course, pharmacists do not work in isolation from other health care professionals. They generally work as part of a multidisciplinary team to a greater or lesser degree. For example, a hospital pharmacist will work with others every day, they will be part of a team of medical experts who work together to provide the best care for patients. On the other hand a community pharmacist may not have as much contact with other health professionals but will still be working with general practitioners and nurses at the very least. It is for this reason that pharmacists need to understand what other health care research is being carried out, how to interpret it and how to incorporate it into their own practice. Thus understanding what research is and how it is done in different disciplines is important because it enables pharmacists to 'borrow' research findings and ways of doing research from others. More about multidisciplinary research will be found in Chapter 2 (Section 2.5).

1.3. UNDERSTANDING THE RESEARCH PROCESS

The most important aspect of doing research is that it is done as well as it possibly can be. If you have not conducted your research properly your conclusions may be unsound, and any recommendations that you make on the basis of flawed results may have negative implications for both pharmacists and their patients.

To minimise the risk of this happening, we need to fully understand the research process and ensure that we conduct our research with 'methodological rigour' (see Section 1.4 and Chapter 2).

The research process broadly involves:
1. identification of the need for research
2. a literature review to find out what research has already been done into the topic of interest and how it has been conducted
3. development of the research question
4. identification of appropriate methodology and methods, e.g. theoretical framework
5. identification of participants
6. design of data collection instruments, e.g. questionnaire
7. obtaining research ethics approval as necessary
8. a pilot study of data-collection instruments
9. data collection
10. data analysis
11. discussion of findings in the context of existing knowledge
12. writing a report and disseminating findings.

All of the above steps are dealt with in more detail in subsequent chapters of this book (the outline of this textbook which is found prior to Chapter 1 will tell you where to find these). However, there are two **key points** about research that should be understood before embarking on the research process. These are the following:
- We need to find out what is already known about our topic of interest
- We need to understand how we know about the research topic and what theories, methods and analysis have been used by other researchers.

In order to understand these key points researchers have large amounts of information available to them through libraries, the internet and the media. It is essential that they can gather information together that is relevant to their research topic both in terms of the topic itself and how research concerning that topic has been conducted previously. The process of gathering information and sifting through it to make sure it is relevant to our topic of interest is called a literature review. The basic principles of doing a literature review are described briefly in the next section. A more detailed description of how to conduct such a review can be found in Chapter 2.

1.3.1. What We Already Know: The Literature Review

Researchers must understand and situate their work within the context. This is most frequently accomplished through a systematic review of the literature which allows researchers a better understanding of the contexts, theoretical frameworks, methods and approaches that have been used in the past. In many cases, the specific topic or problem of interest may not have been studied, but a variation on that theme will most certainly have been reported. Finding this work through a systematic literature search process is important as it can save the researcher valuable time and point him/her in a productive direction.

For novice researchers in particular, the literature review is an essential step in the process of framing a research question. Immersion in the literature can help inform selection of appropriate theoretical frameworks and can help refine and frame the research question. Novice researchers may be tempted to believe that the literature review should only be completed after a research question has been confirmed. Such an approach, however, means that the literature itself cannot play the role it should in helping to develop the question. The literature review should be conducted in a systematic way so that as much of the existing data as possible are included.

Researchers are not expected to cover everything in the world that has been written on their subject, but they should be up-to-date on the foundations of their research topic and theories that have been developed pertaining to it. If research is being conducted over a period of time then the literature review should be updated regularly and at the very least prior to publication. Preparation is probably the most important part of doing any research.

1.3.2. Research Theories and Their Origins

In Section 1 we put forward a definition of research as investigation into an area of interest but that investigation must be done in a way that can ensure that our results can be trusted. This means following certain protocols and rules about how to do research, and these vary depending on the research question we are trying to answer. Research questions are the springboard for research. If we don't ask the right questions about pharmacy practice and medications use, we can't improve patient care or the ways pharmacists do their jobs. In Chapter 2 we give some examples of the research questions that might be asked by our case study pharmacists.

Part of the process of doing research is to develop **theories** or build on theories already put forward by others – for example, that patients with a bacterial infection get better more quickly if they are treated with antibiotics than those who are not. Here we are trying to find relationships between different **variables,** e.g. bacterial infection and treatment using antibiotics. However, there might be other variables that affect the way infections respond to antibiotics amongst different people, so we must account for these when looking at the relationships of interest. For example, researchers might want to ascertain the relationship between patients' ages and their response to treatment with antibiotics.

Thus it is essential that we follow the principles which have been specified for doing different kinds of research. These rules have been developed over time and many of them come from both science and social sciences (see Table 1.1 on page 4). Examining treatment using antibiotics from a purely scientific stance might give researchers information about how many people recover from bacterial infection when treated with antibiotics. This would generally be done using a quantitative approach to research (see Section 1.3.3) which adopts the rules of scientific study including **generalisability** of research findings.

Science and social science provide frameworks or formal structures – a bit like scaffolding – for studying what goes on in a social system (e.g. a pharmacy) and how, for example, going to a pharmacist rather than a doctor for the treatment of minor ailments might affect the broader organisation of society as a whole. This might call for reorganisation of a health system including the allocation of resources. In these circumstances a different approach to research design possibly including qualitative methods (see Section 1.3.4) would be called for.

To return to the example of antibiotic treatment, overuse of antibiotics can lead to antibiotic resistance in the wider population. So the seemingly small act of prescribing an antibiotic for one person can have a profound effect on others. Researchers who work in the area of social sciences including psychology, sociology, economics and anthropology (to name but a few) have developed sets of rules to enable them to conduct their research. For example, an anthropologist would examine a research topic from the point of view of how people live within a particular culture and how this culture affects their susceptibility to illness and its treatment by less conventional means. In this case rules concerning cultural norms would be followed.

There are two words that need to be defined before moving on. These are **methodology** and **methods**. Methodology is the set of principles that underpin the way research is done. This might be whether the researcher uses a quantitative or qualitative methodology. The method is how the research is carried out, such as using a questionnaire to collect data or doing face-to-face interviews. Many methodologies have their roots in the science and social science paradigms and provide researchers with the rationale for doing a piece of research in a particular way. Sometimes researchers use more than one methodology in their research and you will find more about this is our final chapter.

In the next two sections we will introduce some of the different ways of doing research, and each of these is covered in more detail in later chapters of this textbook.

KEY TERMS

Methodology refers to the theory underpinning how and why we conduct our research in the way we do. **Method** is the way we conduct our research.

1.3.3. Quantitative Research Methods

Quantitative research (see Chapters 4 to 11) has its roots in the **positivist** approach to research. This **objective** approach is all about facts and relies heavily on the concepts of **validity** and **reliability** which are dealt with in detail in Chapter 5. Put simply, validity refers to whether the **results** obtained from research meet the requirements of the scientific research methods, e.g. does the questionnaire we are using to measure one of our variables measure what we claim we are measuring. Reliability is whether the way we are measuring something enables us to measure it time and time again and produce the same results. The important thing to remember about this method is that the aim is to collect enough data from enough people to enable us to generalise our findings across a wider population. You are probably quite familiar with quantitative methods of doing research and know that these involve counting, measuring and analysing sets of data, often using statistics to draw conclusions from that data. Some types of research that use quantitative methods are listed here:
- Surveys
- Experiments
- Randomised controlled trials.

Returning to the earlier example of antibiotic use, collecting sufficient information about how many people recovered from their bacterial infection, what (if any) treatment they received, and how long it took can enable us to say with a reasonable amount of certainty that people in general, when treated with the correct antibiotic, will recover. This in turn means that we can plan treatments and interventions that work.

In Chapters 4 to 11 we will take you through how to conduct quantitative research in a step-by-step way, including design of data collection materials, data analysis, setting our findings in the context of existing research and report writing.

KEY TERM

Positivist approach to research assumes that everything is measurable and tends to rely heavily on scientific research methods.

1.3.4. Qualitative Research Methods

Qualitative research (see Chapters 12 to 18) has its roots in the **constructionist** approach to research. This **subjective** approach is not generally about facts as described in quantitative methods but is about understanding peoples' experiences about a particular phenomenon. The approach has its roots in the social sciences when researchers began to realise the importance of understanding how human beings experience and interpret the world. The terms validity and reliability are not used in qualitative research but it is important that the trustworthiness of qualitative data is assessed and in Chapter 12 this process is described in detail. The important thing to remember about this method is that the aim is not to collect large amounts of data from which it is possible to generalise results to a wider population (although it can be possible to make some broad generalisations). Some types of research that use qualitative methods such as interviews and focus groups include:
- Framework analysis
- Content analysis
- Discourse analysis.

Results of qualitative research tend to be referred to as **findings** to help to distinguish the two types of research output. Qualitative methods generally use techniques such as face-to-face interviews or focus groups to draw conclusions about what people think and feel about certain phenomena. Again returning to the antibiotic example, qualitative methods can be used to find out how people feel about taking antibiotics and how much they know about antibiotic resistance. This in turn can inform, for example, how information is presented to patients when antibiotics are being prescribed.

In Chapters 12 to 18 we will take you through, in a step-by-step way, how to conduct qualitative research.

KEY TERM

Constructionist approach to research assumes that there is more to behaviour than can be measured or counted. How people think and feel is important.

1.3.5. How We Communicate What We Know: Writing Up Research

Once researchers have completed their work and have some results to share, decisions need to be made about how best to get these results to the people who can benefit from them.

1.3.5.1. Reports to Funding Bodies

If the research has been funded by an external body, e.g. Pharmacy Research UK, they will expect to receive a report of the research. The form this report takes will vary from funder to funder with some expecting two sides of A4 and others expecting a 25-page document. Once received by the funder the report may be placed on their internet website and hard copies may be sent to interested stakeholders such as the Department of Health.

1.3.5.2. Oral Presentations

Sometimes researchers are asked to give presentations to stakeholders such as patient groups, or to conference delegates. Presentations usually provide a 'snapshot' of part of the research as there would not be sufficient time to tell people everything.

1.3.5.3. Peer-Reviewed Journals

This involves the preparation of an article or paper that conforms to often very strict guidelines that are imposed by journal editors. It can take a long time – a year or more – to get a paper published in this way because the paper is reviewed by people who are experts in the same field as you are working in (thus your peers). Working with others who have experience of writing for journals is important if a paper is to be accepted for publication. Some journals have a higher readership than others and are given ratings such as '**impact factors**' and '**H factors**', so many researchers aim for publication in journals with a high rating. Please see the text box below for a brief outline of how these factors are calculated.

KEY TERMS

Impact factor is the average number of times the articles from a journal published in the last 2 years have been cited in the Journal Citation report (JCR) year. The IF is calculated by dividing the number of citations in the JCR year by the total number of publications in the previous 2 years.

'**H' factor** is based on the number of publications an author has and the number of times each article has been cited. It works only for people working in the same field of interest.

1.3.5.4. Web Pages, Blogs and Social Networking

Researchers work either individually or as part of a group and may have their own website that gives up-to-date information about their research. Some have **blogs** that are followed by interested people including patients and practitioners. These and social networking are excellent ways of reaching many people with your research findings, but remember, once research is out there it can change lives.

1.4. MAKING A DIFFERENCE: RESEARCH IN PHARMACY PRACTICE

As we have seen, pharmacists work in a variety of practice settings that may require them to identify and solve problems and apply principles of practice-based research. Thus any research must fit the setting and the population it is designed to help, so doing rigorous research that is meaningful to the patient population in pharmacy practice must be what drives us. At this point, let us introduce the cases we will be using throughout the book.

CASE STUDY 1

Sandy Sullivan is a pharmacist working in a primary care collaborative practice. In this setting, he works closely with general practitioners (family physicians), nurses, nurse practitioners, and other health care professionals. The practice is responsible for the care of approximately 10,000 patients, most of whom live in the local community and who have been coming to this practice for years. The community itself is quite multicultural and people from different cultural, ethnic, and religious backgrounds may have different health care needs (Further reading: Diversity and Ethnicity in Healthcare). Recently, Sandy has noticed there have been many more young patients (under the age of 25) being referred to him for education and medication counselling related to Type II diabetes. Sandy knows that this is a complex condition involving both physiological and psycho-social issues: diet, exercise and other lifestyle choices are as important for blood sugar control as appropriate use of prescribed medications. As a pharmacist, Sandy knows and understands the importance of good blood sugar control as a way of optimising long-term health care outcomes and facilitating 'healthy aging'. Sandy fears that many of these younger patients are less concerned about their health than they should be, and have a difficult time understanding the long-term health risks they may face if they do not control blood sugars in their teens and twenties. Sandy works hard to meet with patients, customise his counselling and education approach to the needs of his diverse patient group, but he notices that, for many of these patients, there is a deterioration in blood sugar control after working with the team, rather than an improvement as one would hope and expect. Sandy is at a loss to explain this, but recognises that it cannot be business-as-usual for the team. While they are doing what they were trained to do – including education, monitoring, follow-up, routine testing and evaluation of laboratory results – the outcome for his patients is not satisfactory.

As this case illustrates, some pharmacists become interested in practice-based research because of a specific need they have identified amongst their own patients. People become health care professionals because they want to help others and prevent/manage diseases like diabetes. As part of their education and training, pharmacists (like physicians, nurses, dentists and all health professionals) learn to apply evidence and translate scientific research into clinical care. This may be accomplished by, for example, following treatment guidelines and algorithms produced by well-respected professional bodies (such as Diabetes UK and its equivalent throughout the rest of the world), or by applying recently published evidence from clinical trials to a particular patient's needs. Most professionals have a belief that in following these practices and using these approaches, optimal health care for patients will follow. As Sandy has discovered, this is not always the case. Sandy's observations are starting to form a pattern, or a trend, one that can no longer be overlooked. If only one or two patients in this practice experienced a **paradoxical** decline in their blood sugar control, it may be possible to attribute this to random, patient-specific effects. Sandy's observation that 'many' patients seem to be experiencing this means he now has a professional (and personal) responsibility to investigate this further – and move from being simply a consumer of other people's research to being a practitioner who uses practice-based research to understand a disturbing phenomenon. His ultimate aim will be to improve the quality of care provided by the practice. For Sandy this will begin the 'cycle' of research to practice and back to research that we mentioned in Section 1.2.

CASE STUDY 2

Rosi Magruder is an MPharm student at the University of Fazakarly. She is in the fourth and final year of her studies and for her research project, her supervisor has suggested that she and her project group (four other MPharm students) explore whether there is a need and demand for an on-campus pharmacy to serve the needs of the 22,000 students and staff that come to the institution each day, as well as those in neighbouring communities. Rosi herself has often wondered why there is no 'model pharmacy' that would allow students like her to actually be able to practise pharmacy in a way that they have been taught. She and her team wonder if university students and staff – who they assume to be generally healthy – actually need, want and would use a campus-based pharmacy offering the highest quality pharmaceutical care available.

Although Rosi is working as part of a team we will just be following her as she conducts her project.

In this case, Rosi is dealing with quite a different situation to Sandy. For one thing she is still a student and her research does not have anything to do with the direct treatment of patients. While Sandy's situation is focussed on specific, identifiable patients within a practice, Rosi is exploring a situation that occurs at many universities and she wants to explore people's views rather than fixing a potential health problem that she has already identified.

Rosi has already learned a lot about doing research in her third year when she did a research methods module, and she is looking forward to doing some 'real-life' research over the course of a semester.

1.4.1. Research Design, Scope and Impact on Practice

The potential impact of Sandy's work could be significant, and could positively impact the practice of health care professionals and the care of patients. Both cases 1 and 2 illustrate critical concepts all researchers – including pharmacists – must consider. The starting point for most research is an observation, an incident, or some other event in a researcher's life that raises questions of some sort. For both Sandy and Rosi, there is an additional objective. For Sandy, it is quality improvement, an enhancement of the way things are currently being done within his specific contexts. For Rosi, she wants to do well in her project as it accounts for a big chunk of her marks for her final year.

While day-to-day observations are in fact a very powerful source of inspiration for researchers, they do not – by themselves – help researchers with their work. Translating observations into research questions is an important step in the process, allowing the researcher to clarify, specify, and appropriately narrow the scope and remit of the research in a way that is simultaneously meaningful and achievable. A question that is too broad (for example 'how can we make depressed patients feel better?') cannot be answered in a reasonable period of time. While the answer to such a question would, of course, be meaningful, it is not realistic and in Chapter 2 we will describe how to decide on or 'frame' a research question that will provide you with the answers you are seeking. We will frame a research question for each of our case study pharmacists and various ways of answering these questions will be given in each remaining chapter of this book.

Rosi's enthusiasm for tackling her research project must also be reconciled with a 'reality check'. It would be great to have all the time in the world to complete her project but she is time-limited and so needs to have a focussed research question to work with. An effective research question should also clearly be rooted in its own context, not an abstract, universal setting. On the other hand, Sandy's interests are in his patients and in their unique situations, stories and experiences. The work he is undertaking may or may not be relevant and applicable to others in different contexts; that will be for others to decide. Being clear in the scope of one's research – who it will address, who it will impact, and who it may benefit – is an important starting point for creating effective and clear research questions.

1.4.2. Improving the Quality of Health Care

As stewards of pharmaceuticals and the budgets that pay for them, hospital pharmacists face unique and growing pressures to balance different priorities. Pharmacists must, of course, be primarily interested in the wellbeing of their patients, and strive to ensure the most appropriate pharmacotherapy for each individual. Simultaneously, of course, they must also reconcile real-world economic and fiscal realities: around the world, pharmacists are increasingly being asked to 'do more with less' and recommend alternatives that can achieve an acceptable health-related outcome for patients while still minimising costs for governments, employers, insurers and other payers.

Pharmacists are uniquely well-suited for this important but difficult task: no health care system can be sustainable if every prescriber and patient had access to every medication she/he wanted. Focussing on what is actually needed and the most cost-effective and efficient mechanisms to ensure every patient has access to the medication she/he needs is a job well-suited for pharmacists.

Let's consider another case and pharmacy practice context where research may be valuable:

In such situations, the pharmacist's unique pharmacotherapeutic knowledge and skills can be **leveraged** to help frame research questions and objectives in a manner that respects the ethical requirements of the pharmacy profession. Simplistic budget-balancing and cost-saving exercises that do not fully address patient's health and medication-related needs will not, in the long run, address the problem Dorothy's hospital administrators are trying to solve: asking a pharmacist (rather than an accountant) to explore this issue is indeed a prudent and appropriate step. For Dorothy, the challenge going forward will be to apply her skills as a researcher and her experience as a clinical pharmacist in a way that balances many seemingly competing

---

CASE STUDY 3

Dorothy Tseng is a hospital pharmacist and part-time MSc in Health System Improvement working in a community hospital. Recently, the hospital has been struggling with budget issues, and hospital administration has asked the pharmacy department to identify potential opportunities for saving through the drug budget. As a pharmacist, Dorothy is aware that there are many opportunities for quality improvement in prescribing; in some cases, this may result in cost savings, but in other cases, optimal prescribing may actually result in drug expenditure increases even if there are savings in other areas (for example through decreased length of hospital stay). Her experience as a pharmacist has taught her the importance of not thinking of the drug budget in isolation from other aspects of the overall hospital budget, and to never forget the real objective is best possible care for each patient. As part of her MSc degree program, she is required to complete a research-based thesis; her workplace interests and needs have highlighted a potential area of focus for her work.

Through her years of experience and observation in the hospital pharmacy environment, Dorothy recognises that appropriate use of antibiotics is a particular challenge, both from a budget and quality perspective. Antibiotic prescribing is challenging: while best practice indicates that culture and sensitivity tests should be done prior to

prescribing, the practical reality is that it is often difficult to get results back in a timely fashion to support informed prescribing. As a community hospital, there are many time lags and process delays associated with ordering C & S tests, processing them in the lab, and communicating results back to the prescriber. As a result, many physicians rely on their intuition and experience and prescribe antibiotics 'empirically' without C & S test results. Frequently, this means that 'over-prescribing' is done: a more powerful, expensive, broad-spectrum antibiotic may be used just to be safe, when a more conventional, cheaper, and targeted antibiotic may be actually needed. When the results do come back, it can be very difficult to change, discontinue or modify the antibiotic that was initiated: there seem to be few good mechanisms for communication and effective process between the clinical laboratory, the prescriber, and the pharmacy, and everyone in the system seems loathe to change something that appears to be working. As a result, Dorothy believes there are opportunities for improving prescribing, saving money, enhancing process without compromising quality of patient care. As this project will serve double duty (both as her MSc thesis and as part of her day-to-day work responsibilities), Dorothy wants to ensure she approaches this problem and her ideas in a scientific, rigorous and defensible manner.

interests and objectives. Her findings will, no doubt, be controversial and spawn debate and discussion. Rigorous research can yield data that can be useful for defensible projections, to help different stakeholders better understand implications of findings and recommendations that Dorothy may be presenting.

1.4.3. Trying Out Research Skills in Practice

The purpose of conducting any research should be to further our understanding of a field of interest. As we have said earlier, many of the best research ideas come from practice and have the potential to save lives. Community pharmacies exist, as their name suggests, to provide a service to a local community. Often a pharmacy is the first place people go to when they have a health issue. Sometimes the advice they need may just involve reassurance, sometimes they need to be referred on to their GP and sometimes they can be helped by their pharmacist. Pharmacists working in community pharmacies can be isolated from other health care professionals and often have to make decisions about peoples' diagnoses and care on their own. During their studies MPharm students are taught how to respond to the symptoms described by their clients and once in practice this helps them to make the right choices.

Our final case study is another MPharm student who has a weekend job in a community pharmacy.

CASE STUDY 4

Serena Leesi is a 3rd year MPharm student with a Saturday job at her local pharmacy. She really enjoys working with the clients who come into the pharmacy and has got to know many of them who come in regularly. Some of the older clients seem to come in just for a chat and that's OK with Serena as long as the pharmacy is not too busy. Mrs Olive Trolave is one of the clients that Serena has got to know quite well and they are even on first-name terms. Olive is a 56-year woman who has struggled with many health issues, including respiratory disease, high blood pressure and high cholesterol. As she thinks about Olive, Serena realises that there are a number of clients like her who struggle with health issues, and what many of them have in common is that they need to quit smoking. Serena is interested in doing something concrete, practical and meaningful to help patients like Olive through the smoking cessation process. The generic tools and approaches she has learned at the university don't seem to be very effective for some reason.

Some of the approaches to smoking cessation are based on theories about getting people to change their health behaviours. In theory this sounds like a great idea but in practice, changing peoples' behaviours is no easy task. When it comes to smoking, people are often addicted to nicotine, but also smoke to help them get through their everyday lives. The tools and interventions that are designed to help people give up smoking must take into account individual circumstances. Serena knows that Olive has a tough time at home. Her daughter is a single parent who works full time, and Olive helps to look after her grandson by taking him to school in the morning and collecting him in the afternoon. Her health problems sometimes make her very tired so looking after a lively 5 year old can be exhausting. She also worries about her daughter, so sitting down with a cup of tea and a cigarette once they have gone helps her relax.

When Serena first began her studies she couldn't understand why anyone would do something that would be so damaging to their health. Now she realises that life is not so simple and understanding why people do the things they do is important to helping them change. Serena thinks that some of the problems with the smoking cessation approaches she was introduced to at university are that they don't take into account peoples' lives and the reasons why they may find it difficult to change. Research into behaviour change seems to be the way forward, but Serena wonders how much evidence there is for the effectiveness of some of the smoking cessation programmes in place in community pharmacies. Serena decides to read up on some of these theories but realises that she is not going to be able to just send out a questionnaire about peoples' smoking habits. What she needs is to see if she can get permission to talk to some of the pharmacy clients who smoke, to find out more about them.

For both Serena and Dorothy, there is an immediate concern or question about the quality of the research itself. For Dorothy, her findings will lead to recommendations that will have important implications for many people within her institution. These recommendations must be built upon a foundation of the highest-possible-quality evidence, and this fact raises the concern as to whether 'highest-possible-quality evidence' can actually be produced by a single pharmacist (or even a team of pharmacists) at a single community hospital. She may ask '*shouldn't such important decisions be based on REAL research that has been published, peer-reviewed and vetted, rather than on something me and my colleagues do?*' Similarly, Serena may ask herself whether research done on such a small scale can make a difference. Coming from a profession rooted in a scientific education, she has realised that the social sciences can help her learn more about Olive and other people who smoke. Qualitative research methods such as interviews, focus groups, or observations, can yield both valuable and respected data and will be the methods of choice to help Serena to begin to explore smoking cessation.

1.5.   LOOKING FOR THE TRUTH: THE REALITIES AND LIMITS OF RESEARCH

As scientifically trained health care professionals, it may be tempting for pharmacists to believe that unless the best-possible research design is utilised, research findings are either meaningless or severely diminished. Indeed, in everyday conversations one may hear pharmacists and other health care professionals dismissing certain types of research findings because the methods utilised did not conform to a perceived 'gold standard'.

For all four of our pharmacists – Sandy, Rosi, Dorothy and Serena – there is a legitimate and important concern expressed regarding the quality of evidence and how the research they undertake may be perceived and used by others. As students and pharmacists, all four are familiar with the traditional 'evidence chain', or hierarchy that has historically been used to interpret research findings within a clinical context.

The evidence hierarchy (Fig. 1.2) has a long tradition in pharmacy (and health professions education) as a tool for understanding the strength of findings and value of research, particularly within a clinical domain. Historically, the double-blinded, randomised, placebo-controlled drug trial has been viewed as the highest form of evidence, due to its perceived ability to compare alternatives, contain investigator bias, and demonstrate size or significance of differences between alternative options. In a clinical context associated with interventions (such as medication x vs medication y, or procedure a being compared with procedure b) this approach is both meaningful and clear.

It is important to recognise that the use of double-blinded, randomised, placebo-controlled drug trials does not happen quickly, nor is it the first research experiment undertaken with an intervention. Before getting to the stage where such a trial is even an option, researchers must painstakingly undertake many other forms of research. The evidence chain is often visually depicted as a pyramid precisely because there is a step-wise progression towards its peak. It is generally very difficult to undertake higher-level forms of research in a meaningful way without first having undertaken lower-level forms, to confirm or refute initial hunches or hypotheses.

None of our four pharmacists is in a position to undertake a randomised double-blinded placebo controlled trial – not only is such an experimental approach not feasible at their level, it is also not desirable. Without previous research, findings to support the design and development of specific interventions for comparison within such a trial, there is no point in simply selecting random interventions for comparison. Instead, in all four cases, there is significant value in undertaking other, different forms of research as a way of building the evidence chain itself.

Researchers understand that ALL research – including randomised, double-blinded, placebo-controlled research – has limitations. Good researchers understand, accept and (most importantly) articulate these limitations so that consumers of the research can better understand how it may (or may not) meet their unique and specific needs. No

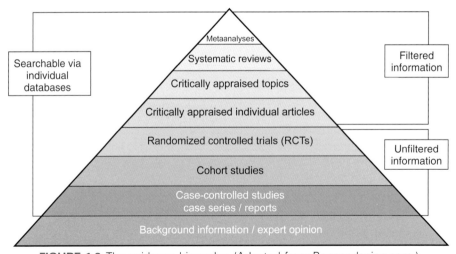

FIGURE 1.2 The evidence hierarchy. (Adapted from Boneandspine.com.)

research method is perfect, and no research findings can ever present 'truth' or an incontrovertible right answer. It is sobering and humbling (but important) for pharmacists and all health professionals to recognise that some of the greatest reversals in clinical practices have occurred precisely because gold-standard research was utilised. For example, randomised, double-blinded, placebo-controlled research that had been peer-reviewed and vetted in the 1980s and 1990s lead to broad recommendations that all women of menopausal age be placed on hormone replacement therapies as a way of preventing long-term health complications, and reducing mortality and morbidity. Pharmacists of that generation will remember the large volumes of prescriptions dispensed during that time of conjugated estrogen products or progesterone supplements. Later, other, different randomised, double-blinded, placebo-controlled, peer-reviewed studies emerged that came to precisely the opposite conclusion – and a clinical practice that had been widely adopted the world over abruptly reversed course.

As pharmacists and as researchers, one must always retain a healthy scepticism of any work that purports to reveal 'the truth'. At best, even the highest-quality research can only provide insights into the phenomena being studied and suggest alternatives for further exploration. Clinicians – or researchers – who follow findings of research with blind certainty often end up regretting actions taken and decisions made. A certain measure of humbleness in the face of the ambiguity and uncertainty that characterises both professional practice and life is usually warranted. If answers were easy to find, someone else would have already found them. Research is important precisely because it can help to address 'messy' issues that defy simplistic conclusions or solutions. The findings of research need not lead to categorical answers or perfect solutions in order to be valuable: indeed research that suggests it DOES lead to such answers or solutions should likely be regarded with

some suspicion. Researchers readily acknowledge their own limitations and the limitations of the research they are undertaking. They seek instead to understand their findings within the specific time, place and context it took place, and avoid suggesting their work may be universally applicable for all time.

For all four of our pharmacists there may be feelings of excitement, fear, dread, and optimism about the work that lies ahead. Most researchers experience the same mixture of emotions as they embark upon new projects. The opportunity to address observations or questions of personal interest or relevance, ones that build upon our own day-to-day experience of the world, can be exhilarating. At the same time, questions of one's capacity to undertake this work, or feelings of self-doubt about one's right to be called a 'researcher' can plague individuals, so much so that they simply stop and instead expect that others more qualified than them will take up this work. Practice-based research is important because the observations and experiences that drive the development of research questions come uniquely from practitioners, and not from professional researchers. While professional researchers can, of course, be an indispensable complement to a research team, the day-to-day experience of professional researchers is removed from the practice context itself. In this way, practitioner-researchers have an immensely important responsibility in identifying and leading the kind of research that addresses real-world situations and real-world problems.

Practitioner-researchers face unique ethical and professional obligations in their work that other professional researches may not experience. It is important to recognise that practitioner-researchers must always adhere to both general research ethics requirements as well as the unique and stringent ethical codes of conduct that govern practice of their profession. At times, this may lead to both difficulty and conflict. More about the ethics of doing research may be found in Chapter 2.

CHAPTER SUMMARY

- This chapter provided an overview of and introduction to some of the fundamental features of research in pharmacy to be found in this book.
- It looked at research in pharmacy practice and discussed why doing evidence-based practice is so important in pharmacy research.

- It introduced the basic principle of research including the history of health care research in general.
- It looked at the distinction between quantitative and qualitative research.
- Finally, it introduced the case study pharmacists who will join you on your journey through this book.

2

Planning Your Research

LEARNING OBJECTIVES

After reading this chapter you should be able to:
- understand the difference between methodology and method
- describe some of the practical issues that face researchers
- describe the ethical issues' importance to research
- understand the basics of conducting a literature review
- write a research question
- explain what a theoretical framework is
- describe the Theory of Planned Behaviour
- understand how the Theory of Planned Behaviour may be applied in pharmacy research

2.1. INTRODUCTION

Pharmacists and health professionals tend to be observant and curious individuals who seek to understand the patterns they observe in day-to-day life. From our observations and curiosity we build mental models, maps and theories for the purpose of explaining what we have observed and predicting behaviours and outcomes in the future. As such, most of us already are researchers of a certain kind, using the world around us as a basis for generating theories and models about the way things work.

While this natural inclination is a good starting point for research, it is rarely systematic, methodical or rigorous enough to be entirely trusted. As human beings, we are all subject to bias, stereotyping and misconceptions. Sometimes we see only what we want to see and overlook evidence that does not conform to our preconceived notions and ideas. As such, more formal mechanisms and controls are needed to ensure a certain degree of rigour, reproducibility and generalisability to our work. Building upon the natural strengths of observation and curiosity, and ensuring the very natural and human tendencies to overlook, stereotype or overemphasize do not cloud our judgement, formal research provides us with methods, tools and approaches that allow us to more effectively, accurately and precisely observe, measure, document and draw inferences about the world around us.

2.2. METHODOLOGY AND METHOD

Before continuing on the journey to become a researcher, it essential to develop an understanding of some of the key concepts and terms that will be used throughout, not only this book, but also the majority of research publications. The first is the difference between methodology and method which was introduced in Chapter 1.

2.2.1. Methodology

Methodology refers to the theory that underpins **why** and **how** research is conducted. Methodology is the theoretical analysis of a set of principles that underpin the way research is done. These principles give researchers a rationale for doing the research in the first place and, more importantly, this rationale is based on as much theory about doing the research that is available to us. For example, you might choose to collect data in a numeric way (how many people say or do things) and this would come from a *positivist methodology*. This will become clearer once you have read through this chapter, and in Section 2.3 you will find more about finding the right methodology for your research.

2.2.2. Method

Method is simply the 'recipe' for doing your research. This recipe will include the original idea for the research such as observing something in practice that you want to find an answer for, or a better way of doing things to improve patient care. This is then followed by a thorough literature review (see Section 2.4) not only of the topic of interest but how research about it has been done in the past.

The method for a piece of research might then proceed as follows:

1. Rationale: Literature review to define research question
2. Participants: Decide who is going to take part in your research
3. Recruitment: How are you going to find your participants and ask them to take part?
4. Data collection: How are you going to collect information from your participants, e.g. by questionnaire sent through the post or online (a quantitative approach), or by interviewing them about their experiences (a qualitative approach)?
5. Data analysis: Are you going to set up a database and input the information from your questionnaire or are you going to code transcripts from interviews with participants?
6. Results: How are you going to set your results or findings?
7. Discussion: How are you going to present the findings of your research and who will your audience be? In other words, who do you want to reach with your research so that they can increase their knowledge too?

Having a method to follow is essential as a guide to doing your research and means that you can be as sure as you can be that your results or findings can be trusted. Remember, the moment you publish your findings either formally (e.g. in a peer-reviewed journal) or informally (e.g. by sharing your research at your Local Practice Forum), peoples' lives may be changed as a result. The aim of conducting sound, rigorous research is to make sure peoples' lives are changed for the better.

2.3. PLANNING RESEARCH

Methodology and method are both included in the planning process. As suggested above, careful planning will ensure that the research is carried out well and that you will not find halfway through that you have missed something important. Take time with the planning of research and discuss your ideas with others both in practice and those working in research. It is also essential that you include stakeholders such as patients, carers, and other health care professionals in your planning. If you are applying for funding from, e.g. UK National Health Service, it will be a requirement that you include patients and carers at all stages of your research. This is called Patient and Carer Involvement and there are a number of organisations that can help with this. You will find lots of information

about this aspect of research in the United Kingdom at http://www.invo.org.uk/. This careful planning will help you to prepare a '**Research Protocol**' which is a document that sets out your research question and how it will be answered. We will refer to the research protocol throughout this book and in Chapter 19 you will find an example of a research protocol that one of our case study students, Rosi, has prepared.

Each chapter of this book covers a different way of doing research. However, regardless of the way research is done the above steps will be included in each. More detail about each of the steps is given in each chapter and related to the particular methodology and method used but the remainder of this chapter focusses on doing a literature review, framing a research question and deciding on which theoretical framework to use. At the end of Section 2.7 a research question is presented for each one of the case studies and in Section 2.8 an example of how to use a theoretical framework for each of the case studies is given. Before moving on to explore the literature review process in more detail there is one aspect of doing research that is of paramount importance and applies to every piece of research you will ever do. This concerns the ethics of doing research and what processes are in place to ensure your research is ethical.

2.3.1. Research Ethics

The issue of the ethics of doing your research is a very important one. Research ethics are the moral principles by which we decide which areas of investigation and ways of conducting research are acceptable and not acceptable. One of the issues you may encounter when you conducted your research project, for example, might be how to recruit participants who have mental health problems or who suffer from terminal illnesses. When it comes to the ethics of doing research things can become very complicated. Decisions need to be made as to what is acceptable for researchers to expect of research participants. There are rules about what we can and cannot do to human beings and animals in the name of research and other rules for the use of human body parts. There are also rules about what researchers can do with the information they collect in the course of their research and this is covered by legislation concerning data protection (see Section 2.3.2).

Readers who have studied psychology may be familiar with the Stanford prison experiment that was conducted in America in 1971 by Philip Zimbardo (http://www.prisonexp.org/). Zimbardo designed an experiment that involved two sets of participants (he called them 'subjects' which is strongly discouraged now) who role-played either prisoners or prison guards. Participants were recruited by advertisements placed in newspapers asking for male college students to take part in research into 'prison life'. The real reason for the research was to explore the interpersonal dynamics involved in the behaviours of the two groups. The experiment (again, it is not appropriate now to talk about experiments on human beings but we can take an 'experimental approach', see Chapter 8 of this book) was due to last for 2 weeks but it was stopped prematurely because of the escalation in behaviour of the 'guards'. The reference provided at the end of this chapter is a commentary by Zimbardo in answer to critics of his research.

SELF-CHECK QUESTION Go to http://www.prisonexp .org/ and read about the experiment conducted by Zimbardo. Consider whether the research was appropriate or inappropriate and why and then read the paper by Zimbardo (the reference for which is given at the end of this chapter).

There are now very strict guidelines on doing research, and it is essential that you obtain approval for your research proposal from an ethics committee. As a pharmacy student or pharmacist your research will most likely come under the banner of 'health services research'. Some ethics committees are run by specific departments in universities and hospitals and have a local role in approving research proposals. Others are made up of people in academia, science, medicine and patients, carers and stakeholders and are appointed by the Health Research Authority (http:// www.hra.nhs.uk/ England only) and other national bodies. If you are conducting a research project as part of your pharmacy training then your supervisor or tutor will generally guide you through this process and take the lead in applying for research ethics approval. This may not be the case in countries outside the UK so please make sure you know how things are done in your own university.

When considering whether it is acceptable or not to expect your participants to do certain things as part of your research, ask yourself how you would like to be treated yourself. For example, how would you feel if you were told the research was about one thing only to discover afterwards that it had a different purpose? Another example might be being asked about very personal issues, e.g. how a young woman might feel being asked about unwanted pregnancy and contraception.

2.3.2. Data Protection

The Data Protection Act 1998 is an Act of Parliament in the United Kingdom which regulates the processing of information relating to individuals, including the obtaining, holding, use or disclosure of such information. The Act

gives individuals rights of access in relation to personal data which is about them – which means that participants can ask for copies of personal data collected by a researcher. It requires that anyone who processes personal data must comply with eight principles, which make sure that personal data are:

- fairly and lawfully processed
- processed for limited purposes
- adequate, relevant and not excessive
- accurate and up to date
- not kept for longer than is necessary
- processed in line with your rights
- secure
- not transferred to other countries without adequate protection.

(See http://www.ethicsguidebook.ac.uk/Data-Protection -Act-111)

Section 251 of the National Health Service Act 2006 (which superseded Section 60 of the Health and Social Care Act 2001) deals with confidentiality of patient information. If research involves patients then they are covered by this Act. If your research does not involve patients but concerns other pharmacists or health care professionals they are still entitled to be treated in the same way, although this is not a legal requirement. Any information you gather as part of your research must be held in complete confidence and so you must not divulge that information to anyone. Below is some of the information that must be kept confidential:

a. Name, address
b. Job title and place of work
c. Any information that might serve to identify participants when research is published, e.g. names of other people or places.

2.4. THE LITERATURE REVIEW

In Chapter 1 we suggested that there were two key points about beginning the research process. These are:

1. to find out what is already known about our topic of interest
2. to understand how we know what we know about the research topic and what theories, methods and analysis have been used by other researchers.

This section outlines the procedure for conducting a literature review to show you how to gather the information you need to help plan your research project.

The Centre for Reviews and Dissemination (CRD) (https://www.york.ac.uk/crd/) is devoted to providing information to support health and social care research, and it is recommended as a resource for all researchers. The CRD website provides detailed information about conducting literature reviews of different kinds. Here we offer some steps to follow to help you to begin the process.

2.4.1.   Getting Started

Starting a literature review can be a daunting task so it is important to be clear in your mind what you are hoping to achieve. If the purpose of the review is to find out about a proposed research topic, e.g. when and how it was conducted and whether there are any gaps in knowledge that you might choose to do some research into. Sometimes researchers do literature reviews to provide others with an overview of the research that has been done on a topic and the CRD website (mentioned above) gives more information about these.

Following the initial review it is a good idea to ask other people who may be interested in your research to be on hand to read papers that you are unsure of or do not fully understand. At this point some quiet reflections on what you think are the expected outcomes of your review will be time well spent.

2.4.2.   Literature Review Protocol

Once the initial thinking is done a Review Protocol should be prepared. This sets out in advance how you will conduct your review and is rather like the recipe we mentioned for the methods used in your research. The protocol is for you to follow as you work through your review and will make the task easier. In Chapter 1 we used the example of some research into treatment with antibiotics and we will use this example again to illustrate the steps of the protocol. The protocol should include the following:

- Specification of the initial research question, e.g. do patients with a bacterial infection get better more quickly if they are treated with antibiotics than those who are not?
- Identification of research evidence, e.g. evidence for this would be research that has been conducted on patients with bacterial infections being treated with antibiotics
- Identification of study inclusion and exclusion criteria using **PICO** elements (see the Key Term box below), e.g. evidence would be **included** if it concerned treatment of bacterial infection with antibiotics and without but evidence concerning viral infection would be **excluded**
- How you are going to identify relevant literature, e.g. an electronic search using databases held by your university library
- How you are going to extract the information you need and draw it into a coherent report, e.g. start a table with headings about the research evidence you find and add the information from the research papers to it. (See example table at the end of this chapter).

> ## KEY TERM
>
> **PICO**: This is a technique used in evidence-based practice to help health care researchers to frame their research questions:
> P = patient, problem or population
> I = intervention
> C = comparison, control or comparator
> O = outcome

2.4.3.   Critical Appraisal

Many pharmacy students will have been introduced to critical appraisal early in their studies, and it is a skill worth learning if you are to do evidence-based practice. The more practice you get of doing critical appraisal, the better able you will be at appraising the research of others. Do not underestimate the importance of this because it is the basis for evidence-based practice.

The CRD recommends the following criteria for critical appraisal of research evidence:

- Was the review question clearly defined in terms of population, interventions, comparators, outcomes and study designs (PICO)?
- Was the search strategy adequate and appropriate? Were there any restrictions on language, publication status or publication date?
- Were preventative steps taken to minimize bias and errors in the study selection process?
- Were appropriate criteria used to assess the quality of the primary studies, and were preventative steps taken to minimize bias and errors in the quality-assessment process?
- Were preventative steps taken to minimize bias and errors in the **data extraction** process?
- Were adequate details, e.g. how many participants there were, how were they recruited, presented for each of the primary studies?
- Were appropriate methods used for data synthesis? Were differences between studies assessed? Were the studies pooled, and if so was it appropriate and meaningful to do so (more about data synthesis will be found in Chapters 11, 19 and 20)?
- Do the authors' conclusions accurately reflect the evidence that was reviewed?

There are a number of tools freely available for use in the critical appraisal of research evidence, and some of these can be found in Research Resources at the end of this chapter.

2.4.4. Identifying Research Evidence

Here are some ways of identifying research evidence:

- Searching electronic databases such as PubMed and Emerald
- Visually scanning reference lists from relevant studies
- Hand searching key journals and conference proceedings
- Contacting study authors, experts, industry, and other organisations
- Searching relevant internet resources
- Citation searching
- Using a project internet site to canvas for studies.

2.4.5. Keeping a Record of References

There are a number of ways of keeping records of the references to research evidence that you find. This is just like the list of references at the end of a journal article but you will be keeping it for your own use. Our advice is to make a record as you go along otherwise the task can be very difficult. Keeping accurate records of all the references you use is one of the ways you can avoid **plagiarism** (intentionally or unintentionally passing someone else's work off for your own).

Again tools for managing references can be found in the Research Resources section.

2.4.6. Study Selection and Data Extraction

Keep copies of all of the studies you select as evidence for and against your chosen topic. You can use the PICOS elements for this and make a table to enter all the information you need from each study. This will include the results of the study, how the study was carried out, how many participants there were and **demographic details** such as age, sex and education of your participants.

2.4.7. Drawing Data Together and Writing It Up

You may find that you need to keep more than one table of the data extracted from your literature review. This is because you may find that you are identifying different types of paper and different types of research. For example, you might want to create a table of studies that use quantitative methods and another for those that use qualitative methods. This way it is easier to compare and contrast different studies. If you do find this useful it is wise to keep these separate but to write up a brief summary of your findings. These will give you the information you need to make the decision to proceed with your research or to abandon the idea. If you proceed, then the literature review summary will end with your proposed research question.

2.5. THEORETICAL FRAMEWORKS

2.5.1. What Is a Theoretical Framework?

A theoretical framework is a diagram or description of how the variables in a research project might 'fit together'. Such a framework (as the title suggests) must be based on theory, and this is where an understanding of methodology is important (see next section). As we suggested in Chapter 1, if research is not based on solid theory both in its research questions and in the way it is conducted, we cannot be sure that our findings are as accurate as they possibly can be. For example, our pharmacist Sandy (Case Study 1) had noticed that the blood glucose levels of some of his younger patients seemed to be poorly controlled. If he just assumed that the fact that he had noticed this in a few patients meant that it was true of all patients, then any intervention he made would not necessarily be accurate. Sandy will need some hard evidence that young people are really not controlling their blood glucose and then try to find out why (Fig. 2.1).

Interestingly, whether we use the term or not, all of us are familiar with theoretical frameworks in our day-to-day lives: briefly, they provide a particular perspective, or lens

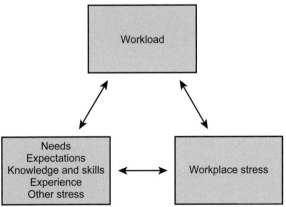

FIGURE 2.1 Example of theoretical framework showing the potential relationship between pharmacists' job satisfaction and workplace stress. The above figure shows that there might be a relationship between pharmacists' workload and workplace stress but we are not sure which direction the arrows will go in. In other words we are not sure what causes what. In our theoretical framework we would include some background theory about workload and stress, possibly drawing on previous research that has been conducted in other areas of health care, e.g. nursing, medicine. The diagram will help us to specify the factors we need to take into account when exploring our research question.

through which we examine a topic. All of us must filter the world we experience in some way in order to make sense of it – without such filters, the onslaught of data from everyday life would become paralyzing. For many of us, the lens (or filter or framework) through which we experience our world has been constructed based upon our own experiences, education, background, values, culture and preferences. Such everyday frameworks exist but are rarely articulated or described. Without them, we would have no way of knowing what matters to us, what is of importance in a particular circumstance, and what can be safely discounted or ignored because it is simply background 'noise'.

An everyday example of how such frameworks influence our thinking and behaviour can be seen in the way interprofessional teams function. We all carry with us a model, framework or mental map about how our world functions; this applies to the physicians, pharmacists, nurses and other health care professionals on a team. Part of this mental map – or framework – involves our understanding of our own role and where we fit in within the hierarchy or pecking order of the team. For many of us, this framework may be constructed and clouded by emotional or psychological issues. For example, if one's internalised framework of professional authority is a pyramid, with the physician on the top and everyone else below, it is likely this framework will lead to a series of behaviours, e.g. deference to authority, unwillingness to correct a physician, lack of confidence in presenting one's views. Conversely, if your internalised framework is built upon the notion of expertise, you will recognize that pharmacists have much more formal university-based education around medications and medication use than physicians. Consequently, the behaviour that flows from this framework will likely be more confident, more open, more willing to challenge and debate medication-related issues. When we fail to reflect upon, critically self-assess, and articulate the frameworks which shape our interpretation of the world, we deprive ourselves of the opportunity to improve and advance.

2.5.2. Borrowing From Other Disciplines

Researchers must use frameworks of a more theoretical nature to facilitate the sorting of data that is part of the research process. Within pharmacy practice research, theoretical frameworks usually come from other disciplines: for example, sociology, psychology, anthropology or economics. These social science disciplines have long established and articulated frameworks for helping to interpret and explain the world around us. In general, researchers gravitate to a particular discipline's theoretical framework out of reasons of personal interest, academic background or

previous experience, though there is no reason to limit oneself to one particular approach.

2.5.3. Practical Application of Theoretical Frameworks

A framework can yield important and interesting insights, but it is impossible to examine an issue using all possible frameworks. Researchers must therefore make careful and informed choices about the frameworks that will guide their work. The selection and articulation of a theoretical framework is frequently the single most challenging aspect of the research question development process, so time and careful attention are recommended. One of the outcomes of a literature might be that you find a new framework for doing some research that can bring new insights into a research pharmacy practice issue. This can be as simple as finding that nurses experience barriers to implementing research in practice and using that information to find out if pharmacists do too.

2.5.3.1. Case Study Example

Consider the case of our pharmacist Sandy Sullivan who has observed in his practice an increasing number of younger patients presenting with type II diabetes. This is an observation that is of relevance to his professional work and also of personal interest to Sandy: as a pharmacist he recognizes this is a problem that requires intervention, but as a person, he is concerned about the lives and futures of so many young people that may be affected by this chronic condition. As he sets out to examine this issue, he will need to identify and articulate a theoretical framework that will serve as a lens for interpreting the environment and what he finds.

He could explore this issue from a **socio-economic perspective** thus examining the issue through the lenses of poverty and disparity and their impacts on diet, exercise and health. Alternatively, he could examine this issue from a **psychological perspective**, through the lens of personal beliefs about illness and health, and influences of peers on behaviours such as eating and physical activity. As another alternative, he could examine this issue from an **anthropological perspective** to understand the role of culture in shaping behaviours that influence health outcomes within his multicultural community.

2.5.4. Right or Wrong?

As the above example illustrates, there are no right or wrong theoretical frameworks: each framework by itself provides an important but incomplete insight into a problem or situation. A single theoretical framework cannot possibly 'explain' everything about a situation or problem, but it can help us to better understand it. Clearly articulating our framework so that readers of our work can understand our perspectives and interests is important. Applying established theoretical frameworks that have stood the test of time, that have been used in diverse settings, and that have an established track record of success in helping us to better understand and interpret problems and situations can go some way to ensuring that our research is rigorous.

Sadly, there are no lists of theoretical frameworks from which someone new to research can choose. If you are a pharmacy student the training you have during your studies will be invaluable in highlighting how much you will need to know about doing research in practice. Once you have started to practice as a pharmacist there may not be very much time to go back and study, so make the most of the resources you have in your department or university. Most university departments collaborate with each other and so you have the opportunity to learn from other disciplines such as social sciences, about how to apply theoretical frameworks.

Examples of theoretical frameworks from psychology are those that concern behaviour change. As pharmacists, one of the challenges might be coming to an understanding of why people do/do not do something if they know it will be bad for them. Why do people still smoke? Why don't they take their medicine . . . get more exercise . . .? To begin learning, consider the recommendations of the Further Reading section of this chapter, as a way of learning more.

We will then give examples of how this framework could be used to help our case study pharmacists plan their research. First, however, we need a research question.

2.6. THE RESEARCH QUESTION

Most practitioner-initiated research begins with observations and attempts to solve real-world problems rooted in a particular work-related context. The day-to-day realities of professional work – whether it is in a clinical patient-facing environment or another area – provides both the inspiration for research and the tools required to undertake a successful project. A critical first step in the process is the importance of actually converting observations and insights into research questions.

The research question is frequently the starting point for pharmacy practice research. It is easy to underestimate the time and difficulty associated with developing a good research question, but experienced researchers recognize this investment of time and energy is essential. Many good ideas for research will founder when research questions are too big, too vague or too complex. In moving from observations to questions, researchers need to be mindful of the principles of framing a good research question.

Good research questions should:

a. reflect a topic of legitimate interest to the researcher
b. be grounded in a theoretical framework
c. build on work that has previously been done without duplicating it
d. provide a fresh perspective on a topic
e. address a topic or problem of relevance
f. be ethically appropriate and defensible
g. clearly define the constructs being used
h. clearly define the variables being examined
i. be scaled appropriately – small enough to be answerable but large enough to be manageable.

2.6.1. Crafting a Research Question

At first glance this list may appear long, but it reflects the importance of taking sufficient time and care at the outset to carefully craft a research question that will form the foundation of a research project. Failure to craft a good research question can lead to problems with the research process itself: poorly written research questions can create confusion, lead researchers into blind alleys or produce findings that are not actually the interest or intention of the researcher.

Good research questions are generally crafted over a period of time in an iterative fashion. Pharmacists new to research in particular may benefit significantly from the opportunity to work with another more experienced researcher to refine ideas and thoughts: 'bouncing ideas' off another person and asking that person to point out flaws, inconsistencies, discrepancies or ambiguities is an essential discipline even for the most experienced of researchers. Few researchers (if any) would have the confidence to craft a research question entirely on their own: to be credible, research must be able to withstand external scrutiny and criticism, and this process usually begins with the research question itself. In the following section we set out some guidance on how your research question should be written.

2.6.2. Interest and Enthusiasm for Your Research Topic

The research question should reflect a topic of legitimate interest to the researcher. Research can be a painstaking and laborious process, particularly when it is done in a rigorous manner. Many interesting ideas and observations that spawn a research question are never followed through due to lack of conviction on the part of the researcher. In most cases, practice-based researchers have a strong personal or professional interest in the question and topic being researcher: this provides the psychological energy and tenacity necessary to withstand the various challenges that all research will present. Novice researchers are well advised to honestly self-appraise their commitment and investment in a topic: disinterest or ambivalence about a topic – simply not caring very much about what is being researched or what the answers may be – is an important cue to reconsider the topic before more time and energy is invested. Knowing you are actually interested in the problem itself and feeling a personal connection to it makes the process sustainable, enjoyable and even exciting!

2.6.3. Building on the Work of Others

The research topic should be grounded in theory (see Section 2.5), and the research question should build on work that has previously been done. For example, it can be useful to partially duplicate work that has been done by other health care professionals, such as nurses and doctors, to allow for comparison with findings from a pharmacy sample. Building on the work of others and using their published work to inform your own is not plagiarism as long as the original work is appropriately acknowledged and referenced. Most research is an accretive process: this means that researchers build upon each other's work over time, even if they are not necessarily working together in a common cause. In virtually all cases, researchers can connect backwards to similar work that has been done by others and can connect forward to support those who in the future will carry on this work. Building on previous work is an important objective for researchers and an important criterion for a good research question.

2.6.4. Providing a Fresh Perspective

The research question should provide a fresh perspective on a topic. For both novice and experienced researchers, there is great enthusiasm and excitement in embarking upon a new project. The thought that it may be possible to contribute to making the world a better, healthier place, is both inspiring and humbling. Novice researchers frequently simultaneously overestimate and underestimate the potential contribution they can make. For the most laudable of reasons, novice researchers may amplify their enthusiasm in a way that suggests it actually is possible to solve the problems of the world: more experienced researchers recognize the complexity of systems, the intractability of many problems, and the value of addressing difficult situations in a step-by-step way. Small steps are still important even if they do not command the interest or attention one anticipates.

Practitioner-researchers are uniquely well positioned to contribute meaningfully because their context is the real-world, patient-facing practice within which problems and solutions meet. Practitioner-researchers bring unique and important experiences and background to problems. While they may lack formal research training, their perspectives are essential and may be something that more experienced non-practitioner researchers actually lack. The partnership of practitioner and professional researchers can be particularly fruitful for both parties and can lead to long-term collaborative relationships.

2.6.5. Relevance of Research Question

The research question should address a topic of relevance, and a literature review will help to determine this. Researchers need other people to help them by either participating in their work, or facilitating access to information or resources. Either way the research question must resonate with others as being something worthwhile that they want to be part of. Working with others is as important to the research process – and the research question – as anything else. While you may be inspired and enthused by your research, others may not find it so engaging. Learning to 'sell' ideas to others is a crucial part of working together.

The remainder of this section is devoted to framing a research question for each of our case studies.

> **SELF-CHECK QUESTION** Before reading the research questions that follow go back to Chapter 1 and re-read Case Study 1. Think of how you might frame a research question for each one. There are no answers for this SCQ but an example of how Sandy might develop his possible research question is given below.

2.7. CASE STUDY EXAMPLE RESEARCH QUESTIONS

The process of crafting a good research question is as much art as science. It requires patience, honest self-appraisal, a critical eye, and the ability to respond well to feedback from others. The best research questions evolve over a period of time, in response to other people's feedback and new insights and findings from the literature and the environment. Do not expect that the first research question you ask will ultimately be the research question that will guide your work: the time and energy invested up-front in shaping and refining a research question will pay off in the end through a more effective and efficient research process.

To illustrate this, let us consider the interests facing one of our four pharmacists from Chapter 1:

2.7.1. Case Study 1: Research Question

Recall that Sandy is a primary care pharmacist concerned about the number of young patients being referred to him for education and medication counselling related to type II diabetes. Sandy has noticed that other young patients' blood sugars have also deteriorated. As a pharmacist this frustrates and alarms Sandy as he contemplates the public health consequences of uncontrolled diabetes amongst younger adults. Sandy's initial recognition of this potential problem has prompted him to consider doing some research that might help identify the problems. Sandy's initial question might be '**How do I design an intervention to improve patients' blood sugar control?**'

As a practitioner, it may be understandable for Sandy to want to begin with the question 'What are we doing wrong?' Although this is a natural question it may not be anything that Sandy and his team are doing wrong that is affecting peoples' blood sugar control.

As a first step, Sandy needs to confirm that his observations (and the conclusions he has drawn from them) are accurate, after all where would be the point in asking his patients about their diagnosis and their blood sugar control, when he has no hard data to show whether or not the **anecdotal** evidence he has is accurate.

He could do this by:

- beginning a literature review looking at data about type II diabetes in young people to see if he can find data to compare with what he is observing in his own practice
- conferring with colleagues within his own practice or in other practices in his city
- confirming through the above means that there is indeed a problem or situation that warrants further work; a single person's unconfirmed perceptions of a problem may simply be skewed interpretation rather than an actual issue.

If after doing some background work Sandy finds that there is something unusual about blood sugar control among younger adults within his practice, it allows him to frame his observation in a more effective manner. It also leads him to recognise that he is dealing with an enormously complicated situation involving multiple stakeholders with different needs and perceptions. First, there is Sandy and the other practitioners in his practice but there are also the patients themselves who may not think they have a problem.

Sandy has noticed during his interactions with young adults with diabetes that many of them do not really seem to think of it as a disease, nor do they perceive any urgency or consequences associated with it. Whatever the reason for this attitude, Sandy has noted how difficult it can be at times conveying the seriousness of the diagnosis to many of his patients.

Rather than defining this as the problem Sandy 'knows' it to be, he begins to wonder if uncontrolled blood sugar 'feels' like a problem to his young patients. What do they think about this? How do they respond to the well-meaning but sometimes unsolicited advice provided by Sandy and his colleagues? Sandy remembers being that age and not necessarily believing, trusting or even listening to what adults told him would be good for him – could it be possible that his patients actually aren't listening and frankly are tuning-out when he speaks to them? As Sandy thinks through this situation from the patients' perspective, a new question emerges for him: '**How do my patients feel about their diagnosis of diabetes and the need for consistent blood sugar control?**' With this re-framing of his interests, narrowing of his question and more clear direction, Sandy now can embark on his own clarifying process to further refine and narrow the question.

2.8. CASE STUDY EXAMPLE THEORETICAL FRAMEWORK: THE THEORY OF PLANNED BEHAVIOUR

The Theory of Planned Behaviour (TPB) was put forward by Ajzen in 1991 (see Further Reading). It is one of a set of models or frameworks that were designed to try to explain human behaviour in a health context. In other words, why some people continue to do things that they know are bad for them and others seem to be able to change their behaviour relatively easily? The core assumptions of these kinds of models are that (a) human behaviour is potentially modifiable and (b) peoples' beliefs about health affect their behaviour over time.

A diagram of the TPB is given below (Fig. 2.2).

The TPB suggests that actions are based on belief that behaviour will:

- lead to outcomes which people value (attitude towards behaviour)
- be valued by others (subjective norm)
- be possible, because people have access to resources (perceived behavioural control).

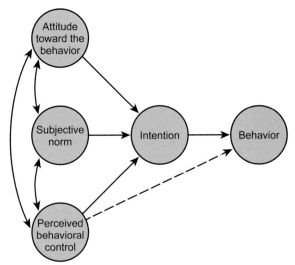

FIGURE 2.2 Theory of Planned Behaviour. From: Ajzen 1991.

The three factors above all predict behavioural intentions, which in turn predict actual behaviours. Perceived behavioural control (PBC), the extent to which we have control over our own behaviour, can have a *direct effect* on behaviour without **mediating effect** of intentions. For example, a mother or father of young children may find it difficult to see how they can fit in a healthy diet around catering for the children and being on the go all the time. They may think they do not have control over their own situation because the children's needs come first. Understanding that there are ways of catering for everyone and providing support to do that may help them to shift their thinking and feel that they do have some control over their situation after all.

Each element of the framework will be described in more detail in Sections 2.8.1 and 2.8.2.

The TPB has been applied widely in health research:

- Smoking, alcohol consumption, sexual behaviours, health screening attendance, exercise, food choice, breast/testicle self-examination.

Not every theoretical framework or model works in all contexts and there are other health-related frameworks, e.g. The Health Belief Model (Further Reading: HBM and Stages of Change), that will do a better job in some circumstances. A significant amount of research has been done using the TPB and on the plus side it has been widely tested and successfully applied. It also incorporates the important cognitive variables that are believed to be involved in health decision-making. Another plus is that it takes into account the roles of social pressure (e.g. what others think of us) and past behaviour (e.g. having tried to give up smoking in the past and failed).

Some criticisms of the model are that intention does not always result in actual behaviour. We only have to think about all those broken New Years' resolutions! It also does not look at peoples' beliefs about the **amount** of control they have over the behaviour in question. There is also some confusion about which order peoples' health beliefs come in and what beliefs cause what behaviour. Having said all this, it is a very good example of a theoretical framework that can help to explain some of the things that make people do the things they do (or not).

Case study 1 (Sandy) is again used to show how the TPB might be used in pharmacy practice research.

2.8.1. Theory of Planned Behaviour: Case Study 1

Sandy's research question is '**How do my patients feel about their diagnosis of diabetes and the need for consistent blood sugar control**?'

Sandy has done his literature search and review and found that how people feel about a diagnosis and how they behave as a result of the diagnosis is affected by many things. A friend who is trained in psychology has suggested he tries using the TPB to help make sense of what his patients might be feeling and explain why some of them are not controlling their blood sugar as well as they might.

Remember, Sandy is trying to understand how his patients feel about having a diagnosis of diabetes and the need for consistent control. So if he is going to use the TPB as a theoretical framework to help answer his research question he is going to have to try and put himself in their shoes.

To make this easier to conceptualise we have one of Sandy's patients, Julia, to help us. Sandy has got to know Julia quite well over the past year and has noticed that she has put on weight recently. He has a chat with her to find out how she feels about her diabetes and its control.

Julia is 26 years of age and was diagnosed with type II diabetes 1 year ago. At first Julia had her blood pressure well under control, though she didn't like being labelled 'diabetic' at her age. Over the past 6 months she has found it harder and harder to stick to the diet that the doctor gave her to follow and thoughts about having diabetes and what the future might hold intrude regularly in her daily life. Julia thinks now that she is going to just get on with her life and eat and drink what she likes. After all she misses out when she goes out for a meal with her friends and can't have what she wants to eat and drink. The trouble is, since she decided to do this she has piled on the weight and her doctor has suggested she might lose a few pounds because it would help with her blood sugar control. She is not sure how she feels about this.

After talking to Julia, Sandy writes down how he thinks Julia might be feeling and using the TPB as a guide, tries to explain her behaviour (Fig. 2.3).

Sandy realises that if he can gather information about all the young people in his practice who have type II diabetes, including those whose blood sugar is well controlled, he might be able to design an intervention for those with poor control and test it to see if it works. His psychologist friend has told him that there is a questionnaire (see Further Reading) that asks people about all of the aspects of the TPB and so he could use this in his research.

There is significant value in adopting an existing, well-validated framework that uses a questionnaire to tap the concepts it holds. Firstly, being well validated the TPB can be used in a number of settings and there is enough evidence in the literature to suggest that researchers can use it with some confidence. There are, however, always limitations to theories and these need to be thought through and acknowledged in any publication of research findings. Secondly, it provides a framework by which to plan your research and highlights the fact that behaviour change is

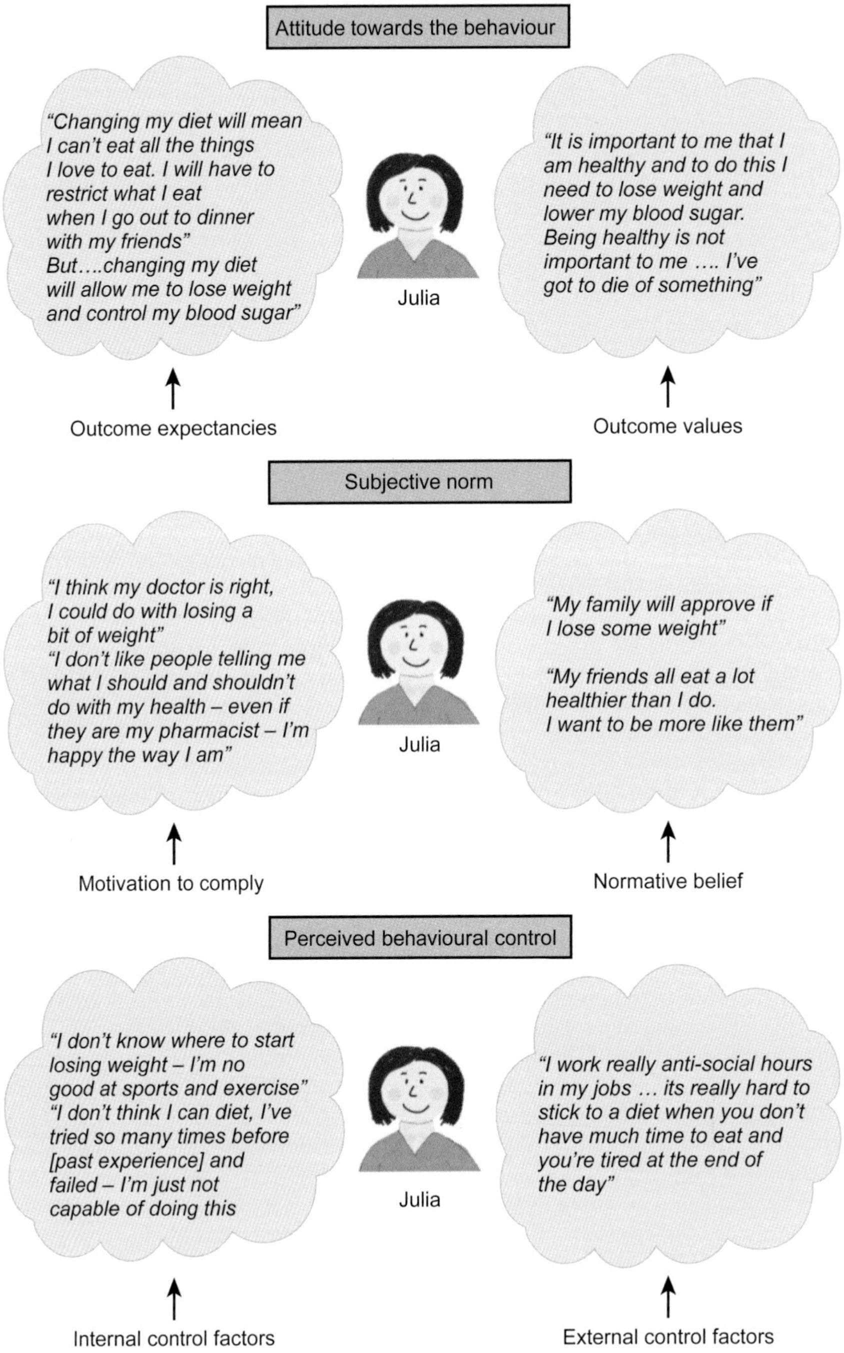

Attitude towards the behaviour

"Changing my diet will mean I can't eat all the things I love to eat. I will have to restrict what I eat when I go out to dinner with my friends" But....changing my diet will allow me to lose weight and control my blood sugar"

Julia

"It is important to me that I am healthy and to do this I need to lose weight and lower my blood sugar. Being healthy is not important to me .... I've got to die of something"

↑   ↑
Outcome expectancies   Outcome values

Subjective norm

"I think my doctor is right, I could do with losing a bit of weight" "I don't like people telling me what I should and shouldn't do with my health – even if they are my pharmacist – I'm happy the way I am"

Julia

"My family will approve if I lose some weight"

"My friends all eat a lot healthier than I do. I want to be more like them"

↑   ↑
Motivation to comply   Normative belief

Perceived behavioural control

"I don't know where to start losing weight – I'm no good at sports and exercise" "I don't think I can diet, I've tried so many times before [past experience] and failed – I'm just not capable of doing this

Julia

"I work really anti-social hours in my jobs ... its really hard to stick to a diet when you don't have much time to eat and you're tired at the end of the day"

↑   ↑
Internal control factors   External control factors

FIGURE 2.3 In each of the above Julia is supposed to be thinking about her choice between two options for each one (attitude towards the behaviour, subjective norm, perceived behavioural control). Courtesy of Dr Hannah Family.

no easy task. If as pharmacists you are aware that the issues that affect the way Julia behaves also affect many of your patients, then you will be able to do research that has better real-life application.

CHAPTER SUMMARY

- This chapter has introduced the terms 'methodology' and 'method'.
- It looked at planning research including ethical considerations and data protection.
- It introduced the basic principles of conducting a literature search including the importance of critical appraisal.

- It looked at how to use a theoretical framework to clarify the things we want to research.
- It looked at how to write a research question using one of our case study pharmacists as an example.
- Finally, it introduced the Theory of Planned Behaviour and gave examples of how this might help to explain patients' health behaviours.

FURTHER READING

Theory of Planned Behaviour
Ajzen, I. (1991). The theory of planned behaviour. *Organisational Behaviour and Human Decision Processes*, *50*, 179–211.

Health Psychology
Morrison, V., & Bennett, P. (2006). *An introduction to health psychology*. Edinburgh: Pearson Education Ltd.

Health Belief Model
Rosenstock, I. M. (1974). The health belief model and preventive health behaviour. *Health Education Monographs*, *2*, 354–386.

The Stanford Prison Experiment
Zimbardo, P. G. (1973). On the ethics of intervention in human psychological research: With special reference to the Stanford Prison Experiment. *Cognition*, *2*(2), 243–256.

RESEARCH RESOURCES

https://www.skillsyouneed.com/learn/academic-referencing.html

Levels of Measurement

3.1. WHAT IS MEASUREMENT AND WHY IS IT IMPORTANT?

As any carpenter (or chef) knows, it is best to 'measure twice and cut once'. For researchers as well, measurement is critical to a successful outcome: without careful consideration of both the instrument used to measure and the nature of the measurement itself, results may be compromised. Measurement is used in both quantitative and qualitative research but not always in the same ways. For example, information collected by means of a questionnaire asking people to say 'Yes' or 'No' to each question is one form of measurement that would provide us with little more than a set of numbers. However, we could also use qualitative face-to-face interviews to explore peoples' feelings about things and then count up the number of times each interviewee mentioned a particular word or phrase. We could then set this in the context of how a group of people viewed a particular life/world event, e.g. what it feels like to be diagnosed with high blood pressure, and get a more complete picture of peoples' experiences.

Measurement is a central component of statistics, and statistics are an important part of our everyday life. Whether we are considering the weather, our bank balances, course grades, or personal health parameters such as blood pressure and temperature, statistics are critical to the collection, organisation, analysis, interpretation, and presentation of much of what we do. Statistics focus on the numerical rather than the qualitative and while this is important, in many cases (as mentioned above) it may present an incomplete picture.

EXAMPLE

If we were interested in understanding how satisfied customers of community pharmacies were with the services and care provided, we could ask a general question such as 'Rate, on a scale of 0 (not at all satisfied) to 5 (very satisfied) the quality of the interactions you have had with a pharmacist' (see below). While such a question would yield valuable quantitative data, it can only partially answer a complex question related to customer satisfaction. This is because the reasons behind the number are not gathered through this question. In other words, if a customer indicates they are not at all satisfied, as providers of health care we should be asking 'why?' See Section 3.2.6 for more information on this type of scale.

Please tell us how satisfied you are with the quality of care you have received from your pharmacist. We would like you to use the rating scale below to rate each of the next 5 visits to your pharmacy on a separate scale. The scale runs from '0' – 'not at all satisfied' to '5' – 'very satisfied'.

Visit 1

0	1	2	3	4	5
Not at all Satisfied		Neither Satisfied Nor Dissatisfied		Very Satisfied	

In Chapter 6 you will find more guidance on the wording to use in the design of questionnaires.

We will be giving you examples throughout this chapter to help you better understand each of the concepts of measurement. In the final section we will look at two of the case studies in depth and apply the principles of measurement to them. This will enable our case study pharmacists to think about the design of their measurement tools to facilitate the most accurate and applicable responses from the participants in their research.

3.1.1. Descriptive Statistics

Descriptive statistics are techniques and procedures used to organise or summarise a set of measurements: as the term suggests, descriptive statistics 'describe' measurements. In the example above, descriptive statistics may provide us with a mean (or arithmetical/mathematical average), a mode (most frequently occurring number) and a median (or middle-point of the data set). These numbers could then provide us with some sense of general satisfaction – and the descriptive statistics utilised would have been a useful tool for helping us to organise, summarise, compare and describe a specific measurement.

If the mean, mode and median were all the same (as one might predict if a very large number of customers of community pharmacists were asked a vague question such as 'Are you happy with your community pharmacy?'), we may start to draw some conclusions from the data about the respondents and their preferences. In Chapter 10 of this textbook you will find more detailed explanations with examples of descriptive statistics.

3.1.2. Inferential Statistics

Inferential statistics, as the name suggests, allow us to 'infer' or 'read-into' the results from a sample, producing broader findings applicable to the larger population from which the sample was drawn. In the example above, the mean and median may be similar but there may be two distinct modes representing two groups of customers – one group that is very satisfied and one group that is very dissatisfied. Mathematically, these two groups may balance one another out and give the appearance of general moderate satisfaction. However a deeper look at the numbers might provide us with further insights that warrant follow-up. In Chapter 11 we will explore inferential statistics in greater detail and find out how we can look more deeply at the numbers.

3.2. CLASSIFYING MEASUREMENTS

Measurement is most typically thought of in terms of quantifiable, observable traits or features of a person or object; for example, the height of a child or a volume of milk required for a recipe.

3.2.1. Levels of Measurement

In statistics, measurements may be thought of more broadly and are more frequently referred to in terms of 'levels of measurement'. When we want to measure something it is essential that we do so in a way that means other people know how they have been measured and that we can measure them again in the same way if we want to. For example, the level of measurement for a child's height would be numeric and could be in feet and inches, metres, centimetres, etc. It is essential that researchers understand the implications of their choices, and recognise that problems might inadvertently arise if levels of measurement are not taken into accounts.

3.2.2. Discrete and Continuous Variables

One frequently used method for differentiating amongst measures is to consider the type of variable involved. A variable may be thought of as the thing that we want to measure (e.g. the height of children) – it changes (or varies) based upon different factors, and in measuring the variable, we hope to get a better understanding of these factors and their influences and impacts. So if we were measuring the height of children at different ages and wanted to look at differences in the height of boys and girls, height, age and sex would all be our variables of interest. Variables are frequently categorised as being either discrete or continuous, and some of the things we measure can only fit one category.

3.2.2.1. Discrete Variables

Discrete variables are measurements that fall into fixed categories: for example, Yes/No or Male/Female. When working with discrete variables, we must take care to ensure the variable of interest is indeed as fixed as the researcher believes. For example, sex variables (Male/Female) which are considered to be fixed may not be as certain as once thought.

3.2.2.2. Continuous Variables

Continuous variables represent measurements that occur along a continuum; while there may be fixed points along that continuum, the variable (measurement) itself can be ever so slightly more or less than that point. Examples of continuous measurements include temperature and height.

The measures we use must align with the variables of interest; in general (though not always) **nominal** and **ordinal** level measures tend to be utilised where the variable of interest is discrete, while **interval** and **ratio scale** measures tend to be utilised where the variable of interest is continuous.

Further details about these different types of measures are provided below.

3.2.3. Nominal Measures

Nominal measurement (also known as '**categorical measurement**') is most appropriate in circumstances where the item of interest clearly and distinctly clusters into identifiable, discrete groupings. Examples of nominal measures may include, for example, age ranges or answers to 'Yes/No' questions. Implicit in the use of nominal measurement is the idea that there is no specific connection or relationship between 'Yes' and 'No' – there is a clear and distinct difference and individuals understand how they stand. In the example above, a nominal measurement question may be 'Are you satisfied with the quality of service and care you receive from your community pharmacy? – Yes or No'.

In situations where the choice is indeed clear-cut and the respondents are indeed decisive, nominal measurement may be appropriate. In the last example above, it may not be so appropriate. As you may have already realised, nominal measurement may 'force' respondents to pick an option that does not completely and accurately characterise their true experience. While nominal measurement has the advantage of simplicity and seems to frame things definitively, we must be careful in using and interpreting nominal measurement. There is a danger that nominal measurement inappropriately forces a certain kind of response and we might be missing what people really think. Using nominal measurement to categorise chronological age ranges may be appropriate, as there is no risk of forcing an incomplete response – there is generally no argument about how old a person it is. In other circumstances (for example categorising individuals as 'male' or 'female', or based on race/racial categories) it is essential to recognise that individuals themselves may resist traditional simplistic categorisation. In other words, some people do not want to be labelled as one thing or another. Nominal measures are most valuable at helping researchers find indications of differences between individuals and groups; nominal measures by themselves are not helpful in indicating the direction or magnitude (amount) of that difference.

3.2.4. Ordinal Level Measures

Ordinal measures are used when the objects of measurement have an inherent connection or relationship with one another. It is sometimes referred to as rank-ordering. For example, ordinal measurements are used when assigning awards in an athletic competition (e.g. first vs second vs third place). Ordinal measurement has a qualitative component to it, insofar as 'first' is generally accepted to be better than 'third'.

EXAMPLE

If we were interested in finding out the age range each one of our participants was in we could use a nominal scale to do this. By putting participants into age ranges it means that we don't need to have their exact age. If we had 200 participants who answered the age question we would need some way of categorising them so that we could use age range to compare with, say, the number of times people visit a pharmacy.

Our question might look something like this assuming that all of our participants are aged 18 years or older:

Please indicate which age range you are in by ticking the relevant box below:

☐　18–23
☐　24–29
☐　30–35
☐　36–41
☐　42–47
☐　48–53
☐　54–59
☐　60–65
☐　66–71

Over 72. Please give your age here_____

We have chosen to use a range of 5 years for each category but you can extend or reduce that range to suit your needs.

3.2.5. Understanding Differences

Ordinal measurement helps us to understand that there are differences, in this instance, between the pharmacies being studied as well as pointing to the direction of that difference (e.g. better or worse). Ordinal measurement does not, however, provide us with an indication of the amount or magnitude of difference. In many league tables, sporting events and popularity contests, the difference between first, second and third place is frequently vanishingly small. Nonetheless, most of us will remember who won a gold medal whilst forgetting the bronze medal winner who was a fraction of a second behind.

3.2.6. Likert Scales

One particular type of ordinal measurement should be highlighted. Likert Scales are a frequently utilised tool that can be used to enable individuals to assess things that are essentially qualitative, in a quantitative manner. Likert Scales are frequently used in health care practice (for example, 'on a scale of 1 to 10 with 10 being the worst pain imaginable, how much pain are you in?') and in practice-based research

EXAMPLE

Let us return to our example related to measuring satisfaction of customers with community pharmacy services. We may ask research participants to name/ identify all the pharmacies they have used over a period of time then rank them from best-to-worst in terms of service, care, quality, etc. These results in turn could be used to generate league tables or popularity charts to guide customers in knowing which other people believe are the 'best' and 'worst' pharmacies.

To do this we could begin with a list of pharmacies – we will just call them 'Pharmacy A', Pharmacy B' etc.

The question might look something like this:

Below you will find a list of pharmacies in your area. We would like you rank these in the order of 'best' service with '1' being the 'best' and '6' being the 'worst'. Please only use each number between '1' and '6' once.

☐ Pharmacy A
☐ Pharmacy B
☐ Pharmacy C
☐ Pharmacy D
☐ Pharmacy E
☐ Pharmacy F

If a participant thought that Pharmacy C was the 'best' then they would put '1' in the tick box for Pharmacy C and so on.

EXAMPLE

To help us to understand the magnitude of the difference we could ask people to score each pharmacy out of 10 for service and such a scale would look something like this:

Below you will find a list of pharmacies in your area. We would like you to rate these out of 10 for the level of service they provide.

☐ Pharmacy A
☐ Pharmacy B
☐ Pharmacy C
☐ Pharmacy D
☐ Pharmacy E
☐ Pharmacy F

If a participant thought that Pharmacy C provided a really good service they might give them a score of '10' in the tick box. Using this measurement scale all pharmacies could score 10 whereas in the previous example we are forcing participants to indicate differences in rank, even though some of them may be equal in the service they provide.

(for example, 'on a scale of 1 to 10 with 10 being the best pharmacist imaginable, how good is your pharmacist?'). It is important to acknowledge that questions such as these, despite being framed in a quantitative/numerical way, are actually qualitative and subjective – the assignment of a number to an essentially qualitative experience (such as pain or satisfaction) does not fundamentally change the nature of the experience to a quantitative one. With a Likert Scale the basic difference *between* the numbers on the scale is assumed to be the same but not the *size* of the difference. Further, each individual will interpret this type of 1–10 scale based on their own experience only. Therefore, it is not reasonable or statistically possible to compare responses across different individuals. The fact that Sam rates his pharmacist as '8' and Joanne rates the same pharmacist as '4' does not mean that, on average, that pharmacist is a '6'. Similarly, if Sam rates his pain as '8' and Joanne rates her pain as '4' it does not mean that Sam is in twice as much pain as Joanne. All we can possibly conclude is that if the next day Sam rates his pain as '4', he may be in half as much pain as the day before, with no reference at all to Joanna's pain. Recognising that Likert Scale responses only represent ordinal (or rank-ordering) measurement is important, as there is a tendency to distort or amplify the significance and meaning of such data. Finally, a Likert scale is used alongside other questions – in other words, in a questionnaire that has a number of questions that relate to each other in some way. The answer to each question or 'item' in the scale is added together (summed) and then the mean scores are calculated for each set of answers. Further reading on these and other types of scales can be found at the end of this chapter.

3.2.7.   Likert-Type Scales

Just to makes things even more complicated there are also rating scales that are used in similar circumstances to Likert scales but they are not true Likert scales. The difference is when a scale is used for a single item in amongst other questions, using different levels of measurement, it is a Likert-type scale (again, see Further Reading for more on Likert and Likert-type scales). So, a Likert-type question might be used in a questionnaire to collect information about respondents' demographics (see Section 3.2.8 for an example of a Likert-type scale).

3.2.8.   Interval Level Measures

Interval measurement uses a scale which represents quantity and scaled units ('intervals') to facilitate truer comparisons between items being measured. Temperature scales (Fahrenheit and Celcius) are examples of interval measures, where 0 is not necessarily the absolutely lowest value but simply a point on a scale. Like nominal and ordinal measures, interval measures are useful for describing differences; like ordinal measures, but unlike nominal measures, the interval measure can also indicate the direction of differences (higher or lower). Unlike both nominal and ordinal measures, interval measures can actually be used to indicate the magnitude or amount of difference between measures, and consequently can provide us with different insights into things we are measuring.

Consider, for example, the difference between 10 degrees and 25 degrees. The information provided by that type of measurement ensures we dress appropriately for the circumstance. Had temperatures been reckoned as a nominal measure only (e.g. Warm vs Not Warm), we would likely dress inappropriately far more frequently as the subjectivism and lack of specificity of only two temperature categories would be insufficient to guide our behaviour. Similarly, if temperature were reckoned ordinally, where 'first class weather' was >25 degrees, 'second class weather' was 15–25 degrees and 'third class weather' was <15 degrees, we would likely dress somewhat more appropriately than with nominal temperatures but still there would be too great a range within each category to be truly helpful. The continuous quality of interval measures facilitates the more nuanced understanding of an important phenomenon – like weather – which in turn can be more helpful at shaping our responses.

EXAMPLE

Consider our previous example of measuring customers' satisfaction with community pharmacists' services. An interval scale measurement of this phenomenon may ask 'How frequently does the pharmacist provide you with advice about your medications?' using a 0 to 10 or more scale to indicate such frequency in a given time period. While superficially this may resemble a Likert Scale (insofar as there is a 0–10 scale involved), note the important difference: interval measurement in this case is directly connected to the question being asked (frequency of an activity) which is an observable, verifiable behaviour with less subjectivity than that associated with generic satisfaction questions. In this instance, if Sam answers '8' and Joanne answers '4' it means that Sam has received advice twice as often as Joanne (since the interval scaling represents equal increments or units). See Section 3.2.8 for an example of this type of scale.

3.2.9. Ratio Scale Measures

Ratio measurements are similar to interval measurements in that they also present quantities using scales (equal increments or units); the major difference for ratio measures is the meaning of 0. For ratio measures (such as physical measurements, e.g. height, weight or blood pressure) 0 represents an absolute bottom below which no measurements can occur. It is not possible to have negative height, weight or blood pressure. The availability of an absolutely bottom (or starting point, or 'floor' below which no measurement is possible) means ratio measurements can be interpreted and compared against one another in a more meaningful manner. Thus, ratio measures not only indicate differences between things being measured, but also the direction of that difference, the magnitude/amount of that difference and with reference to an absolute bar or starting point.

EXAMPLE

Using the example of satisfaction with community pharmacists' services we could ask customers to tell us how many times a week they visit their pharmacy. This question asks respondents to respond in a 'measurable way' and the measure has a true zero. Sometimes the question is presented in an 'ordinal' way with ranges but the ranges can still be treated as a ratio scale measure when doing data analysis.

3.3. MEASUREMENT ERRORS AND THEIR CONSEQUENCES

The quantitative nature of measurement – and the resultant number that is reported – can be powerfully seductive to many of us. Numbers provide us with an illusion of certainty and accuracy, when in fact all measurement is a combination of multiple factors that may include 'noise' or errors.

3.3.1. True Score Theory

True Score Theory is a powerful model that helps us to understand that all measurements – no matter how painstakingly undertaken – will be subject to variation and error. Mathematically, True Score Theory is depicted as:

$$X = T + e(x)$$

where X is the observed measurement (or score), T is the hypothetically 'true' level and e represents random error. Random errors are critical features of measurement because they are a reality of life, and failure to consider random errors (or at least the possibility that random error may contaminate or influence a measurement) frequently leads to problems.

3.3.2. Random Error

Random error is generally defined as any factor that is neither predictable nor controllable that can influence or affect measurement. Examples of random error include the influence of mood on final examination grades: as any student knows, one's psychological state of mind (or mood) immediately before and during an examination can wreak havoc on memory, problem-solving and other important factors influencing successful test taking. Despite completing all homework, readings and assignments in a timely and complete fashion, a student may experience a random event. For example, travel problems, an argument with parent or significant other or getting wet feet after being caught in the rain, immediately prior to an examination might make the student feel so uncomfortable that it could affect their performance in the exam.

Random error may inflate or deflate performance on any specific occasion thereby affecting measurement. The same day you experience wet feet prior to an examination, your neighbour may have won a small prize in a lottery, thereby inflating her performance. The critical feature of random error is that over a group of individuals – a **sample** or a **population** – it may have a sum of 0: in other words there are as many ups as downs. As a result, random error may add variability to measurement data but does not actually or necessarily affect the mathematical average/mean measurement for the group. The overall distribution (or spread) of measurements across the group may be broader due to random error, but the average itself may remain unchanged.

3.3.3. Systematic Error/Measurement Bias

In contrast to random error, we must also consider systematic error, also referred to as measurement bias. Systematic error results when an external, uncontrollable but somewhat predictable factor influences measurement. Consider the case of a group of students taking an examination. If, every half hour, a church bell rings loudly right outside the exam room and it distracts students, this may result in an across-the-board (or systematic) lowering of scores for everyone. Unlike random errors, systematic errors are generally always either positive or negative.

True score theory reminds us all to be modest and realistic about the **power** of any measurements we take. Even if it were theoretically possible for any instrument (such as a ruler, a survey, or a caliper) to truly and with 100% accuracy measure a variable of interest, true score theory reminds us that there will always be random and systematic error that may be beyond our control. As a result, all measurement is, at best, merely approximation rather than absolute certainty. True score theory also reminds us of the critical importance of ensuring we utilise appropriate strategies that will help us to mitigate – or minimise – measurement errors as best as possible.

3.3.4. Mitigation Strategies

Examples of mitigation strategies include pilot testing of all instruments/ways of measuring prior to utilisation:

- **Pilot testing** allows researchers to actually observe performance of the measurement tool in the real world, under controlled conditions and circumstances where the results do not matter significantly. Results from pilot testing can allow researchers to adapt their tools in a way that recognises the real-world impacts of random and systematic error.
- Thorough **training** of those actually using the measurement tool. While it may be self-evident to some, individuals have different conventions or rules for using simple tools like a ruler. Ensuring consistency in the way in which a tool is used can help reduce sources of error.
- Finally, one of the most important techniques researchers use to mitigate measurement error is the principle of **triangulation**. This means using different (multiple) measurement tools to measure the same thing. In triangulating, we are better able to manage the risk of systematic errors as well as random errors by using different tools and different times to measure the same phenomenon. For example, we might use a questionnaire to ask pharmacy students if they would like to have some revision classes prior to their exams. This would tell us how many students said they would or would not like this. We could then run the classes and ask them after the exam if they thought the extra classes made a difference to their performance in the exam. We could triangulate this by taking their actual scores in the exam and comparing these with attendance at the extra classes. There are different methods of triangulation and for more information about this please see the further reading at the end of this chapter.

3.4. RELIABILITY AND VALIDITY

True score theory also forms the foundation of a critical concept in measurement: reliability and validity. While these terms are sometimes (wrongly) used interchangeably and other times kept so separate as to imply they are unrelated, the reality is that reliability and validity are crucial characteristics that must be considered any time a measurement tool is used and measurement is taken.

Reliability is basically whether the way we have measured something measures it accurately time and time again. Validity refers to whether the measure we are using does actually measure what we think it is measuring. These concepts are extremely important in research design and conduct because we must be sure that we are measuring what we say we are measuring and that we can do this over time with the same results. It also means that other researchers can see what we have done and replicate our work in different settings. This can improve the validity and reliability of our measure. In Chapter 5 you will find lots more information about validity and reliability.

3.5. LEVELS OF MEASUREMENT AND STATISTICS

As discussed previously, the notion of continuous vs discrete variables of interest defines the level of measurement and the tools we can use to undertake such measurement. Discrete variables are sometimes referred to as 'dichotomous' or 'binary' to emphasise there are a limited number of categories of 'answers' or measurements possible, as opposed to continuous which indicates variables with many possible values.

When working with discrete variables (typically nominal measures or ordinal measures with less than four 'answers'), binomial theory will apply. **Binomial theory** provides a basis for specific groups of statistics (for example chi-square or logistic regression) that can be used as procedures to examine the data in question. In other words, if we measure a variable in a certain way there is a statistical process for analysing the data we produce. In contrast, with continuous variables (typically ordinal measures with more than four 'answers', interval and ratio measures), **normal theory** will apply. Examples of statistical procedures used with normal theory include ANOVA, regression, correlation and t-tests. See the 'Research Resources' section at the end of this chapter for more about statistical tests.

3.5.1. Parametric and Non-Parametric Data

The nature of measurement utilised governs the type of statistics and statistical tests that can be applied. In general, nominal and ordinal data are considered **non-parametric** while interval and ratio data are considered parametric. The term '**parametric**' means that the data resembles the parameters or features of the general population that has been sampled and 'non-parametric' means that there is no such resemblance. For example, when doing research into the effectiveness of antibiotic treatment it would be impossible to do a study that included everyone in the UK who was taking antibiotics. Practically, of course, we do not have sufficient time, resources, or money to track everyone in the country who is taking antibiotics! The only realistic way to proceed is to collect data from a smaller number (a sample, or a 'subset') of people who are taking antibiotics to enable us to understand the whole population of interest. Some of the information we collect will be in the form of means and standard deviations and these are what we call the 'parameters' of our data. Because we cannot collect data

from all of the people on antibiotics we can calculate these parameters using the data from our subset. Parametric data can be analysed in a wide variety of ways and are generally considered to be more powerful than non-parametric data. Parametric data can be more readily mathematically manipulated (for example, added/subtracted/multiplied/divided) to facilitate greater analysis than **non-parametric** data.

Levels of measurement, parametric and non-parametric data and choice of statistical methods can be found in Chapter 11. However, it is important to mention here that you should be thinking early on in your research about how you are going to design your measurement tools and how you are going to analyse the data.

3.6. MEASUREMENT AND QUALITATIVE RESEARCH

Qualitative research involves measurement that is (by definition) not about numbers. It is a time-honoured and important research tradition that cannot be quickly summarised here. Instead our objective is to provide a brief introduction to the way in which qualitative measures work and to point you to other chapters in this textbook and other resources that may be helpful.

Qualitative measures can be particularly helpful for several reasons:

a. **To develop a deeper or more nuanced understanding of an issue**

Most researchers recognise that many topics (particularly in the social sciences) defy simple categorisation. For example, questions related to religion, human sexuality and reproduction, parenting, or justice, defy nominal, ordinal, interval and ratio measures. Human beings generally hold complex, sometimes contradictory opinions on such questions, and their actual behaviours may range from the merely inconsistent to the completely hypocritical when compared to their stated opinions. Many problems that health services researchers look to address (for example, smoking cessation or safer-sex practices) present with an inherent contradiction. People intellectually KNOW what they should do yet (for a variety of different reasons) seem not to actually do what they know to be right. Health care professionals are frequently tasked with the challenge of addressing such complex – yet utterly human – contradictions.

In the previous chapter we introduced the Theory of Planned Behaviour and gave an example of how this might help us to understand why people do the things they do concerning their health. Qualitative methods can also be useful in trying to better understand such issues. Unconstrained by the need to utilise traditional and highly bound nominal, ordinal, interval or ratio measures, and further removed from even the constraints of dichotomous and continuous variables, qualitative research can allow researchers to actually focus on the 'stories' individuals tell about their lives, their experiences, their behaviours and their beliefs. While such stories may not be applicable or generalizable to everyone else, they can provide a rich source of data about some individual's experiences and can be useful therefore in prompting further kinds of research.

b. **To generate new theories about complex situations**

Many researchers use qualitative measurement techniques to become better acquainted and more familiar with the people, situations, and phenomena they are interested in. The value of 'living with' your data and becoming immersed in it (and with the people who produce that data in the first place) is often cited as a reason to undertake qualitative research. All too frequently, well-intentioned but naïve researchers may believe it is possible to leap to an evidence-based solution if only we generate the hard-numbers to back up an approach. Particularly in the social sciences and health services, the reality of most situations is far more complex than this, and researchers (as well as policy makers) need to remember that simplistic cause-effect theories and interventions may actually make situations worse. Qualitative research can frequently help sensitise researchers to the risk of over-reach in their work, and can help them to understand the multiple divergent (and sometimes contradictory) perspectives different individuals and stakeholders have. From these perspectives come new opportunities to generate new theories and subsequently test hypotheses.

c. **To let participants speak for themselves**

A valuable attribute of qualitative research is the opportunity it provides to the participants in the research to speak for themselves. Recall when we discussed nominal and ordinal measures, the risk we highlighted of 'forcing' answers into discrete categories when the true answers simply defy simplistic categorisation? Even using interval and ratio measures requires a commitment to a certain form of quantitative measurement that forces definitions that may be unwarranted. Qualitative measures allow the participants' words to stand on their own, without necessarily requiring the kind of arbitrary categorisation required in quantitative research.

For some, the price of using qualitative measures as opposed to quantitative ones is the trade of depth, detail and richness with generalisability. So long as the sample from which you have drawn your data is demonstrably representative of the population, it becomes possible to apply statistical tests to interpret data and start to draw defensible findings that are generalizable to the broader population. The cost of this generalisability is in the details.

The detail that is found in most qualitative research has been described as both a blessing and a curse. On the one hand it provides depth, nuance and a realism that is simultaneously bracing and enlightening. There is a true sense of commitment to and connection between researchers and participants with this sort of research (and, in some forms of qualitative research, participants and researchers are one and the same). Conversely, the volume of data generated and the question of what to do with it, how to manage it and how to actually analyse it can be very challenging: we will provide more information on all these issues in qualitative research in later chapters.

3.7. DIFFERENCES AMONGST PEOPLE WHO TAKE PART IN RESEARCH

In Chapter 2 we introduced the term 'demographics'. Demography as a discipline concerns statistical data about the characteristics of a living population of people. For pharmacists this could include all people in the United Kingdom who visit a pharmacy, or all people who are treated for hypertension. We can cut our '**population**' down to a manageable size for research purposes and choose a population from our own environment such as people with hypertension who collect their medicines from XX pharmacy or people who attend the hypertension clinic at XX hospital. In Part 2 of this book you will find more about quantitative research and Chapter 7 deals with research participants. However, we need to start thinking about our research or study population right from the inception of our research question. This is because the number of people in our study population and what we want to know about them will affect the methodology and methods we use in our research. For now we will return to a basic characteristic of people who take part in our research and how we might measure it.

3.7.1. Age

One of the characteristics of a population that is relevant to almost all health care research is age. Pharmacists, in particular, are interested in age because the very young and the very old can respond to medications in quite a different way from say people in early adulthood. For example, the dose of a drug will need to be carefully calculated for a baby or young child so that they receive the correct therapeutic dose, that is, a dose that is enough to treat their condition but not so much that it causes harmful side effects or overdose. The way our bodies metabolise a drug (the way it is moved through our body) comes under the subject of **pharmacokinetics** which you will already have learned a lot about. To calculate the correct dose of a drug we need to know certain other things about our patients, such as body weight, and we will also need to know their exact age. For example, is our child patient closer to the age of 2 than 3?

Using the example above of patients with hypertension who attend XX hospital outpatients it is important to think through what effect age has on people with hypertension, both in terms of their body's response to the medication, whether they have other medical conditions (**co-morbidities**) and how they feel about taking medication, e.g. do they relate being on medication to getting old? How we are going to use age in our research study will determine how we or our participants record it. In Chapter 6 we will look at how to set up a database on which to enter our research results, and we need to take into account how we ask questions so that these can be entered readily onto that database.

There are a number of ways to measure age:
1. Ask people to tell you how old they are in years or years and months.

'What is your age?' _____years _____months

If we take this option and we have 100 participants then it will be necessary to enter the age of every single participant on the database. As a result, when we run our analyses we will have potentially 100 different answers, unless we have participants who are the same age in years and months. If it may be useful at some point in the research to know an individual's age in years and months then this method can be used and the research can then place the ages into ranges on the database. More about this in Chapter 6.

2. Give participants a set of age ranges and ask them to put a tick in the box that most closely represents their age. For this example we will assume that we have checked the clinic database and the youngest patient who attends the clinic is 20 years old and the oldest is 68.

'Below you will find a set of age ranges. Please indicate in the box provided which age range corresponds to your own. Please tick one box only.'

20–25 [ ]
26–30 [ ]
31–35 [ ]
36–40 [ ]
41–45 [ ]
46–50 [ ]
51–55 [ ]
56–60 [ ]
61–65 [ ]
66–70 [ ]

The above is just one example of how to divide up the age ranges, but these can be broadened or narrowed according to the needs of the research.

3.8.   CASE STUDY EXAMPLES

During your study design you will need to start to think about how you are going to measure the phenomena of interest to you. This is not as easy as it sounds because for each level of measurement you choose there are rules about what you can do with your data once it is collected. We touched on this in Section 3.5 of this chapter, and you will find more about levels of measurement and statistical tests in Chapter 11.

In this section we will again use two of the case studies to help you understand better how to decide on the level of measurement for your study. As we said at the beginning of this chapter, measurement is critical to a successful outcome. Without careful consideration of both the instrument used to measure and the nature of the measurement itself, results may be compromised.

3.8.1.   Sandy – Researching the Control of Type II Diabetes

Sandy is the practice pharmacist who has noticed that the blood sugar of some of his younger patients with type II diabetes is not as well controlled as it should be. In Chapter 2 Sandy began to consider how he might frame his research question and began with the first draft as '**How do I design an intervention to improve patients' blood sugar control?**' After thinking this through Sandy realised that prior to designing an intervention he really needed to understand how his patients actually felt about their diagnosis and the control of their blood sugar. He therefore revised his question to: '**How do my patients feel about their diagnosis of diabetes and the need for consistent blood sugar control?**'

Since then Sandy has found time in his busy practice to do some more thinking and realises that he should back track in his thinking. What would be the point in asking his patients about their diagnosis and their blood sugar control, when he has no hard data to show whether or not the **anecdotal** evidence he has is accurate. Sandy decides to design a preliminary study to collect information about the blood sugars of all of his patients with type II diabetes. He will then be able to see whether patients in the younger age groups have better or worse control over their blood sugar then the older age groups. He can do this by asking his patients to keep records on their blood sugar over a period of time, but he will have to work out how to measure potential changes in blood sugar so that he can compare the age groups in a meaningful way. At the end of this preliminary study he should be able to say with some certainty whether the younger participants in his study have better or worse control over their blood sugar. In other words, whether there is actually a problem that is affecting younger patients, and that the effects he has been noticing are not just random.

3.8.1.1 Background Work

Sandy does some background reading and discovers that advice regarding optimal blood sugar levels for people with type II diabetes varies. He decides to use the UK guidelines from The National Institute for Health and Care Excellence (NICE) because it is based on previous research. The guidelines for people without diabetes are that their blood sugar should be in the range of 3.5–5.5 mmol/L before meals. Two hours after meals this should be less than 8 mmol/L. However, Sandy knows that the target range for people with type II diabetes is slightly higher at 4–7 mmol/L prior to meals and less than 8.5 2 hours after meals. (There are guidelines such as this for other countries too so if you are studying outside the United Kingdom please check what these are.)

Sandy needs to know what his patients' blood sugar levels are over time and then he can compare these with age and gender. There is so much to think about, e.g. the measuring equipment used by his patients, time of day they take the blood test, dietary changes, stress, infection and so on…. He decides that he can only think about one thing at a time and for the moment concentrates on the level of measurement he is going to use.

3.8.1.2. Rationale for the Chosen Level of Measurement

Sandy has looked up his book on statistics from university and refreshed his memory on levels of measurement. He knows that the measurement of blood sugar uses a **continuous** scale because the numbers on the scale are on a continuum – they could in theory go from infinity to infinity! The scale is not **discrete** – that would mean putting blood sugar into separate boxes and that wouldn't work (though when it comes to asking patients their sex this would be a discrete variable because people can only be 'male', 'female' or 'neither' if they did not wish to say.

Sandy reads on and finds that ordinal and nominal level measures are not used for continuous variables so that just leaves interval level or ratio scale. Below are the key points he considers:

- Interval measurements are useful for describing differences and he wants to look at the differences in peoples' blood sugar levels.

- Interval measures use a scale which represents quantity and scaled units ('intervals') to facilitate truer comparisons between items being measured. Blood sugar is measure by the quantity of glucose in a litre of blood.
- Interval measures can also indicate the direction of differences (higher or lower). Sandy wants to know whether the younger people in his practice have higher or lower levels of blood sugar, so this seems to fit the bill too.

BUT, looking at the guidance on ratio scales Sandy finds that they do all the things that an interval scale does but they have a true zero. People cannot have a minus level of blood sugar and so Sandy can present the question to his participants in an ordinal way in the form of a range. Sandy finds that this can still be treated as a ratio scale measure when it comes to doing his data analysis. With ratio scales '0' represents the absolute bottom below which no measurements can occur. This is important in statistical terms and explanations are given in Chapters 9 and 11.

Based on this decision-making process Sandy decides to create a **ratio scale** as follows:

Before Meals

1	2	3	4	5
Less than 5 mmol/L	5–7 mmol/L	8–10 mmol/L	10–13 mmol/L	Over 13 mmol/L

2 Hours After Meals

1	2	3	4	5
Less than 5 mmol/L	5–6 mmol/L	7–8 mmol/L	9–10 mmol/L	Over 10 mmol/L

By taking the ranges in the scale beyond the recommended 8.5 mm/L Sandy can see just how many of his participants have higher than desirable blood sugar.

3.8.2. Dorothy – Researching the Hospital Drug Budget

We did not frame a research question for Dorothy's topic in Chapter 2 so we will do that now to help to decide on the best level of measurement for her needs. This will illustrate how the activities embedded in the research process build on each other to ensure a successful outcome. Recall from Chapter 1 that Dorothy is a hospital pharmacist who is studying part-time for an MSc in Health System Improvement. She has been asked to reduce the drug budget due to recent austerity measures. As a pharmacist, Dorothy recognises that mindless cutting of budgets could compromise patient care and instead she wants to frame this as an opportunity to optimise and improve the quality of prescribing within her institution. Dorothy recognises that a hospital is an incredibly complicated environment and that numbers (such as drug costs) do not tell the entire story. While typical hospital budgets segment costs based on departments, she realises the hospital as a whole operates as a system. A "saving" in the drug budget due to premature discontinuation of an antibiotic may inadvertently produce a bacterial resistance leading to a follow-up A&E visit – which would cost the institution much more than simply ensuring rational prescribing in the first place. Dorothy has attended several conferences and spoken to many administrators, and recognises that it is not advisable to tackle something as large and complex as the overall hospital "drug budget" as a single entity.

3.8.2.1 Background Work

Dorothy has reviewed the expenditures across the hospital – and across her neighbouring institutions – over the past 5 years, and has noted a few areas of particular interest. Anti-infectives (including antibiotics and antifungals) continue to be a significant driver of costs within hospitals, both in terms of medication costs and nursing time required for administration to patients. **Anecdotally** she has been told by her pharmacists that there appears to be little rhyme or reason to the prescribing practices of some physicians. Sometimes they will prescribe antibiotics without taking culture-and-sensitivity tests, and even when these tests are done and results available they are very slow to make changes. Further, there has been a steady rise in bacterial resistance (for example vancomycin-resistant enterococcus, or methicillin resistant staphylococcus aureus) across the country.

3.8.2.2 The Research Question

Based on these observations, Dorothy recognises there may be an opportunity to undertake a programme of Antimicrobial Stewardship. This is an inter-professional collaboration designed to encourage optimal prescribing which frequently has the benefit of reducing overall health care (including drug) expenditures (see https://www.nice.org.uk/guidance/qs61/chapter/quality-statement-1-antimicrobial-stewardship).

Rather than simply say *'There is no more money for drugs'*, Stewardship programmes focus on education and support for practitioners, to ensure best possible prescribing and administration of costly and powerful antibiotics. Dorothy had recently visited a colleague at another hospital who had initiated such a programme and was impressed with the outcomes. This colleague, however, was brutally frank with her in terms of barriers and challenges to implementation. Many physicians were resistant to the idea of their prescribing being 'second-guessed', many pharmacists lacked confidence to be able to articulate rationales for recommending changes. Furthermore, many nurses were frustrated with the lack of clarity around who was actually responsible for prescribing and monitoring antibiotics.

Dorothy believes there may be value in exploring implementation of an Antimicrobial Stewardship programme in her hospital, but she wants to proceed carefully in an inclusive way to prevent the problems she has observed elsewhere. She believes such a programme may indeed result in cost savings, but her greater interest is in reducing antibiotic resistance and in optimising prescribing to improve patient care. As she thinks about her research question, she begins with: **'What are the barriers and enablers to implementation of an antimicrobial stewardship programme in my institution?'**

3.8.2.3 Rationale for the Chosen Level of Measurement

Dorothy arranges to meet with her colleague who has already implemented a Stewardship programme in her hospital to find out how she designed her study and collected her data. Her colleague says that she enlisted the help of a biostatistician friend who helped her decide on the best way to design her study. She advised Dorothy that it needed a significant amount of thought because her findings may be the impetus for changes to be made across the hospital, and perhaps even beyond into primary care. It also requires a significant amount of careful advanced planning. A clear understanding of the problem you are trying to solve should help structure a clear and coherent research question, which in turn should allow for development of a method and data gathering tools (such as surveys or questionnaires) which are focused and precise. Working with a biostatistician or person with experience in this area right from the outset is an important way of building quality into your research process. Most of all the research needed to be as rigorous as possible because the lives of patients could depend on any changes made.

Dorothy realises that to answer her research question she needs to ask members of the multidisciplinary health care team involved in antibiotics prescribing, their views on the implementation of an Antimicrobial Stewardship programme.

Dorothy does some more reading and discovers some information about Likert Scales. Below are some of the points she considers:

- Likert Scales are used to ask respondents to a questionnaire to answer a qualitative question in a quantitative way. It is often referred to as an 'attitude' scale. Dorothy wants to find out what peoples' attitudes are to the Stewardship programme.
- Likert Scales are essentially subjective experiences examined in a quantitative way but these experiences are not changed by being 'measured' quantitatively.
- Dorothy wants to collect as much 'attitude' information from as many people as possible so the Likert Scale seems to be the best way of collecting that information.

BUT, each respondent's attitude towards the subject in question will be perceived differently to another's. Dorothy wants to explore those differences, but she will have to be careful that she takes this into account when she designs her questions and analyses her data. After considering the use of a Likert Scale and taking advice from her colleague, Dorothy decides to use the scale.

It is often possible to find a validated questionnaire that has been used in other research. Sometimes the authors of the questions will allow you to make some minor changes to make them appropriate for the group of people you are interested in. For example, the link that follows is to a questionnaire that has been used in the USA prior to implementing an Antimicrobial Stewardship programme: http://www.shea-online.org/Portals/0/GNYHA_ Antimicrobial_Stewardship_Toolkit_FINALv2%20 Dec2011.pdf

This is an example of 'borrowing from other disciplines' (see Chapter 2, Section 5.2), and you will find more about the reliability and validity of questionnaires in Chapter 5.

In Chapter 6 you will find detailed information about how to design a questionnaire and all the things that need to be taken into account. At the moment we will just deal with the level of measurement issue as this will form the basis of Dorothy's questionnaire. The example given below is just one question that Dorothy might include in her questionnaire to illustrate how the scale looks. An important point is that, although Dorothy has an overall research question, when using a scale to measure attitudes towards something each scale is used to measure just one aspect of the topic in question so is in effect asking a series of mini-questions.

EXAMPLE

Below we ask you to tell us how much you agree or disagree with the statement. Please indicate your answer by using the scale where '1' = Strongly Disagree and '5' = Strongly Agree. Please only use option '3' if you have no feelings either way.

'Antimicrobial Stewardships programmes improve patient care':

1	2	3	4	5
Strongly Disagree	Disagree	Neither Agree Nor Disagree	Agree	Strongly Agree

CHAPTER SUMMARY

- This chapter has concentrated on the different ways we can measure the things we are interested in in our research.
- It looked at measurement error and its consequences for research findings.
- It introduced the basic principles of reliability and validity.
- It looked at how to use statistics on the things we have measured.
- It looked at how to explore the characteristics and differences amongst people who take part in research (research participants).
- Finally, it used the research of two of our case study pharmacists as examples of how to decide on which measurement levels to use.

ANSWER TO SELF-CHECK QUESTION 'What type of measurement is best used for age and why?':

Nominal measurement (also known as 'categorical measurement') is most appropriate to measure age because age clearly and distinctly clusters into identifiable, discrete groupings. Implicit in the use of nominal measurement is the idea that there is no specific connection or relationship between the groups and each person can only be in one age range.

FURTHER READING

Scales of Measurement and Triangulation
Steiner, D. L., Norman, G. R., & Cairney, J. (2014). *Health measurement scales: a practical guide to their development and use.* Oxford, England: Oxford University Press.

RESEARCH RESOURCES

https://www.discoveringstatistics.com/.This is a link to Andy Field's website that accompanies his book.

Field, A. (2016). An Adventure in Statistics: the reality enigma. London: Sage.
The National Institute for Health and Care Excellence (NICE) https://www.nice.org.uk/.
Diabetes UK https://www.diabetes.org. uk/?gclid=COew7_K18dECFc617QodGlMAGg.

4

Introduction to Quantitative Research

LEARNING OBJECTIVES

After reading this chapter you should be able to:
- understand the key principles of quantitative research
- describe the positivist and scientific approaches to research
- understand the process of quantitative research
- describe some of the situations where quantitative methods work the best

4.1. INTRODUCTION: WHAT IS QUANTITATIVE RESEARCH?

Quantitative research has historically dominated the work (and thinking) of pharmacists and other health care professionals. As the term suggests, quantitative research is focused on numbers, and uses mathematical tools and methods to make sense of our world. Integral to the use of quantitative methods is the presumption that, through numbers and their analysis, it becomes possible to understand and interpret a broad array of processes and phenomena of interest to researchers. In this chapter we will be introducing a number of terms that are used in research, and definitions will be given for each one. This chapter is just an introduction to quantitative research and when we would use it. All of the principles we discuss will be explored in greater detail in later chapters because the whole of Part II of this book is about quantitative research. You will find signposts on the way and further reading at the end of each chapter. Some of our case study students and pharmacists will also appear in practical examples of how the quantitative research might be used to answer some of their research questions. Quantitative research can be broadly placed into two categories: descriptive and experimental.

4.1.1 Descriptive Quantitative Research

This generally involves the observation, measurement and mathematical interpretation of the natural world without any type of significant interference by the researcher. In other words we are interested in finding out what is happening to a group of people. For example, we might want to find out how many people visit their community pharmacist, how often and why they make their visits. Under these circumstances we would be describing a pharmacy practice issue as it happens. Surveys are one of the most frequently used types of descriptive quantitative research tools used. Respondents who take part in this type of research will usually be asked to answer questions about themselves, what they do, how they think and feel and very much reflects these phenomena at one point in time.

4.1.2. Experimental Quantitative Research

In this type of research researchers generally focus on deliberate interference within a system or process through manipulation of one or more key elements. Participants might be invited to take part in such an experiment because they have, for example, a particular illness and might be divided into two groups – one that has a type of treatment and one that does not. For example, our case study pharmacist, Sandy, might use such a technique to look at the effects of a pharmacy-supervised diet programme for young people with type II diabetes who want to lose weight. To do this he would have two groups of young people – one group that took part in the diet programme run by the pharmacist and one group who did not. Sandy could keep records of the participants' weight and see whether his **intervention** (see key point below) in the pharmacy made a difference to how much weight (if any) his participants lost. The purpose of this type of research is to observe, measure, then mathematically interpret what effect different **treatments** (see key point below) have on an outcome of interest. At the end of Sandy's research he would be able to say whether a pharmacist-led diet programme improved participants' weight loss.

Clinical trials used to develop and assess the efficacy and/or effectiveness of new or alternative treatment options are an example of this form of quantitative research, and this type of research will be examined in Chapter 8.

KEY TERMS

Intervention: An intervention in health or clinical terms is any action that is carried out with the aim of improving, maintaining or assessing peoples' health. Sandy's intervention is to see whether a diet programme helps people lose weight and improve their diabetes control.

Treatment: Treatment in this context means the interventions that Sandy incorporated into his patients' care which could also include reducing, increasing or changing a drug. It can, however, mean that nothing was done to some patients, as in Sandy's group who did not join the diet programme.

Whether one is interested in descriptive or experimental (sometimes referred to as **interventional**) research, data collection using either approach is broadly similar (and will be discussed below). The way in which one interprets and analyses data, however, will vary based on the researchers' aims and intentions, and the design of the study itself.

4.2. QUANTITATIVE RESEARCH: KEY PRINCIPLES

Quantitative research is used when we are interested in understanding how, when and by how much something is changing or happening. Quantitative methods allow us to apply principles of measurement to our observations which can facilitate comparisons between groups or allow us to track how a process or system evolves over time.

In other words we need to answer these simple questions:

• How much?
• How many?
• How often?
• To what extent?

In this section you will be introduced to the tradition of positivism which is the basis for quantitative research, and the '**scientific**' method.

4.2.1. The Positivist Approach

A foundation principle for most quantitative research is the idea that **observer bias** and expectation must be controlled so as not to unduly interfere with the research process. In other words researchers must be careful that they do not let their own ideas about the outcomes of their research

affect the actual outcomes. We all want our research to show what we think and hope it will, but that is not the case in the real world (see 'Objectivity' below).

The extent to which the expectations or biases of the researchers themselves interfere with the process, cloud the interpretation or inadvertently skew the research is of significant concern to those who believe that objective, universal truths are possible and do exist, and the central objective of research is to uncover these truths (**positivists**). To these **positivists** (and most (though by no means all) quantitative researchers), data can and should be a true representation of the object of interest, untainted by the researcher's biases and interests.

There are four key principles of high quality, positivistic quantitative research:

1. **Empiricism** is a philosophy that states that knowledge (and wisdom) comes only or predominantly from sensory experiences. It emphasises the importance of objective evidence over feelings or beliefs, and in particular values the type of sensory experiences and evidence that are features of a typical experiment. Empiricists have implicit faith in the power of **observation** to both find answers and solve problems, primarily because of their belief that answers in fact DO exist and problems in fact DO have solutions.

2. **Measurement tools** in quantitative research must be precisely developed and described, in order to facilitate **reproducibility** (see d, below). The instrument we choose to use in an experiment is of critical importance, whether that instrument is a caliper, a survey, a ruler or a glucometre. Researchers need to confirm and to demonstrate that their instruments are reliable, stable and capable of reproducible measurements. Where other instruments (such as surveys or other written tools) are used to capture data, they too must conform to the same principles of reliability, stability and capability of ensuring reproducible measurements. In Chapter 5 we will explain in more detail the concept of 'reliability'.

3. **Objectivity** is the principle that suggests researchers must strive to eliminate any and all personal biases that may interfere with the way data are collected. Examples of typical methods used to maintain objectivity including double-blinding of a clinical trial, in which both physician and patient are unaware of whether the patient receives a medication or a **placebo**. Because they believe objectivity is possible, positivists believe it is essential in ensuring good-quality research.

4. **Reproducibility (or replicability)** is the principle that emphasises the importance of others being able to reproduce a researcher's work in a way that produces substantially similar results and outcomes. Reproducibility is considered a virtue as it reinforces the empiricist notion

that right answers exist and solutions to problems can be found. The more frequently and consistently different researchers using the same approaches arrive at the same conclusions, the closer we are to establishing truth. This is one example of the **validity** of a measure used in research, and in Chapter 5 we will explain the concept of validity in more detail.

As may be evident, not all researchers believe all these principles are necessarily virtuous or even possible in all circumstances. Most quantitatively oriented researchers, however, strive to meet these ideals as a way of reassuring themselves of the quality of their processes and significance of their work.

4.2.2. The 'Scientific' Method

The empiricist underpinning of most quantitative research has produced a widely described and accepted model of what 'scientific' research should involve. This has been named the Scientific Method (though many social scientists may, quite rightly, strenuously disagree with this characterisation).

The Scientific Method has, at its core, the notion that our everyday observations of our world produce questions, speculation, ideas and, eventually, an hypothesis. The term 'scientific' is meant to reinforce the concepts of empiricism, measurement, objectivity and reproducibility that underlie the method. In most circumstances, it is described as an ongoing process for gaining a better understanding of our world.

The Scientific Method usually begins with the natural inquisitiveness and curiosity that characterizes human experience. In our day-to-day world, we see, observe, hear and notice things around us, which causes many of us to develop an idea – or an hypothesis – about why things are the way they are and how things can be changed or improved. We then use these hypotheses as a basis for formulating predictions about how future events may occur. However, before we can rely upon our hypotheses for predictive value, we must subject them to testing to ensure, in fact, they are correct and can be reasonably relied upon for this purpose. This hypothesis testing is at the core of the scientific method. The mechanisms of hypothesis testing involve measurement, objectivity and reproducibility.

In Chapter 8 we look at the experimental method and hypothesis testing in more detail.

4.3. QUANTITATIVE RESEARCH: THE PROCESS

For those readers who enjoy a rule-governed life, quantitative research is for you. There are sets of principles that are specified for virtually everything we want to achieve by using these methods – some more complicated than others. In this section we will follow the process of doing quantitative research highlighting some of the things that must be done if we are to adhere to the scientific principles.

4.3.1. Sampling

In Chapter 3 we introduced the topic of research participants or respondents and that another term for choosing the people who take part in our research is 'sampling'. This is because our participants are a 'sample' of everyone in our given population who, for example, has the illness or is receiving the treatment we are interested in. We undertake quantitative research in order to test hypotheses and consequently develop predictions about future behaviours within a group. Frequently, our group is a large, diverse and **heterogeneous** cluster of individuals who may have some similarities but who are likely to have many more differences amongst them. This group is the 'population' that we talked about in Section 7 of Chapter 3. Examples of a research population of interest might be left-handed people, patients with Alzheimer's disease or nurse-practitioners working in community care centres.

As described previously in Chapter 3, quantitative researchers try to control or at least minimise factors which may bias the outcome of a study. This becomes particularly important when considering that in the majority of circumstances involving quantitative measurements, we must deal with a sample rather than an entire population. Factors that might bias the outcome of the study are often related to the sampling technique used.

Probability sampling makes the assumption that the researcher has access to everyone in the population and that all those people have an equal chance of being selected to take part. There are three issues associated with probability sampling that we will mention here – **sampling error**, **random sampling** and **sampling bias**. Chapter 7 of this book is devoted to choosing your participants and sampling issues including inclusion/exclusion criteria, and random/non-random sampling methods.

The methods we use to select the sample population for a study are important in helping to reduce bias. For example, the sample Sandy chooses may not be as representative of his study population of young people with type II diabetes as he thought and this would bias his findings. In other words, he could not be sure that his findings really did reflect what was going on in all young people with type II diabetes.

4.3.2. Data Collection

The way data are collected will depend largely on the design of the research. With quantitative studies, because we are collecting numerical data, we need to have as much of this as possible. If you have decided to conduct a study that requires the collection of large amounts of data then the simplest and most cost effective way is to collect it either from already existing records, e.g. records of patients' blood pressure held by GPs, hospital doctors or in community pharmacies, or from information provided directly to the researcher by the patient. In Chapter 6 we will explore some of the ways you can collect quantitative data from patients.

Briefly, quantitative data can be collected in the following ways:
- Information collected from patients' medical records
- Questionnaire administered by the researcher
- Self-completed questionnaire
- One-to-one
- Face-to-face

SANDY – RESEARCHING THE CONTROL OF TYPE II DIABETES

Remember that Sandy has been noticing more and more patients being diagnosed and treated for type II diabetes within the practice. He is concerned because so many of these patients are young, (under 25 years of age) and their diabetes does not seem to be well controlled. His first thought was that he is doing something wrong in spite of the fact that he had made sure that he and the health care team are following guidelines and providing the care required. Sandy works through the problem and decides that he needs to get some evidence for what he is observing in practice. There are two things that he needs to do and for both he decides that he needs good hard evidence in the form of numbers to really be sure about his patients' conditions.

First he needs to:

a. confirm his casual observations are actually true and supported by some kind of evidence from the practice itself

b. determine the magnitude of the problem.

Let's look at how quantitative methods can help Sandy achieve these first two objectives. The best way to do this is to write down all the things that could be measured in order to answer the question 'Are my observations true?'

Sandy has noticed that there seem to be more young people being diagnosed with type II diabetes and that their diabetes is not well controlled.

What Needs to Be Measured?

1. Blood glucose

2. Age

3. Date of diagnosis.

Each of these three variables can only be measured in a numerical way. In Chapter 3 Sandy did some background work on how to measure blood sugar so you could return to that now and remind yourself of what he did. When Sandy did his background work he realised that there might be some differences in diabetes incidence and control between males and females and so he can add 'sex' to the list of variables. There may be other things that need

to be measured during the course of the study and these can be added at a later date. For now we just need to illustrate how quantitative methods are really the only way that Sandy can collect evidence for his assumptions about his patients with type II diabetes.

Study Sample

The patients who attend Sandy's practice are just a small sample of all people who attend GP practices nationwide. Of the people who attend the practice those with type II diabetes are smaller in number yet again. To compare age and sex with date of diagnosis and blood sugar levels we need to have a selection of people from Sandy's practice. The best thing Sandy can do is to include everyone in the practice who has type II diabetes and then describe that sample population. So Sandy's study population would be:

'Patients from one GP practice with a diagnosis of type II diabetes'

As suggested earlier, there are some issues about sampling that need to be acknowledged and accounted for as far as possible. The way Sandy's study population is identified and selected may introduce some bias into his study. One of these may be that the size of his sample may be too small to draw any conclusions that could be applied to the wider population of people with type II diabetes.

Data Collection

Sandy is fortunate in that all of the information that he needs is available from the patient medical records held by the practice and so he does not need to recruit participants to his study at the moment. This will make things easier in some ways and it will certainly make sure he has a larger sample size than if he had to ask for people with diabetes from his practice to take part in the study. However, this is going to be a time-consuming task and later on in this section we will come back and find out how Sandy collected his data and what he is going to do with them.

- Telephone
- Post
- Electronically, e.g. web-based or email.

More often than not, the method chosen for quantitative data collection comes down to how we can collect as much data as possible, as quickly as possible and in the most cost-effective way. Data collection takes time and effort and so you need to choose your method wisely. As you move through the chapters of this book you will find different methods described in detail.

Let's pause here and have a look at how out one of our pharmacists and one of our students might use a quantitative approach in their research studies.

Let's take another example of quantitative research from our case studies.

ROSI –STUDENT PROJECT INTO DEMAND FOR AN ON-CAMPUS PHARMACY

We introduced Rosi in Chapter 1, and here is the background to her project.

Rosi Magruder is an MPharm student at the University of Fazakarly. She is in the fourth and final year of her studies, and for her research project, her supervisor has suggested that she and her project group (four other MPharm students) explore whether there is a need and demand for an on-campus pharmacy to serve the needs of the 22,000 students and staff that come to the institution each day, as well as those in neighbouring communities. Rosi herself has often wondered why there is no 'model pharmacy' that would allow students like her to actually be able to practice pharmacy in a way that they have been taught. She and her team wonder if university students and staff – who they assume to be generally healthy – actually need, want and would use a campus-based pharmacy offering the highest quality pharmaceutical care available. Rosi's task is to find out the best way to collect the data for the project.

For her MPharm project, Rosi needs to determine the optimal method of gathering these data, analysing and interpreting them, and then making sense of them for the rest of the research team. To do this she should begin by deciding what needs to be measured.

What Needs to Be Measured?
Just some ideas to begin with:
1. Information about who is on campus, e.g. job, department, age, sex, whether they have any health conditions requiring medication
2. What prescription medication they take
3. What over-the-counter products they use
4. How often they visit a pharmacy off-campus
5. What they visit their pharmacy for
6. Whether they think it would be a good idea to have a pharmacy on campus
7. Why they think it would be a good idea or not.
   This study is a little more complicated than Sandy's

because it has more elements. Some of the information is best collected using quantitative methods and some requires a more qualitative approach – for example the answers to the 'why' questions. We will look at the methods used in qualitative research in Part III of this book so for now we will concentrate on how quantitative methods may be used.

Rosi can collect information about questions 1 and 2 from two sources. The university website can provide the number of students and staff, and she can use a questionnaire to collect information about the people who take part in the research (participants). Questions 2 to 6 could also be included in the questionnaire.

Study Sample
The sample for this study will be anyone who studies, works or visits the university.

There are some challenges that will be faced by Rosi and her project group that Sandy did not have because he was able to obtain all of his data from the practice records. Rosi and her team are going to have to find a way of recruiting patients to their study and will have to include information about recruitment when the study is finally written up. This will include whether all participants in the above group were invited and whether or not they had to volunteer. Participants in research who volunteer introduce a different kind of bias in that they may be the people who use a pharmacy more regularly because of a health condition.

Data Collection
Rosi decides that the quantitative data collection is going to have to be done by sending out a questionnaire to all people who volunteer to take part in the research. The design of questionnaires is covered in Chapter 6 so we will leave this for now and move on to our choices about what to do with information or data once we have got them.

4.3.3. Data Treatment

The term 'data treatment' refers simply to what we are going to do with our data once they have been collected. Although the term sounds simple the process of deciding how to treat research data should be carefully considered. That decision-making needs to begin as early as when researchers are reviewing the literature concerning the topic of interest to them. **Data analysis** is part of the data treatment process, and how the data are analysed will depend on how they were collected in the first place. For example, if we used a questionnaire to collect data we would need to think about how the questions were asked to provide answers that we could enter on a database. In Chapter 6 we look in detail at how to design a questionnaire, and the specific methods used to deal with data collected in different ways may be found in Chapters 8 to 11.

We also have to think through the statistical analyses we want to perform so that our database 'works'. This involves understanding what sort of data we have and the rest of this chapter looks at how we categorise the things we want to measure to provide us with answers to our research question

4.3.4. Characteristics of Our Data

Quantitative research is based on the idea that whatever we decide to measure will vary between individuals, and may vary within any specific individual before or after a particular event or intervention. For example, not everyone experiences side effects to medications and sometimes those who do experience side effects may find the side effects change under certain conditions. Similarly, people who do not normally experience side effects may begin to do so if their state of health changes. So, there are many things about people that we need to take into account when doing research and these things or 'characteristics' are called '**variables**'. These variables are the main focus of quantitative research. Variables of interest can include any characteristic. For example, in examining the experience of young adult patients with type II diabetes in his practice, our case study 1 pharmacist, Sandy, may focus on his patients' sex, their dietary habits, or their exercise routines. Variables can take many forms, but in general, a variable of interest must be specific, observable, measurable and describable.

This becomes particularly important when we consider the issue of how we describe the processes involved in our research (operationalisation). One way of doing this is to use a theoretical framework as described in Chapter 2. Sandy might decide to map out the potential relationships at work in his study to make sure he hasn't missed anything and to help with his data analysis. A simple framework for Sandy's data might look like Fig. 4.1:

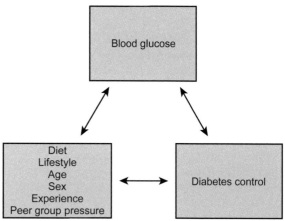

FIGURE 4.1 Processes involved in Sandy's research. The above figure shows that there might be a relationship between control of diabetes and a number of factors such as diet and lifestyle. Sandy cannot be sure which of these factors (if any) has an effect on blood sugar and diabetes control so the arrows show a potential two-way relationship. In his theoretical framework Sandy would include some background theory about diabetes and its causes, possibly drawing on previous research that has been conducted in other areas of health care, e.g. nursing, medicine. The diagram will help Sandy to specify the factors he needs to take into account when exploring his research question.

4.3.5. Describing Variables

A vaguely or generally described variable such as 'dietary habits' is not helpful to a researcher. A more specific variable should be used instead (for example, total calorie intake >2000 calories/day). If we define a variable too broadly, the focus of the research will be lost and we are likely to become overwhelmed by an array of confusing or **confounding variables** that interfere with our understanding of the process of interest (see Section 4.3.5). For example, if 'dietary habits' were not further defined and specified, Sandy would have to make an endless series of subjective judgements about what constitutes 'good' or 'bad' dietary habits, and this would be a significant threat to the reproducibility and objectivity of his work. For Sandy's study, examples of confounding variables that may confuse or cloud data analysis may include seasonal variations in food availability (e.g. in the Northern Hemisphere, fresh fruit and vegetables may be less available or more expensive in the winter time and as a result, many individuals find their diet shifts towards more processed/refined foods). Studying an individual's diet from April to October vs from October to April will likely result in different food consumption patterns because of this confounding, seasonal variable.

Many times in quantitative research, we are using an experimental or **comparative study** design method. We will deliberately and in a controlled way manipulate one variable of interest to test its effects and influences on other variables. In such studies, the variable being manipulated is called the **independent variable**. The impacts and effects that result from the manipulation of the independent variable are called the **dependent variables**. For example, as Sandy considers his population of young adult patients with diabetes, he may draw on a sample from his accessible population to undertake an experiment. He may provide some of these individuals with a glucometer and education in how to use it, while other individuals in the group may not get this new intervention. Sandy is wondering if this intervention may increase his patients' awareness and, as a result, delay onset of a diagnosis of diabetes. In this case, the independent variable is the glucometer and education programme; the dependent variable will be time to initial diagnosis of diabetes.

The issue of confounding variables must be carefully considered here. For example, if within Sandy's population and sample there are a large number of non-English speaking individuals, then the nature of Sandy's education programme will need to be examined. Unless the programme can meet the linguistic and health-literacy needs of patients, it cannot be effective and consequently its value as an independent variable in this study would be significantly diminished. Another example of a confounding variable may be socio-economic status: even if a patient receives and understands the education provided, they still must have the economic wherewithal to actually take action to improve the readings they get from the glucometer. These might be making dietary changes that have a cost implication, like buying fresh fruits and vegetables rather than the often cheaper prepared foods and crisps. Without a careful assessment of each patient's ability to actually implement the education Sandy provides, the risk of confounding variables interfering with study objectives will be significant.

4.3.6. Differences in the Processes

In your study it is important to recognise the processes that are going on in your area of interest in its particular setting. Identifying the variables in play, e.g. the age, sex and dietary habits of Sandy's patients with diabetes, and correctly defining them will make all the difference to the design of the study and the collection and treatment of the data it yields. You can use the levels of measurement described in Chapter 3 to further refine your study design. Using a framework to make a visual plan of your variables and how they relate to each other can help you to make decisions about what

information you need to collect and how, in order to meet the objectives of the study. Quantitative research produces raw data that will require organisation and interpretation to analyse. Statistical methods will help establish the differences between the variables and the parts they play in the processes you are interested in. Sometimes we may just want to describe what is going on in a process and for this we would use **descriptive statistics** and in Section 4.4.1 we will show how Sandy can use these to begin to illuminate the characteristics of his study sample. Later on Sandy and our other case study students and pharmacists will use **inferential statistics** to help decide whether the data collected actually demonstrate the expected differences and patterns or not. The type of statistics that can be used will be further described in more detail in Chapters 10 and 11.

4.3.7. Measurement of the Differences

When designing a research study that is going to be treated quantitatively it is essential that it is possible to *measure* the differences in the processes of interest. In Chapters 1 and 2 we described a research study that investigated whether patients with a bacterial infection get better more quickly if they are treated with antibiotics than those who are not. In that example we are trying to find relationships between different variables, e.g. bacterial infection and treatment using antibiotics. Remember, there might be other variables that affect the way infections respond to antibiotics amongst different people, so we must account for these when looking at the relationships of interest. Here are some of the questions that should be considered:

- Are the processes to be measured clearly specified?:
  What is the bacterial infection?
  What antibiotics are being used to treat the infection?
  When were the participants first diagnosed?
  How old are the participants?
- How do we intend to measure the processes?:
  Taking a blood test to identify the organism causing the infection
  Recording when antibiotics were started, dose, form, strength
  Change in health of the participants including presence or absence of infection
- What changes are taking place in the participants?:
  How many participants are getting better?
  How quickly are they recovering?

4.4. SANDY

Now we will return to Sandy and look at how he might deal with his data. Sandy has identified the information that he needs for his study and has decided that he needs to set up a database. This will help him to understand the format that each variable is measured in and help him to decide what to compare with what. So, before setting up the database Sandy looks at what information he has and what he wants to compare with what. This means he is thinking about how he will eventually analyse his data (see Section 4.3.3).

4.4.1. Data Collection

Sandy knows that he can collect all of the data he requires for the first part of his study from patients' medical records. He has the permission of his practice colleagues to do this. After a discussion with one of the doctors in the practice he makes a list of all the variables that he wants to compare in order to meet his study objectives. Sandy knows that he will need to set up a database that will enable him to describe what data he has, e.g. how many people there are with type II diabetes and what their age and sex is. Below is a list of the variables Sandy has identified so far, you can go back to Fig. 4.1 and see these variables in Sandy's research framework:

1. Blood glucose
2. Age
3. Date of diagnosis
4. Sex

There are also some other variables that might be interesting to explore to help to understand what is going on with the patients with diabetes:

5. Weight
6. Height
7. School/university/employed
8. Family history of diabetes.

There may be other variables that you can think of that Sandy might include – these are just an example of a few. Sandy needs to extract these data from the patients' medical records. Fortunately for him, the practice he works in has full electronic records so he should just be able to do some searches of the database and come up which the information he needs. Sandy now needs to set up a database and in Chapter 6 we will show you how to do this.

4.4.2. Data Treatment

We know already that the **data treatment** for this part of Sandy's study is based on principles of quantitative research. Sandy has now extracted all the data from the records and has an entry on his database for each patient in the practice with type II diabetes. He can now begin to explore some of the variables and see how they related to one another.

4.4.3. Characteristics of the Data

Sandy has discovered 298 patients on the practice records that have type II diabetes and he has set up his database to contain the following:

- Patient identifier (this will be in numeric form in the order Sandy enters their details on to the database, e.g. patient 1, 2, 3.......)
- Age
- Sex
- Work status (school or university or employed)
- Family history
- Weight
- Height
- Data of diagnosis
- Blood glucose (there will be more than one entry for each patient).

Self-Check Question   Have a look at the variables above and see if you can classify what type of data they are and how you would measure them.

4.4.4. Descriptive Statistics

As stated earlier, descriptive statistics are exactly as they sound. They are used to 'describe' the characteristics of your **dataset**. The statistics package you use will give you the opportunity to do this and so you can find out how many people on your database are in different age groups, how many of each sex – in fact all of the variables listed above. Descriptive statistics are an important first step in our data treatment because they enable us to visualise patterns that might be present amongst our group of patients. Indeed, Sandy might even find that there are more patients in the younger age range being diagnosed with type II diabetes. Descriptive statistics will also give us the **central tendency**, e.g. how the scores for Sandy's 298 patients are distributed from the lowest to the highest, and what the central point of this distribution is in terms of **mean**, **median** and **mode**. Sandy will also be able to look at the **spread** of his scores. For example, if there are a greater number of younger patients with diabetes, when he looks at the table for the spread of scores for the variable age, they will be bunched together at the bottom end of the table. The next step in the analysis will be for Sandy to see if he can 'infer' anything from the data using **inferential** statistics. This will enable him to make some generalisations about his patients compared to the rest of the population. In Chapter 10 you will find more about descriptive statistics and Chapter 11 is devoted to inferential statistics.

4.5. WHEN DO WE USE QUANTITATIVE METHODS?

Many pharmacists and health care professionals in general are intuitively drawn to quantitative research, methods and data due to their traditional scientific/mathematical orientation. The certainty of numbers, the relative ease with which numerical comparisons can be made, and the power of statistical testing all lead many of us to believe quantitative research is inherently more 'scientific' or true than alternative forms of research. As we will see in Parts III and IV of this book, this is not always the case: while there are of course circumstances when quantitative research may be the most appropriate choice, there will also be circumstances where it is not only inappropriate but potentially misleading – if we slavishly abide by the numbers alone. Particularly in the context of health services research and human participants, we must recognize and acknowledge the inherent 'messiness' of any research involving people, their health, their behaviours and their attitudes.

Thus, researchers must be mindful and deliberate when deciding to use quantitative research methods, and not simply use them as a default or go-to standard of practice. For example, it may be tempting to consider the problem of diabetes as a lack of exercise. Further, it may be tempting to try to address this issue by simply asking patients, 'On a scale of 1 to 5 (with 5 being extremely certain and 1 being not at all certain), how certain are you that you will exercise for 30 minutes sometime in the next week?' A question like this (which asks patients to translate their intentions into a quantitative scale) will yield a mathematical answer that may be amenable to statistical treatment. However the actual value or meaning of these numbers will be very small as the notion of 'intent' is so subjective and open to interpretation. Worse, within the context of a study, the participant may have a strong need to save face or please the researcher and may consequently upwardly inflate their intentions – again, significantly compromising the value of the numerical result.

Knowing when – and when not – to use quantitative research methods and numerical data is a critical skill for researchers, and recognizing that not everything that can be measured with numbers should be measured with numbers is important. The strong and generally natural inclination many pharmacists have for quantitative data may lead us to over-rely or over-emphasise these forms of research, which may inadvertently lead to a distortion in our analysis of objects of interest.

4.5.1. When Your Research Question Asks 'How Many?'

In health services research, frequency of an occurrence is an important starting point for understanding a phenomenon of interest. For example, the prevalence of a specific diagnosis can provide important clues as to what is significant for a specific population. Quantitative research methods are particularly well suited to these sorts of questions and to providing researchers with a numerical foundation for understanding frequency, prevalence, concentration, spread, distribution, density and other important health-related constructs. Many important general and public health questions depend upon clear data that illustrate the extent of a condition or diagnosis within a population, or the degree to which certain interventions (e.g. vaccinations) have been up-taken by the population at large. While numbers may not tell the whole story, in cases such as these, quantitative data set the foundation for understanding importance, significance and impact.

4.5.2. When There is a Numerical Change

Quantitative data are also essential to understanding how a process may evolve over time and in response to different circumstances. Particularly in the context of health, illness, wellness and disease progression, it is important to track changes over time as this may provide important insights into mechanisms by which conditions evolve. Baseline and tracking systems provide researchers with an opportunity to mathematically describe variables of interest over a period of time. The 'baseline' represents the initial or first formal measurement of a variable of interest, and is frequently numerically described as Time Zero (t0). Baseline data are critical to help establish changes over time and to understand the magnitude, rapidity, severity and importance of change. Tracking systems allow for measurements at different, defined points in time (numerically represented as t1, t2, t3, etc.) in order to facilitate comparisons between variables at different points on a time continuum. For epidemiologists and others interested in public health, this is an extraordinarily powerful tool to numerically describe the evolution that occurs within a population.

4.5.3. When You Want to Find Out What and How Many Other Factors Affect the Change

Consider for example the public health issue of childhood obesity. Recognizing the knock-on effects on health in adult life (with respect to cardiovascular health, diabetes risk etc.), it is important for health care professionals, policy makers, and the general public to understand the dimensions of this issue. Without real data, we cannot answer questions such as: ARE childhood obesity rates actually increasing (or are we simply more observant than in the past)? How quickly is this change occurring? Is childhood obesity increasing faster in cities, rural, or suburban areas? Is it concentrated in certain ethno-cultural groups? etc. Answers to these questions – which involve monitoring and tracking over time, with reference to a pre-established base point – can provide us with insights into possible solutions that are targeted to specific causes and needs.

Baseline and tracking systems are invaluable quantitative tools to establish that changes have occurred and to quantify their magnitude and rapidity. Well-constructed quantitative research can also aid us in understanding the factors (or variables) affecting the changes. With good long-term tracking systems built upon a solid baseline foundation, it becomes possible to mathematically depict the evolution that occurs within a population and to begin to draw cause-effect inferences or associations between variables of interest. This is a powerful tool that, for example, led epidemiologists to understand the link between smoking and lung cancer, or climate-change scientists to understand the association between human polluting activities and global warming. While it is tempting for a researcher to hope (expect?) that his/her own research will be similarly impactful, it is essential to understand how difficult a task this is, and how many layers of controls are required within the research to make such conclusions.

Community pharmacies are in a particularly important position to monitor public health issues. Sales of certain over-the-counter medications can be an early warning indicator of public health issues in the community. Establishing a monitoring system for these medications can provide invaluable information to public health officials regarding emerging issues. In a well-publicized example from Canada in the 1990s, community pharmacists in a rural farming community noted a rapid increase or spike in sales of over-the-counter anti-diarrheal medications such as loperamide. The rate of change and the magnitude of increase were significant enough for these pharmacists to contact public health officials who investigated. Shortly thereafter, it was determined that the local aquifer which supplied drinking water for the community had been contaminated by *E. coli* due to run-off contamination. Without the alert response of these pharmacists to follow-up on the change they had noted and measured in their practice with respect to sales of over-the-counter products, it might have taken weeks or months before this situation was seen as a public health issue, not simply an embarrassing personal issue. The research these pharmacists did was simple but effective: comparing changes over time in sales patterns and volumes across pharmacies of a specific category of drugs. Their findings, however, expedited the identification of a major public health risk in the community.

For most of us, research may illuminate or surface an association, or link, between factors and variables of interests. A power – and significant danger – of quantitative research is its potential to suggest cause-effect connections between dependent and independent variables. As we will see in Chapters 11 and 12, correlation is not necessarily causation. To say an intervention 'causes' a specific change requires a much higher burden of proof than to say that intervention is linked with, or associated with, a change. Quantitative research is uniquely well suited to establishing causal proofs, but it is important to be mindful of the fact that just because quantitative research is done does not necessarily guarantee causality.

4.5.4. When You Want to Test an (n) Hypothesis

Central to the Scientific Method is the notion that observations lead to hypotheses, and that hypotheses can be tested to establish their predictive value. Why is this so important? First, within the positivist paradigm, the testing of hypotheses (when done in an objective and reproducible manner) provides the greatest assurance possible of accuracy and validity. Quantitative research using appropriate statistical analytical methods provides us with the best possible mathematical approximations of the object of our interest. Second, hypotheses help us to explain our world, particularly the phenomena and situations that, at first glance, may appear somewhat confusing or contradictory. Methodical and rigorous quantitative research helps us to focus on reasons and root causes, rather than our emotional or subjective responses to such situations. Finally, hypothesis testing, at its best, allows us to better understand the cause-and-effect relationships that influence our observations of the world or, at the very least, helps us to establish the non-causal associations and relationships that start to explain how our world operates.

It is important to recognize that hypothesis testing does not necessarily or always prove our hunches, nor does it always yield conclusive results. This too can be valuable information for a researcher: when your hypothesis fails a test, many valuable and important lessons can still be learned that will help re-shape or re-orient the hypothesis for future testing. So-called negative results should not be interpreted as failure, but instead as simply the next step in the research process. Unfortunately, particularly within some academic environments, there is a tendency to want to avoid reporting or sharing of negative results for fear of giving the appearance of error or defeat. Failure to report negative results deprives you and the rest of the community of an invaluable opportunity to learn and to reconsider; it is, in fact, just as legitimate an outcome of research as a confirmatory, positive result.

CHAPTER SUMMARY

- In this chapter we have outlined some of the key principles of quantitative research.
- It has described the positivist and scientific approaches to research.
- It has outlined the processes of quantitative research and the variables at play in a research topic.

- It uses Sandy and Rosi's research to illustrate how they might use these principles.
- Finally, it describes some of the situations where quantitative methods work the best.

ANSWER TO SELF-CHECK QUESTION Have a look at the variables above and see if you can classify what type of data they are and how you would measure them.

See Chapter 3 for more explanations.

Age = Nominal data. Measurement would be Yes/No answers

Sex = Nominal data. Measurement would also be Yes/No answers

Work status (school or university or employed) = Nominal data measured using Yes/No answer. Note here that Sandy could ask his participants to indicate all that apply because they may be at school but have a part-time job.

Family history = Nominal data if Sandy is asking if there is a history of type II diabetes in the family. Again measured by Yes/No answers.

Weight = Interval data because we can compare differences in terms of heavier or lighter and we can also say how much heavier or lighter one measurement is than another. Sandy would probably just keep a record of participants weight over the course of the research and then use statistics to work out if the change in weight was significant (see Further Reading and Research Resources at the end of Chapter 3).

Height = Interval data. As for weight above.

Data of diagnosis = Simply measured by the date of diagnosis but Sandy could use this to work out how long his participants had had diabetes for.

Blood glucose (there will be more than one entry for each patient) = Again interval data for the reasons given above. Sandy would take regular measurements of blood glucose or ask his participants to keep a record of their own blood sugar.

5

Validity and Reliability: How Do You Know You Are Measuring What You Think You Are Measuring?

LEARNING OBJECTIVES

After reading this chapter you should be able to:
- understand problems inherent in making accurate measurements
- understand the key principles of validity
- understand the key principles of reliability
- understand how the concept of triangulation can be applied to pharmacy practice research
- consider the advantages of using previously validated measures

5.1. INTRODUCTION

In conducting pharmacy practice research we are attempting to find out things about patients, pharmacists and medicines set in the context of wider health care research. In much of this research it will be necessary to *measure* some of the variables we are interested in, e.g. blood pressure, weight, attitudes towards medicines or medicines adherence. It is essential that we know that we are measuring these things accurately because if at the end of our research we find out that we were not then all of that hard work is wasted. Even more serious would be if we did not realise that our measurements were inaccurate and we based a new pharmacy intervention on the findings. The '**gold standard**' of research is that we know that we are measuring what we think we are measuring; in other words the measurement tool we are using provides us with a **valid** measure. The other standard is that the valid measure we are using will do the same job over and over again, in other words the measurement tool is **reliable**.

Before we look at **validity** and **reliability** in detail we will briefly recap some of the essentials about measurement. This is because the validity and reliability of our research measurement tool is heavily dependent on the principles of measurement.

5.1.1. Measurement

As we described in Chapter 3, measurement is central to much of the work of researchers in the health professions. While the specific type of measurements used will vary depending upon the research we are doing, the quantification of a process, phenomenon or event is a frequently used tool for understanding and making comparisons. Measurement is not simply important to research; it is arguably the cornerstone for much of modern society. Everything ranging from salary decisions to academic grades, to the cost of goods and services is directly connected to some form of measurement. Think of how often we make judgements about a person's success according to how much they earn or how many As they achieved at school.

As measurement has grown to become more important to the effective functioning of society, there has been progress towards the notion of standardisation in measurement, ultimately leading to the current International System of Units (known as SI). The SI system reduces all measurements to mathematical combinations of seven base units: kilogram, metre, candela, second, ampere, Kelvin and mole. With the exception of the kilogram (which is defined in reference to an actual object housed at the International Bureau of

Weights and Measures outside Paris), most of these measurements are based upon globally agreed references. This consensus has evolved over time as a way of providing a common and agreed upon vocabulary for describing something as important as distance.

5.1.1.1. The SI System

The SI system is the generally agreed upon standard in the natural and health sciences, but there are alternative measurement systems that continue to be used in parallel to SI, particularly in everyday use and language. For example, the British system of Imperial Units may still be referred to when people discuss their body mass in terms of 'stones' rather than kilograms. In the United States, their US customary units convention may still be invoked, even within a health sciences context. For example, in the United States, cholesterol values are frequently still expressed as milligrams per decilitre (mg/dL) while in Canada, the UK, Australia and most other countries, they are expressed as millimoles per litre (mmol/L). This difference in measurement and reporting systems can produce serious negative consequences if one is unaware of these different conventions.

The units of measurement are only one (albeit very important) aspect of measurement that researchers must consider. Given the reliance we place on quantification and the faith we place in numbers to guide our decision making, understanding measurement, measurement errors, and mechanisms to ensure rigour and accuracy in measurement and reporting are essential for all researchers.

5.2. THE PROBLEM OF ACCURATE MEASUREMENT

Those who work in the area of measurement theory and sciences (called metrologists) begin with the understanding that all measurement is, by its very nature, only an approximation of reality. This can be demonstrated by two theories from science and social science. The **Heisenberg Uncertainty Principle** states that here is a fundamental limit to the precision with which certain pairs of complementary physical properties can be known with absolute certainty. First described within the field of physics and quantum mechanics, it states that it is impossible to know with absolute certainty both the position and the momentum of a subatomic particle: the actual act of measurement itself will distort one or the other. Some scientists believe that this and the other effect described in social sciences literature – **The Hawthorne Effect** (see below) – are both nothing more than the observer or experimenter effect which states that measurements cannot be made without actually affecting the system itself.

THE HAWTHORNE EFFECT

In the social sciences, this is sometimes referred to as the Hawthorne Effect, named after a seminal study that was undertaken at the Hawthorne Works factory in Chicago in the late 1920s. In these famous studies, the employer (Hawthorne Works) was interested in determining whether workers would be more productive (and consequently more profitable for the company) if they were provided with higher or lower level of lighting by which to work. The first rounds of research seemed to suggest the answer to the question was clearly yes: as lighting levels in the factory were adjusted, productivity did indeed improve. However, these productivity gains were short lived because as the studies concluded, they reverted back to baseline levels. Subsequent researchers recognised the transient and illusory changes that had at first been found in levels of production were simply a result of the confounding that occurs when researchers fail to realise that the act of observation itself changes a process. Knowing that they were being watched, and knowing that others were interested in their behaviour, the workers in the factory unconsciously changed their behaviours to please the researchers/managers. Once the observation period was over, they returned to their normal patterns. Think about how many times you have sat up straight and got on with your work when you realised a lecturer or manager was watching you.

The Heisenberg Uncertainty Principle, the observer or experimenter effect, and the Hawthorne Effect are all important examples of the limits of measurement. Knowing whether we are measuring something real or simply others' attempts to please us as researchers is one component to consider. Another comprises the actual limitations of measurement itself and the fact that we simply cannot know all factors about a process at the same time. The act of measurement itself changes the thing being measured, and researchers must always be mindful of this in the context of presenting results and findings. Please see the second half of Section 5.3.4 on systematic error or measurement bias.

5.3. MEASUREMENT AND HEALTH

So, now we have another problem. If measuring things with accuracy is so difficult then given the uniqueness of human beings and health and illness, things get even more complicated. In the health sciences, where there is a strong premium and value placed on the quantification of results, understanding that measurement is not always what it seems is important. For most health professionals – including (and perhaps especially) pharmacists – there is a strong intrinsic faith in the 'power' of numbers. Notions of 'evidence', 'certainty', and 'confidence' are crucial in guiding decision-making, and numbers have historically provided health professionals with the assurance they were doing the 'right thing'. As we shall see shortly, this faith in measurement and numbers, while not entirely misplaced, may be somewhat over-reaching. Measurement itself is always and inherently simply an approximation of truth, not the truth itself. Recognizing the various ways in which researchers may inadvertently or unconsciously influence an outcome (as in the Hawthorne Effect) or the simple fact that in measuring one variable of interest we lose control of measuring another important variable (as in the Heisenberg Principle), it is essential we always remain appropriately humble and modest about the power of measurement to truly answer important questions.

5.3.1.   What Are the Consequences if We Get It Wrong?

Within clinical practice ensuring that practice is evidence-based is very important. This evidence is frequently presented in the form of quantitative data. Evidence is the cornerstone for individual treatment decisions made by clinicians, as well as broader managerial decisions such as formulary selection. Evidence is relied upon heavily in making society-wide decisions around, for example, whether pediatric immunizations should be mandatory for school-aged children.

5.3.2.   The Need for Evidence

The need for evidence and the value health professionals place on it is understandable. After all if treatments are put in place that we do not know work, patients may die. Health professionals are frequently called upon to distinguish between patients' (and their own) opinions/beliefs and scientific facts; evidence provides the way in which to sort these things out. One contemporary controversy is the debate about the value of pediatric vaccinations. To a typical parent of today with no exposure to or experience of conditions such as diphtheria, tetanus or polio in their lifetime, the emphasis placed on early vaccination might be meaningless. This is because many of the potentially fatal childhood illnesses of the past have been eradicated and so the real-life consequences of such illnesses are hard to visualise.

Some of those opposed to vaccination see any evidence for vaccination as being distorted by pharmaceutical companies interested in maximizing sales of their product. Thus, even when the evidence is there it is hard to get people to accept it. Individuals have their own beliefs about health and illness that are not always based on evidence but on something they have grown up to believe. For example, a person may object to taking a red tablet because a family

member died after being given red tablets. Pharmacists need to understand these beliefs and use the evidence for or against treatment in order to help patients with taking their medication. This is a good time to introduce Serena Leesi, our pharmacy student who has a Saturday job in a local community pharmacy.

CASE STUDY EXAMPLE

To refresh your memory from Chapter 1 here is a recap of Serena's situation.

Serena Leesi is a 3rd year MPharm student with a Saturday job at her local pharmacy. She really enjoys working with the clients who come into the pharmacy and has got to know many of them who come in regularly. Some of the older clients seem to come in just for a chat and that's OK with Serena as long as the pharmacy is not too busy, Mrs Olive Trolave is one of the clients that Serena has got to know quite well, and they are even on first name terms. Olive is a 56-year-old woman who has struggled with many health issues, including respiratory disease, high blood pressure and high cholesterol. As she thinks about Olive Serena realises that there are a number of clients like her who struggle with health issues, and what many of them have in common is that they need to quit smoking. Serena is interested in doing something concrete, practical and meaningful to help patients like Olive through the smoking-cessation process. The generic tools and approaches she has learned at the university don't seem to be very effective for some reason.

Serena needs to have a look at the evidence for and against different smoking-cessation tools and has a lot of planning to do if she is to gain a better understanding of the ones used in pharmacy practice. There are three main strands to her research:

1. Review the methods of smoking cessation that have been used in health care that have a track record of success. This will enable her to decide whether they are tools that actually do help people quit smoking (validity) and that they do so time and time again for a variety of patients (reliability)
2. Identify the smoking cessation methods that might work best for patients like Olive
3. If allowed, Serena could talk to some regular patients who come into the pharmacy about how they feel about quitting smoking (we will follow this up in Chapters 16 and 17).

For now Serena will concentrate on looking for evidence of the validity and reliability of the tools that have been used to help people stop smoking, particularly in the community pharmacy setting.

Let's go back to the theory and look at how researchers can obtain evidence for health care interventions, some of which may be applied in pharmacy practice.

5.3.3. Measurement and Evidence

Measurement, when done well, is perhaps the most powerful tool we have to correct misconceptions and to reduce the influence of feelings and opinions in decision-making. However, the reality is that when we get measurements wrong – when we ignore or forget the lessons of Heisenberg and Hawthorne – there may be consequences for our research findings. One of those lessons, if you remember, is that when we measure one thing we may affect or distort the measurement of another. In a community pharmacy setting a pharmacist might be running a weight loss programme to help reduce the blood pressure of hypertensive patients. The problem is that if one is overweight and is asked to get on the scales then this can send one's blood pressure sky high. Therefore, although the measurement of weight may be accurate the measurement of blood pressure may not be and a wrong conclusion might be drawn that weight loss increases blood pressure!

THE WHITE COAT EFFECT

Some people are particularly sensitive to having their blood pressure taken with the result that their blood pressure can rise when measured. The cause of this is difficult to assess. It may be that some people associate going to a health centre or hospital with unpleasant experiences which increases their anxiety, which in turn increases their blood pressure. If we are not careful, this can result in inaccurate blood pressure readings and the possibility that people are treated unnecessarily for hypertension. Research suggests that the white coat effect is seen more frequently in older rather than younger patients and in women more often than men. A solution to the potential inaccuracy is to ask people to take their blood pressure at home and keep records. This is because the white coat effect appears to be associated with clinic visits.

In the above case, the wrong conclusions might be drawn because of the inferences made about the relationship between weight and blood pressure. This highlights the need to look at all of the variables in the situation and over time, to ensure that the assumptions made and interventions put in place are based on sound measurement. Below is a real-life situation that happened in the 1990s and 2000s that gives an example of how assumptions can be made, when the effects of medicines have not been measured for long enough.

HORMONE REPLACEMENT THERAPY (HRT)

One of the most important recent examples of the consequences of 'getting it wrong' was the overuse of HRT for post-menopausal women in the 1990s and 2000s. HRT is a strategy for supplementing or replacing naturally occurring hormones. During menopause, the reduction in circulating estrogen and progesterone that naturally occur during this phase of a woman's life may also produce a variety of issues, including hot flushes, psychological mood swings and lack of interest in sexual intimacy. A generation ago, HRT was proposed – and studied – as a way of managing these natural age-related changes and providing relief of these symptoms. During this time, many studies appeared measuring the improvements in day-to-day functioning experienced by women on HRT. Over time, these findings became so prominent that HRT began to be seen by many physicians (and women) as just as natural as menopause itself. Why endure the consequences of menopause when, through the power of HRT, one could age more gracefully and comfortably. In many parts of the Western world, HRT was considered standard 'treatment' for menopause, the idea being that all women should be placed on HRT once they approached menopause as a matter of routine. As more and more women began to use HRT, and as data from studies accumulated over a longer period of time, negative findings began to emerge. While HRT indeed was useful for symptom control, with long-term use there were increased risks of cardiovascular complications and heightened risks for certain forms of cancer. Today, we have a better understanding of the role and value of HRT and it is no longer considered 'required treatment' for the 'condition' of menopause. A more sophisticated risk–benefit analysis is required before embarking on HRT, along with a clear pathway for prescribing to maximise benefits and minimise risks. Still, for close to a decade, millions of women around the world received HRT – and today, we would recognize that this was inappropriate and perhaps for some of them even dangerous. In this case the example is more about making sure you measure everything and don't just go for the short-term measurements. In the previous example we highlighted the importance of interpreting blood pressure measurements with caution, in this example of HRT the measurement of menopause symptoms didn't directly have an impact on the measurement of cancer rates – it was that cancer rates were just not measured in the first place.

The implications from the above examples for Serena's research are clear. She needs to really critically appraise the research that has been done on smoking cessation to find out which tools have the best evidence of success. It seems to Serena that it would be irresponsible to use a smoking-cessation tool unless there was real evidence that it worked. People who are trying to quit smoking put a lot of effort in and Serena wouldn't want this to be in vain.

5.3.4.   What Are the Consequences if We Get It Right?

As we have seen, researchers and health professionals have significant responsibilities in both producing and using evidence. Without a clear understanding of the inherent limitations of measurement itself, we risk making suboptimal choices and decisions that can adversely affect individual patients.

However, when we take these issues into consideration, and recognise both the strengths and limitations of measurement and the tools we use to gather numerical data, we are in a very strong position to add to the evidence base and enhance the data upon which good decisions are made. It is important to note that the HRT story evolved precisely because scientists who understood the importance of good measurement undertook **longitudinal** (long-term) studies and it was these data that eventually overturned our initial clinical decisions and practices. For our student pharmacist, Serena, this is a good lesson to learn. Perhaps she needs to take into account the long-term effects of smoking-cessation programmes and will look for research studies that have tracked peoples' progress over time to see if they were successful at giving up in the long term. The fact that no measurement is perfect, that all measurement is approximation, does not mean that measurement itself is a flawed concept and thus should be discarded. Though it may be imperfect, measurement is one of the best tools we have for getting closer to understanding processes and events. Recognising the inherent imperfections and limitations of any form of measurement is an important first step. Not only are the tools we use for gathering numerical data always going to be in question, the way in which we actually interpret, analyse and apply our findings must also be scrutinized closely.

In the remainder of this chapter we are going to focus on two key aspects of measurement that are crucial: **validity** and **reliability.** As we saw in Chapter 3, True Score Theory helps us to better understand the limitations of measurement, and in particular the notion of measurement error. True Score Theory alerts us to the facts of **random error** and **systematic error**. Random errors are those factors that, in an unpredictable manner, may affect measurement. While the manner in which the measurement may be affected is unpredictable, the fact that random error exists and must always be accounted for is very predictable! Random error is sometimes referred to as 'noise' to highlight the fact that it may contribute variability to the overall data collected but it does not actually affect the overall average, since randomness can and does occur in any direction. In contrast, systematic error (sometimes referred to as **measurement bias**) tends to be either consistently positive or negative and consequently will actually affect or influence the overall average. Systematic errors may be a function of the researcher/observer, the measurement tool itself, or the process by which the data are gathered. A classic example of systematic error is the old-style intelligence ('IQ') tests that asked children to answer questions about sports they may simply know nothing about (due to family, cultural or other background reasons) and then equated this with baseline intelligence.

True Score Theory provides us with greater insight into the limitations of measurement; it also provides us with insights into specific techniques to minimise or mitigate measurement errors, and in particular those errors associated with measurement tools themselves. Reliability and validity are critical considerations for all researchers to consider in designing and implementing high-quality research.

5.4.   VALIDITY

The issue of validity is particularly important within the realm of health sciences and diagnostic testing. Many important decisions are based upon results from diagnostic tests and in pharmacy we use medications to treat individuals who, test results indicate, have high blood pressure or high cholesterol. We also use machines to measure blood pressure. As a result, clinicians (and patients) must have the utmost confidence that the tests themselves are actually measuring what we think they are measuring and doing it accurately.

5.4.1.   Validity: What Is It?

Validity is a concept of similar importance to reliability with respect to measurement and errors. Simply put, validity may be thought of as the extent to which a measurement tool measures what it says it measures. The validity of a measurement tool designed to measure a person's height can be relatively easily established by using other tools (in this case rulers) to check that the original height measurement tool was measuring height. However, once we start to think about the *attitudes* of pharmacy customers to having their height or weight or anything else measured, the validity of our measurement tool (in this case a questionnaire) is more difficult to ascertain.

EXAMPLE

Consider Sandy's young patients with diabetes. It is likely that they will have been given the equipment to self-test their blood sugar and the equipment must be quick, easy to use and give as accurate a reading as possible. People with diabetes rely on these machines to give them an accurate measure of their blood sugar so that they can keep their blood sugar under control. Sandy needs to be using a similar machine to ensure that when he does tests on the same patients he knows that both machines are measuring blood sugar and measuring it accurately. The machines can be **calibrated** to make sure they are doing this. Whether or not the blood sugar machine is measuring blood sugar accurately is the *validity* of the measurement tool.

5.4.2. Consequences of Ignoring Validity

Another condition that is dependent on valid measurement is serum cholesterol. Health care professionals make important decisions based on findings of cholesterol tests. Patients are started on medications (usually for life) with sometimes significant adverse effects, and the health care system pays an enormous amount of money to keep serum cholesterol levels below a certain magical threshold number. Clinicians and patients must always consider the validity of tests, their results and the decisions that flow from test results. They must be confident that the tests that are used to measure cholesterol levels are actually measuring cholesterol. The ability of a blood test to measure cholesterol and not something else must be established – that is the validity of the blood test for serum cholesterol. The consequences of ignoring the validity of our measurement tool is that some patients may be started on medication unnecessarily and some may not be given the correct medication – all because the test kit used was not measuring cholesterol in the way it should have been.

As with reliability, there are different types of validity, and in the following section we will explain those and give some examples of where they might be used. Each of these apply, not only to measurement instruments, but also to the actual design and implementation of the research process itself.

5.4.3. Face Validity

Face validity is an expression used to describe a relatively simple and common way researchers establish the validity of their work: on the *face* of it, does this measurement

instrument/tool/research process make sense? Sometimes referred to as 'the smell test', face validation is the method by which researchers assess the suitability of a process or measurement instrument, and by which they satisfy themselves that the process/instrument indeed does measure what we are setting out to measure.

There are many levels of face validation that are possible. At its simplest, an individual researcher simply reflects honestly and self-critically on their work to ensure that their intention is aptly matched by their proposed processes and tools. While this is a crucial form of validation, it is necessary but generally insufficient. Higher forms of face validation typically involve some sort of critical, external, peer review process, in which knowledgeable individuals not directly involved in the research itself are asked to reflect, comment, and critically appraise processes and instruments. In this approach, one relies upon the objectivity of external experts to ensure the research 'passes the smell test': does it make sense?

While there are methods for formalising and quantifying face validation processes, these are typically less important than the face validation activity itself. External scrutiny of one's work through peer review is one of the best ways of enhancing its quality, value and validity.

Let's return to our community pharmacy where the pharmacist is helping people with high blood pressure and who are overweight, to lose some weight in order to lower their blood pressure. One of the issues we raised earlier was that when people are about to have their weight measured they may get anxious and this anxiety may increase their blood pressure temporarily. To assess how anxious the patients are, the pharmacist could design a questionnaire to see whether or not patients were anxious about having their weight measured and what the level of anxiety was. The pharmacist could assess the face validity of his/her measure of anxiety by asking simply the patients whether they felt the questionnaire was measuring their anxiety.

5.4.4. Content Validity

Content validation is a process of examining a measurement instrument more closely to ensure that it actually covers an appropriate and representative sample of what one hopes to measure. Consider the example of a typical university-based examination in a pharmacotherapeutics course. The course may focus on cardiovascular therapeutics, so a student within the course may reasonably expect that the measurement instrument used for the course (the final examination) would cover content relevant to cardiovascular pharmacotherapeutics. If a major component of the examination focuses on questions related to geriatric depression, students may reasonably (and rightfully) complain that the measurement lacked content validity, as the test did not actually measure students' knowledge within the content domain itself.

Content validity is about fairness and transparency and answers the question we have been talking about all through this chapter. We make no apologies for asking it again – 'does the measurement actually measure what we say it is going to measure?' It might be assumed that a student with a grade of 80% in a course titled 'Cardiovascular Pharmaco-therapeutics' mastered 80% of the material in the course. If, however, the exam questions were externally reviewed and the reviewer saw that 50% of the examination covered geriatric depression, it calls into question the validity of the entire assessment process.

Content validation is critical for all researchers. An important component of content validation is sampling of our population of interest (see Chapter 4). Consider again the case of a cardiovascular pharmacotherapeutics examination. If this test had 100 questions, 95% of which covered angina, it would not be thought of as having content validity. This is because while angina is a cardiovascular issue and it is important, there are many other important cardiovascular issues that should be tested (e.g. hypertension, congestive heart failure and hyperlipidemia). A lecturer/teacher with a personal interest in one topic may **skew** the test measurement in a certain direction by putting in more questions about angina and that undermines content validity.

5.4.4.1. External Benchmarks

Content validation most frequently makes use of an external benchmark to match or confirm that the measure being used accurately reflects or represents the object being measured or the subject of the research. For example, in designing an examination for a cardiovascular pharmaco-therapeutics course, a tutor may first want to consult established, objective data regarding the distribution and prevalence of cardiovascular conditions in the country. They might then design a course based on these weightings (e.g. for this example, 30% of the course focuses on hypertension, 25% on angina, 20% on hyperlipidemia, 15% on CHF and so forth), and then ensure that the final examination reflects the emphasis taken in the course. Designing a course and examination in this manner is not just fair and transparent; it is also reliable (because an instructor at another school using the same methods would end up with a similar syllabus and examination).

This analogy extends to any kind of research activity. Researchers need to ensure that the process they are using to identify the content of interest, and the tools they use to measure it, have some objective grounding in the reality of the context itself.

EXAMPLE

Sandy may be interested in gaining a better understanding of the reasons behind his observation of the growing numbers of young, diabetic patients in his practice. If, however, he was politically minded, he may make the argument that government health policies are responsible for the rise in type II diabetes. Consequently he might decide how people vote in a general election is linked to the issue of diabetes and make an examination of local voting records. This would be his external benchmark. Sandy would, of course be wrong to do this because there would be no content validity in this method. It is unlikely that voting for a particular political party is going to have any effect on the development of type II diabetes, so this idea would not be grounded in reality!

5.4.5. Criterion-related Validity

One important method for demonstrating validity involves comparisons of findings or *results* to other external benchmarks. The key difference between criterion-related and content validity involves comparisons with findings/results themselves.

Two main examples of criterion-related validity include **concurrent validation** and **predictive validation**. Predictive validation involves assessment of results today with results from a future, related type of test. For example, one could reasonably assume that academic success within a university-based pharmacy degree programme should predict success on registration exams. Thus, all other things being equal, a student who receives 80% on a course-based examination in cardiovascular therapeutics could be reasonably expected to do better on a national licensing examination in this area than a student who scored 50% on that same test. Note that in this example, we are talking about similar measurement systems (written tests). We are not comparing performance on a written test with performance in practice, or in a clinical setting. If the course-based test has predictive validity, then, in a few years' time when the student takes the national registration test, there should be some association or correlation between scores then and scores now.

The pharmacy equivalent of this would be success in the pharmacy degree and success in the pre-registration examination.

Concurrent validity uses a similar principle, but involves current (or contemporaneous testing) rather than future testing. In the example above, one might reasonably assume that a student who scores 80% in a cardiovascular pharmacotherapy examination has mastered the fine art of 'how to succeed in pharmacy school'. The skills necessary to succeed in one pharmacotherapy examination should not differ significantly from any other similar examination. Thus if a student were taking cardiovascular pharmacotherapy at the same time as taking infectious diseases pharmacotherapy, one could expect that (all other things being equal), similar grades would be received on examinations. If this is the case, one could suggest the examination demonstrates concurrent validity: different instructors, different content but similar processes and tools yielding similar results.

As with face and content validation, criterion-related validation utilises the principle of external benchmarking as an important tool to reassure researchers and consumers of research that tools and processes are indeed measuring things that we think they are measuring. The value of going outside oneself or one's immediate research team and seeking confirmation in an objective way, from uninvolved experts or well-accepted benchmarks, is the essence of the validation process.

5.4.6.   Construct Validity

Perhaps the most challenging form of validation involves a critical examination of the focus of the research activity itself: construct validation. To many, construct validation is the most important and overarching type of validity to consider, with face, content and criterion-related validity subsumed within it.

Construct validity speaks to the appropriateness of drawing inferences, framing conclusions, and making decisions based on the results of research and measurement. Technically, constructs are described as **'latent variables'**: they are abstractions created to help us better describe, define, or conceptualize complex ideas that are neither real nor tangible. Consider the construct of 'intelligence' which we talked about in Section 5.3.4: all of us have some notion of what intelligence means but rarely do we actually discuss and debate the particular details. Intelligence is important insofar as many significant life decisions (including admission to academic programmes, hiring choices, promotion decisions) frequently use the construct of 'intelligence' as a way of justifying reasons for one decision as opposed to another. Intelligence is something that is not concrete or tangible, and may be difficult to observe: are 'book smart' people who lack common-sense intelligent? Does performance on an examination or course provide indirect or proxy evidence of 'intelligence'? Some individuals may be very academically intelligent while others may have an intelligence focused on practical problem solving or motor skills. Given the importance we place on intelligence as a criterion for making important decisions about the course of people's lives, it is perhaps surprising the underlying definition or nature of

intelligence itself (or the 'construct' of intelligence) is so rarely discussed by the general public.

Clinicians and health services researchers may encounter threats to construct validity far more frequently than we recognize or articulate. Consider the construct of 'depression', or 'illness', or 'wellness'. There are, for example, many physiologically healthy individuals who express dissatisfaction or unhappiness. Without clearly articulated and accepted operational definitions of words such as these (which attempt to encapsulate very complex human behaviours), there is a significant risk of making inappropriate treatment decisions.

Consider the following example: when is shyness simply a charming personality trait and when does it become a debilitating medical condition? Social anxiety disorders – the inability of some individuals to make and sustain interpersonal relationships with others due to intense psychological discomfort – can be life-altering and real medical conditions, but they exist on a continuum of human behaviours ranging from bashfulness to awkwardness and nervousness. At what point should it be considered merely part of the diversity of the human experience as opposed to a medical condition requiring pharmacotherapeutic intervention? Without a clear understanding and general agreement/acceptance of the construct itself by the public, decisions around treatment, intervention and medical vs social supports are very challenging to make.

Construct validation is frequently misunderstood as simply proclaiming a clear definition of an ambiguous term. Some researchers believe that by creating an 'operational definition' to alert readers to what they believe is meant by a construct, they have addressed the need for construct validation. While operational definitions are necessary to enhance clarity and allow readers to make their own conclusions, construct validation is usually far more complex than this. It usually requires a systematic, multifaceted and years-long effort to generate discussion, dialogue, debate, and eventually build consensus on the meanings of words we take for granted.

Most researchers are simply not able to invest this time and energy to achieve construct validation. In most cases, researchers are best advised to simply acknowledge this explicitly as a limitation of their work, and to appropriately and mindfully contextualise research questions, methods, measurement instruments and (most importantly) findings in a way that ensures, in this case, that readers understand there is only one true way of understanding a concept.

5.5.   RELIABILITY

We use the term reliable in day-to-day language to describe something (like a car) that is dependable. It is also used frequently to describe something that is trustworthy (for example, the news). Within a research context reliability is a crucial characteristic of both a measurement instrument (for example a survey) and a research process/study design (for example a double-blinded randomized placebo controlled trial).

5.5.1. Reliability: What Is It?

Reliability may be best thought of as consistency in measurement or replicability in findings if everything that we have done remains the same, e.g. the same laboratory conditions, room temperature or people with the same condition. A measurement is considered reliable when we get the same result over and over again. Even better, the reliability of a measurement is enhanced when other people using our tools and processes get the same results we do. Why is this important? Reliability speaks to both dependability and trustworthiness of the researchers, the measurement instruments, and the process. If different people at different times using the same instruments and approaches on the same objects arrive at the same measurements, this provides general reassurance to everyone that what we are measuring and reporting is indeed as close to the 'truth' as possible, given the inherent limitations of measurement described previously. A reliable measurement system (or **assessment tool**) is the crucial method by which consistency in measurement is achieved. An example from pharmacy practice might be when measuring a person's weight in our community pharmacy intervention to help people lose weight and reduce their blood pressure. We need to be sure that our weighing scales are going to measure people's weight in the same way time and time again and the same goes for the accuracy and consistency of our blood pressure measuring machine (**sphygmomanometer**). An assessment tool could also refer to a questionnaire to be completed by our patients trying to lose weight and how they feel about various issues concerning their weight.

When we set out to measure anything, as mentioned earlier, there is always going to be an element of error. The challenge becomes how to assess and put into context this measurement error: and the only way we can assess whether the measurement tool we are using is reliable or not is to use statistics. In Chapter 9 we will explain how to choose the right statistics for your data, including assessing reliability. For now we will outline some of the different types of reliability.

Specific types of reliability to consider that deal with internal consistency issues include inter-rater reliability and test-retest reliability and these two concepts will be discussed in the following section. In some cases, there may be situations where two or more different researchers or individuals are involved in measurement. The extent to which there is agreement or correspondence between these individuals' measurements is referred to as inter-rater reliability.

5.5.2. Inter-rater Reliability

Consider for example a situation where a community pharmacy chain wants its customers to give answers to a questionnaire administered by pharmacists by telephone. The way different pharmacists asked the questions or if they became involved in a conversation in the middle of the questionnaire, could affect the answers given by the customers. This means that the different pharmacists, by not administering the questionnaire in the same way would be reducing inter-rater reliability. So, our pharmacists might be interpreting what the customers say in a different way and there is a lack of consistency of measurement between two independent observers (the pharmacists). Most typically, inter-rater reliability is described using an 'r' coefficient; r values greater than 0.8 (meaning that there is 80% agreement/consistency between raters) is usually considered acceptable.

5.5.3. Test-retest Reliability

In other situations we are more concerned about the stability of measurement over different points in time. For example if a pharmacy student were to take an examination in the morning one would hope/expect his/her grade would be the same as if the examination were taken in the evening. Time of day should not (in theory) influence academic performance. However, we also know some people are morning people and others don't wake up until noon, etc. If there is a performance difference on the exact same examination taken by the same person at different times or days, we become concerned about test-retest validity and try to identify what other confounding variables (e.g. students' sleep–wake patterns) might be influencing the measurement. This can be a concern; if there is a difference in test-retest measurements, then researchers (and students) need to take into account the confounding variable in their measurement practices and protocols.

5.6. TRIANGULATION

As the previous discussion has suggested, validity is an important, complex and very messy factor to consider in research design and measurement. Demonstrating validity of processes and instruments can be more cumbersome and time consuming than actually undertaking the research itself. Mindful of this, and borrowing from the fields of land surveying and seafaring, many researchers prefer to opt for a method known as triangulation to address validity issues. Within surveying fields, triangulation is a process by which a single point in space can be determined through the convergence of measurements taken from two or more other, distinct, different points. Rather than directly measure one point in space, surveyors and sailors use multiple measurements of different points to cross-reference one another, thereby increasing confidence in the final result.

Within health services and pharmacy practice research, this principle of triangulation is equally important. It is one of the most powerful techniques available to allow for substantiation and cross-verification of data. For researchers, triangulation refers to the use of several different, complimentary research methods and instruments to study the same event or phenomenon, then pooling the findings and results to arrive at the closest approximation possible of the truth. It also prevents overreliance on one perspective or set of instruments/tools that may inadvertently produce blind spots for the researcher: building triangulation into a study design enhances both credibility and quality of the outcome.

Frequently, triangulation involves mixed-methods type research, in which both quantitative (e.g. a survey) and qualitative (e.g. interviews with key informants) methods are used concurrently to study a phenomenon. Findings from one approach inform the interpretation of findings of the other approach in an iterative manner. Moreover, since different measurement instruments are required for qualitative and quantitative approaches, this may reduce problems with systematic measurement errors even if it does little to address random errors. Increasingly mixed methods research is gaining prominence within the health services research context, partly in recognition of the challenges associated with reliability and validity in single-methods approaches. Using mixed-methods as a tool for triangulation does not excuse the researcher from still carefully considering issues of reliability and validity with each individual method used; however, within the context of a mixed-methods study, this form of triangulation can be a powerful tool for overcoming the weaknesses, biases and limitations inherent in single-method research designs and measurement instruments.

5.7. USING PREVIOUSLY VALIDATED MEASURES

For most pharmacy practice researchers, the challenges of starting and running a research study are significant. To make life easier and to avoid a lengthy validation process for the measure we have designed ourselves, the alternative is to use a measure that has been previously well-validated. In most cases, both novice and experienced researchers are encouraged to consider using measurement tools and instruments that have been previously validated, used and reported in the literature. Do not underestimate the unique

challenges introduced when using other's work: you won't be able to simply cut-and-paste. First and foremost, you need to consider the context within which the original measurement instrument was used and validated, and the extent to which it corresponds to your context. For example, a measurement tool examining patient's satisfaction with the health care system that was developed and validated in the United States may not 'fit' in the United Kingdom: the health care systems and national cultures are so different that a validated tool from the United States may not demonstrate the same reliability and validity when used in the United Kingdom.

Even when using previously validated measures, there may be a need for some small modifications: for example, drug names may vary from one country to another, spelling of certain words (e.g. 'colour' vs 'color') may be different, etc. Small editorial changes such as these may not affect the validation of the instrument; however, when researchers begin to significantly alter items on a questionnaire, interview prompts or other aspects of the measurement tool in order to better 'fit' their context of interest, they need to be mindful of the fact that after a certain number of changes, the previously validated instrument may no longer work as originally intended.

It is also essential to understand the context within which the measurement instrument was actually used in the original study. For example, if a validated interview questionnaire guide is being used, were the interviewers in the original study trained in a specific way to use the guide...and can you train your interviewers in that same manner in order to ensure that, even if you are using the exact same interview questionnaire guide, it is being used in as close to the same way as the original as possible?

In all cases, when using previously validated instruments, it is essential to establish contact with, receive permission from, and seek advice and input from the original authors of the instrument itself. Their experience in developing and validating the instrument in the first place for their context will be invaluable for those contemplating its use in a different context. It is a matter of academic integrity that you contact the researcher who designed the original research and in some cases not doing so can result in legal action being taken against you or your institution. This is because many researchers copyright their work and by using it without their permission you would be breaching this.

A thorough literature review could potentially yield previously validated instruments that may be of relevance to your work. Systematic appraisal of these potential instruments for your context and work is part of the preparation process that is integral to the commencement of any research project. All researchers, however experienced, should resist the ego-temptation of wanting to develop and name their own survey, instrument, tool or other measurement. Using previously validated tools and judiciously adapting them for your context is by far the best method of addressing the many challenges associated with reliability and validity discussed in this chapter.

CHAPTER SUMMARY

- In this chapter we have outlined some of the key principles of validity and reliability used in quantitative research.
- Some of the problems we face when trying to make accurate measurements and the consequences if we get our measurements wrong have been outlined.
- Serena and Sandy's research has been used to illustrate how they might use the principles of validity and reliability.
- Finally, triangulation and how this might be implemented is described.

FURTHER READING

There is no specific further reading for this chapter; most books on statistics cover the concepts described. Andy Field's website that we referred to in Chapter 3 will also provide you with valuable resources https://www.discoveringstatistics.com/.

6

Planning a Survey, Designing Your Questionnaire, and Setting Up a Database

LEARNING OBJECTIVES

After reading this chapter you should be able to:
- explain what a survey is and the key principles of survey design
- describe different types of survey and explain when each type might be used
- describe how a survey can be conducted and the strengths and weaknesses of each one
- describe different survey formats
- understand what a questionnaire is and how it might be administered
- understand the key principles of questionnaire design
- describe different types of questions that can be used in a questionnaire

6.1 INTRODUCTION

Surveys are amongst the most frequently used research tools in health services and pharmacy practice research. Survey research is a data gathering and analysis methodology most frequently used to assess participants' thoughts, opinions, beliefs or feelings. In some cases, survey research can be used to assess participants' behaviours and actions, but this will frequently rely upon self-reporting which introduces inherent bias or potential error. In everyday life, we are generally most familiar with surveys used to assess voter intentions during elections, or opinions about public policy issues. In most cases, surveys use questionnaires that consist of a series of set/specific questions which are 'given' to the participants. Survey questionnaires can be administered in person (through an interview format), over the telephone, online using electronic distribution methods such as email or the internet, or through the mail.

Surveys are frequently used in health services (including pharmacy practice) research for three main reasons:
1. First, surveys tend to provide us with quantitative results which can be useful for making comparisons and drawing conclusions in a way that is both familiar to and comforting for health care professionals.
2. Second, surveys are a cost-effective way of collecting data from large numbers of people. The main costs are incurred at the design and testing stage of planning a survey but after this it becomes cost- and resource-effective to include additional participants. This gives us the opportunity of increasing the number of participants if we choose to.
3. Third, surveys can be pilot tested and validated in a rigorous manner to ensure they conform to requirements and expectations of the researcher and those who will be consuming the results of the research.

Not all surveys are created equally: as we shall see in this chapter, survey design is as much science as art. Designing effective, fair and meaningful questions for a survey is a challenging and essential task that will fundamentally affect the quality of the data collected. There are many surveys that demonstrate bias, deliver leading questions, or use ambiguous terms or phrases that produce data that are ultimately unreliable, invalid and consequently meaningless. In this chapter, we will review processes for ensuring robust survey processes and clear question development which will contribute significantly to a high-quality outcome.

It is frequently tempting to use results of surveys to draw sweeping conclusions about an entire population of interest. For example, during an election, the media may breathlessly report on political candidates' standing in the polls, and draw inferences about the general population's intentions, desires, and expectations from survey data. Surveys will frequently collect demographic data about respondents, such as their age, sex, geographical location, income level and education so media interpretations of research results may focus on one or more of these. While surveys can be useful to allow for detection of a relationship between different variables (for example, sex of a respondent and opinions regarding desirability of universal child care) it is always important to remember that just because there is a relationship between two variables does not mean that one causes the other. Simply because a survey uncovers or points to a trend amongst certain types of respondents with respect to an outcome of interest does not prove **causality**. The correlational data that is generated through survey research can be valuable and significant if interpreted correctly. However, more sophisticated statistical techniques may be necessary to move beyond the level of association, relationship, or correlation. These are known as inferential statistics, and we introduced them in Chapter 3. The whole of Chapter 11 is dedicated to these types of statistics with step-by-step guidance on how to use them. As with all research methods, it is essential to be accurate in terms of collection, analysis and presentation of data, and to only draw conclusions from the data that are truly there.

Survey questionnaires are typically administered to a representative sample of a population of interest. That is a subset of the general population broadly similar to the larger population in terms of demographic characteristics. When this is achieved, researchers can make inferences from the survey results about the thoughts, feelings, attitudes, opinions and beliefs of the broader population of interest. As will be discussed shortly, those using survey methods must be conscious of the importance of sampling techniques, as this will determine the **generalisability** of findings to the broader population.

6.2 DIFFERENT SURVEY TYPES AND WHEN TO USE THEM

In our daily lives, we see surveys used to determine all sorts of things. For example, universities in the United Kingdom participate in a National Student Survey which provides detailed information about what students think of their place of learning; hospitals ask patients about their satisfaction with out-patient clinics, and community pharmacists may ask their customers about the services they offer. Such surveys provide valuable information about the provision of services and give organisations the opportunity to improve and develop in the direction the consumer prefers.

Within professional pharmacy practice there are many circumstances where surveys are appropriately used. For example, if a pharmacist were trying to build a business and wanted to better understand the needs and wants of the local community, she/he may distribute a survey to local health care providers and customers. Alternatively, if a hospital pharmacist wanted to evaluate the success of an educational programme she/he had delivered, and what could be done for quality improvement in the future, a survey of participants in the programme could be helpful. Those in the pharmaceutical industry frequently rely upon surveys in the context of market research to determine what consumers want and what they are willing to pay for.

In general there are three major categories or types of survey research that are used: cross-sectional, successive independent samples, and longitudinal type research:

1. Cross-sectional survey

A representative sample of a population of interest is studied once, for example, a public opinion poll prior to an election. This approach would provide a 'snapshot' of public opinion at one point in time and place.

2. Successive independent samples survey

This involves use of multiple random but representative samples from a population at different times. This approach can be useful for examining *changes* in opinions, beliefs or attitudes within a population, but not for changes *within* individual participants because a different representative sample is used each time. As a result we cannot actually identify reasons or causes for individual changes in opinions over time, just that there has been a change. This approach might be used to track societies' evolving opinions towards important social issues such as same-sex marriage.

3. Longitudinal studies

These involve surveying the same random and representative sample at multiple different points in time. In this approach, researchers can track both the evolution of a group's thinking, attitudes or opinions, and the way individuals within that group have changed. Such surveys are logistically complicated (since individuals will move, die, drop out or simply disappear from the view of the researcher) and expensive to operate as they occur over a longer period of time. Examples of major longitudinal surveys include aspects of the Framingham Heart Study which examined long-term, ongoing cardiovascular health of the residents of Framingham Massachusetts. Beginning in 1948, over 5000 adult subjects enrolled, and now the study is on its third generation of participants (grandchildren of the original cohort). The same participants are contacted on a periodic basis and asked to complete questionnaires regarding diet, smoking, exercise and other lifestyle choices, and these results are then matched to those participants' health outcomes with respect to blood pressure, cholesterol levels and incidences of major cardiovascular illness. This study produced the Framingham Risk Functions that are used today. The study has its own website which can be found at https://www.framinghamheartstudy.org/ and makes for interesting reading.

As can be seen, survey methods are broad and diverse, and strongly depend upon both the researchers' interests and goals, and availability of time and resources to facilitate completion. They can be used in a variety of different contexts and for different purposes but regardless of context or purpose it is critical that the measurement tool used (e.g. the **questionnaire**) is both reliable and valid (see Chapter 5) for the stated purpose.

6.3 CONDUCTING A SURVEY: THE QUESTIONNAIRE

Within a survey, the questionnaire is the most commonly used tool for eliciting information from participants. A questionnaire is simply an instrument to gather data from participants, usually using a question-answer format.

Questionnaires allow for tabulation of results, electronic management of data through use of databases, and (depending upon the types of questions asked) the ability to statistically interpret findings. Designing a questionnaire and writing individual questions takes time and attention. Before beginning it is imperative that the researcher has a clear understanding of his/her objectives; a clear research question and a solid understanding of what kind of evidence is needed to fulfill the purpose of the study; and to know not only the purpose of the research but how the information gathered will be used, analysed and synthesised. People participating in research that uses questionnaires are also called '**respondents**' because they are responding to questions. We will use that term for the remainder of this chapter.

6.3.1 What Are Your Goals, and Who Can Help You Reach Them?

In most cases, survey methods and questionnaires are used to describe a population (for example, customers in a pharmacy and what services they value and are willing to pay for out of their own pockets). In some cases – that may require a very different study design and questionnaire format – the goal is to make comparisons between different groups of individuals (for example, those who use pharmacists for minor ailments needs vs those who continue to rely upon family physicians). In other cases, questionnaires are used to simply elicit specific feedback around a targeted question from a specific group of individuals, and to learn more about their wants and needs (for example, asking customers of a pharmacy if they actually appreciate a 'call-back' from

a pharmacist several days after receiving a new prescription, to determine if there are any questions or needs).

Once the specific research goals and objectives are finalised, this will likely provide guidance as to the target population for the study. Here are some questions that need to be answered:
- Who are the people you need to hear from in order to answer your questions?
- What criteria separate those who should be included in your survey from those whose responses will not be helpful to you?
- Can you survey an entire population? If the target population that is identified is small, readily accessible, and willing to be involved, it may be possible to actually survey the entire population.

For example, if a pharmacy owner is wondering about the best way to allocate holiday time amongst the staff in the pharmacy, everyone will have strong incentive to participate and have their voice heard, and this is a relatively small number of individuals. When the target population is large, less motivated to be involved, and harder to reach, a sampling strategy will be required to ensure a representative subset of the target population is involved in the research. Working with research participants and building random samples will be discussed in Chapter 7.

Let's rejoin our hospital pharmacist, **Dorothy**, as she continues to work out how to conduct the research for her Master's thesis. When we left Dorothy in Chapter 3 she had decided on her research question which is:

> *'What are the barriers and enablers to implementation of an antimicrobial stewardship programme in my hospital?'*

Dorothy has realised that having a clear understanding of the problem she is trying to solve should allow for the development of a method and data gathering tools (such as surveys or questionnaires) which are focussed and precise. Dorothy will include the rationale for how to gather her data in her research protocol (see Chapter 2, Section 2.3 'Planning Research'). Remember, this is just one example of how a survey-based research project *might* be developed.

One thing that is for certain is that there are a significant number of people with different knowledge and skills involved in the use of antimicrobial drugs. It will, therefore, be necessary for Dorothy to design her questionnaire so that it contains core questions that can be answered by all staff groups. She will also have to allow space for questions about things like testing for infections and the implementation of policies.

We will now have a look at the theory of questionnaire design, and Dorothy will join us at different times throughout the remainder of this chapter.

Dorothy's Goals

Dorothy wants to find out about the feasibility of beginning an antimicrobial stewardship programme in her hospital. This is an inter-professional collaboration designed to encourage optimal prescribing which can have the added benefit of reducing overall health care (including drug) expenditures. This will be her overall goal but there may be other goals she wants to meet along the way. In research the primary goal is often described as the 'Aim' and the other goals are described as the 'Objectives'. The overall goal indicates what Dorothy's overall aim of her research is and the objectives will help her to organise how she is going to achieve her aim. Dorothy's aim comes directly from her research question, and the aim and objectives are set out below.

Aim:
To identify the barriers and enablers to implementation of an antimicrobial stewardship programme in XX hospital.

Objectives:
1. Describe the attitudes of the interprofessional team towards antimicrobial stewardship
2. Compare the views of doctors, nurses, pharmacists, microbiologists and others involved in the antimicrobial prescribing decisions made at XX hospital
3. Identify barriers to implementation of an antimicrobial stewardship programme
4. Identify the enablers to implementation of an antimicrobial stewardship programme
5. Develop a draft programme
(......again there may be other objectives but this gives an idea of how they might be set out).

6.4 QUESTIONNAIRE DESIGN

As you may have realised by now, the design of the questionnaire to be used in our survey is fundamental to the success of our data collection. Once the survey has begun and questionnaires have been distributed it will be too late to add or delete questions. To help you get this right the first time here are some questions you should ask.

6.4.1. What Kind of Information Are You Trying to Collect?

In designing a questionnaire and constructing individual questions, it is important to be clear about the kinds of data that you are trying to collect. At least four different categories of information can be differentiated; items on a questionnaire should clearly delineate what kind of data are being collected:

a. Knowledge and awareness: what do participants know and how well do they understand?

This category of question is focussed on the foundations of understanding: what do people know, is it correct/incorrect or accurate/inaccurate? An example of this kind of question in **Dorothy's** questionnaire might be:
- 'Which antimicrobial drugs do you prescribe?' or
- 'Penicillin V is used to treat _____'.

Although prescribers have different preferences, in general specific antimicrobials are used in specific circumstances. Thus the above questions have right and wrong answers that are objectively determined and are not subject to opinion. It can be very useful to ask knowledge questions in a questionnaire to establish if respondents have a common, accurate foundation in facts. For example, the knowledge that health care professionals have will inform their opinions, beliefs and attitudes towards antimicrobial prescribing and thus their subsequent behaviours.

b. Beliefs and opinions: what do respondents feel about what they know and understand?

This category of question is focussed on the psychological state of mind of respondents. As a result, these questions represent an amalgam of knowledge and feelings, facts and emotions. While individuals may 'know' something to be true and understand it, they may also have had a previous experience with it that creates an emotional response that in turn may produce an opinion, attitude or belief. For example, a pharmacist in Dorothy's study may have experienced a situation where a patient had a fatal reaction to an antimicrobial which may have made him more cautious about the prescribing of antibiotics. The pharmacist may know that such a reaction only happens to 1:1,000,000 patients but the connection between what he knows to be true and what he has experienced can sometimes result in surprising or illogical behaviour; perhaps the experience was so difficult the pharmacist cannot disassociate it from prescribing decisions. It is important that when writing questions for her questionnaire Dorothy is mindful of the types of questions she is asking and how their responses might be 'coloured' by emotion. An example of such a question might be '*Which member of the health care team is most knowledgeable about antimicrobial prescribing?*' which asks respondents to make a judgement based on their own feeling about others' knowledge.

c. Behaviours and actions: what do people actually do with what they know and what they feel?

Behaviourally oriented questions ask respondents to report on what they have done in the past in a specific situation and to say how they may respond in the future to a hypothetical situation. Asking participants to respond to hypothetical scenarios of 'how would you respond in this situation' can be challenging, as can interpretation of the responses, because just because someone says they intend to do something doesn't mean they actually will when the situation arises (think about New Year's Resolutions!).

Look back to Chapter 2 and remind yourself about the Theory of Planned Behaviour. This works for health care professionals as well as patients.

Examples of these sorts of questions include 'Think about the last time you considered the cost of an antimicrobial drug?' (a question about something that has been done in the past) or 'Would you consider cost in the future when prescribing an antimicrobial drug?' (a question about future intentions).

d. Attributes and characteristics: what people are

An important category of questions to consider are those which allow researchers to stratify participants based on specific demographic factors such as age, education level, occupation, income, sex, etc. These attribute questions are of interest in helping to generate predictive models of how others not sampled in the research may be expected to behave. The assumption here is that demographic characteristics have a strong influence on knowledge, beliefs and, subsequently, actions, and that by finding relationships between demographic characteristics and these other factors it becomes possible to more accurately predict how the population as a whole will behave in a certain situation. An example of this category of question in Dorothy's questionnaire might be, 'Where did you train as a pharmacist/doctor/nurse?'

Dorothy knows that she must gather information about her respondents somewhere on her questionnaire. This can come at the beginning or the end. At the end of this chapter you will find a copy of the demographics pages of Dorothy's questionnaire. (See Appendix A) For now, we are going to leave Dorothy's questionnaire and look at some other examples from pharmacy practice to demonstrate how different types of question can be used.

6.4.2   What Are You Going to Ask?

Once you have decided what information to collect, you need to start thinking about how to collect it: what questions are you going to ask? In designing a questionnaire aligned with your research aims and objectives, and being sensitive to the needs of your participants, it is essential to keep the following points in mind:

a. Do not ask a question unless it has a specific use and relates directly to your research purpose. Collecting excess, unnecessary information adds to the time required to complete the questionnaire which will be a disincentive for participants. It also costs the researcher time and money and can result in information overload. Ethically, it is also a dubious practice as it potentially invades the privacy of the participant for no good reason. Avoid the temptation to ask 'nice-to-know' questions, and ensure that every question serves a clear purpose directly linked to the research objectives.

b. As the questionnaire is being developed, it is usually helpful to consider what you as a researcher will actually DO with the results to a specific question:
*   How will data be analysed?
*   How will it be organised so that you can compare responses to different questions?
*   How will information be managed?
*   How will participants' responses and personal information be protected and kept confidential? (see Chapter 7, Section 7.3.1).

These kinds of considerations can help you to winnow down unnecessary questions and ensure the questionnaire stays razor-focussed on the objectives.

6.4.3   How Are You Going to Ask?

Whatever type of questionnaire you decide to administer, consideration needs to be given to how questions are asked and what expectations we have about how they will be answered. It is important to remember that just because a researcher understands a question and interprets it in a certain way, not all respondents will do the same. Conducting a pilot study to see how your questionnaire 'works' is a useful way of finding out and correcting any format issues. The people who take part in the pilot study can provide valuable information about interpretation and also the length of time taken to complete the questionnaire (see Section 6.7). One of the things pilot participants can be asked to do is to provide feedback on any questions that might be ambiguous or difficult to answer, e.g. leading questions or asking two questions in one ('**double-barrelled**'). This provides the opportunity to revise the questionnaire to ensure that respondents can answer it easily. Let's look at some of the question formats that can be used.

6.4.3.1   Dichotomous Questions

These are questions that yield only one of two responses (such as 'Yes/No' or 'Pass/Fail'). Surveys using dichotomous questions force respondents to pick one answer or the other, with no opportunity for nuance or context. An **advantage** of such questions is the relative ease of data management and interpretation. Conversely a **disadvantage** of such questions is the forcing of an answer from a participant that isn't altogether accurate or reflective of what they really think. For example, asking a dichotomous question such as 'Are you in favour of abortion?' takes a complex and difficult question and reduces it to only two choices. Some individuals may not be able to summarise their views in such a stark manner and for others, the circumstances of individual cases will be important to consider. Forcing an individual to answer this question, framed in this way, will result in poor data collection and will compromise quality of analysis. All the researcher will be able to say is how many people said they were in favour of abortion and how many were not.

6.4.3.2   Categorical Questions

These are questions that will have responses that 'fit' into one of several categories. For example, if gathering demographic information related to age, one may ask respondents to report their age based on categories such as <20, 21–30, 31–40, 41–50, 51–60 or >60 years of age. In other cases, response categories may use word labels such as 'very satisfied, satisfied, dissatisfied, very dissatisfied'. Categorical questions provide greater opportunity for respondents to accurately label their responses in a way that is more meaningful for both researcher and participant. In some cases, categorical questions may still force respondents to answer. For example, the satisfaction scale above did not provide an option for respondents to say 'neither satisfied nor dissatisfied'. When selecting and naming categories, it is important that researchers clearly understand the implications of their decisions with respect to framing of categories.

6.4.3.3   Closed-Ended Questions

These are questions that require respondents to select from a set of options. An example question may be:
'Which of the following medications do you take for your
    blood pressure?':
    Beta blocker (e.g. atenolol)
    Diuretic (e.g. furosemide)
    Calcium channel blocker (e.g. nifedipine)
    ACE inhibitor (e.g. ramipril)
    Other (please specify)
    None of the above
    In this example, respondents are asked to select from a comprehensive menu of options, which include an 'other please specify' category as well as a none-of-the-above category to acknowledge that the question may simply not be applicable in all cases.

6.4.3.4   Open-Ended Questions

In some questionnaires respondents can be given the opportunity to use their own words to respond to questions. Open-ended questions are those questions which cannot be answered with simple Yes/No type answers. In an open-ended survey question the objective is not to lead respondents or plant ideas through the wording of questions. Instead, the researchers are hoping to approximate as closely as possible the real feelings, thoughts, opinions and attitudes of respondents by allowing them to use their own words. This can help researchers to understand more about how patients feel about their diagnosis, how it affects their lives or any other information that is important to the patient. In this way patients can be helped to manage their condition more effectively. An example of this might be:

'How do you feel about your recent diagnosis of high blood pressure?'

Space will then be left for the respondent to write as much or as little as they wish in answer to the question. Some patients find it difficult to accept that they have a health problem that needs to be treated with medication. This is because pre-existing beliefs about illness and health can have a significant effect on our attitudes towards a diagnosis and subsequent treatment (see Chapter 2).

Open-ended questions introduce a variety of logistical challenges in terms of data management and analysis, and can sometimes produce enormous volumes of words depending upon how much respondents want to share. Further, the words themselves may be challenging to interpret as individuals may use certain terms (e.g. *'I feel fine'*) that mean different things to different people. However, open-ended questions do provide researchers with unique opportunities to better understand the real thoughts and opinions of participants rather than leading them through a checkbox exercise of forced questions. For this reason such questions are particularly suited to qualitative research which is the subject of Part III of this book.

6.4.4   Setting the Tone

Having determined the category of questions to be constructed, it is important to know how best to actually write (or 'word') questions in a way to ensure clarity, minimise ambiguity, ensure accuracy, encourage honesty, and eliminate potential bias:

a. Make sure the instructions on how to complete questions are accurate and easy to understand.

b. Use the simplest words possible: Do not 'talk down' to respondents but ensure you are clear and succinct. For example, do not use the term 'gastrointestinal distress' when 'stomach ache' is what you actually mean.

c. It is important to be specific: vague descriptive terms will frequently result in ambiguity and misinterpretation, compromising the accuracy of responses and the overall reliability of your questionnaire. Carefully scrutinise each

EXAMPLE

If a researcher were interested in asking a question about uptake of a pharmacy service such as a minor ailments programme by the local community, there are various options:
a. Open-ended, unstructured question:

'What do you think of the idea of pharmacists diagnosing and providing treatment recommendations for minor ailments (such as pink eye otherwise known as conjunctivitis and cold sores) without referring a patient to the doctor?'

While this may be an easy way to ask a question, and may elicit deep and valuable information about patients' preferences, and their view on the status of pharmacists and physicians, information collected in this way will not be easy to analyse. The variety of words, terms and ideas that will emerge – while interesting – will be challenging to manage. Most likely, information gathered this way will need to be categorised and summarised first, then analysed. Such questions may be useful for stimulating thinking about a topic, eliciting creative solutions, or for probing for more details.
b. Closed-ended question with structured response:

'In the last six months, how frequently did you access a pharmacist for minor ailments consultation for the following conditions?'

	0 times	1–2 times	3–4 times	>4 times
Pink Eye				
Cold Sores				
Unexplained Rash				

While this question may be complex to answer (as it requires the respondent to interpret a chart and select the correct box for completion) it has the advantage of generating clear, specific, '**retrospective**' data that will be easy to manage and useful for analysis – assuming the respondent is able to decipher the table and answer it accurately in the first place! A problem with questions that ask people to think back is that they may not be able

to remember the number of visits they have made to their pharmacy, and this can lead to **recall bias** of the respondent. An alternative and easier way of presenting closed-ended questions with structured responses is the traditional Yes/No:

'In the last six months, did you access a pharmacist for minor ailments consultations for the following conditions?'

	Yes	No
Pink Eye		
Cold Sores		
Unexplained Rash		

Closed questions such as these are generally preferred by researchers because they are clear, provide useful data for analysis and are easy to manage. Care must be taken to ensure they do not inappropriately force respondents to answer questions in an inaccurate way, and that the presentation of the question itself is not overwhelming or burdensome.
c. Closed-ended questions with unordered responses

This style of question may be useful in eliciting beliefs and opinions from respondents in a non-leading way. For example:

'For which of the following conditions would you follow a pharmacist's recommendation without seeking another opinion from a physician?' (circle all that apply):

Pink Eye
Cold Sores
Unexplained Rash

This question makes data management and analysis relatively straightforward. A variant of this format of question is the partially closed-ended question in which an 'other' category, with an opportunity to specify, is included in the question to encourage participants to share opinions and beliefs that may not necessarily have been captured in the selections already listed.

question to ensure it is appropriately specific without being burdensome. For example, to return to Dorothy's research, a question such as 'Do you think antimicrobial stewardship programmes improve patient care' relies on the respondents knowledge of such programmes and may not be based on a valid experience of how programmes do or do not improve patient care. We also have 'improve' and 'patient care' to deal with! A more suitable question might be:

EXAMPLE

'What do you think are the possible outcomes of an antimicrobial stewardship programme?' Please list your answers in the space below.

This wording leaves the respondent to list positive and negative outcomes and does not lead them to think that all outcomes are good by using the word 'improvements'.

d. Do not use jargon or abbreviations that will not be understood by participants: unnecessarily complex medical terminology, short forms that are only familiar to health care professionals, or abbreviations that some may take for granted but will be confusing to other respondents.

e. Be cautious about the way personal characteristic questions are presented: recognise that participants may be sensitive about responding to certain questions. What may be a straightforward question to you as a researcher about ethnicity or race may provoke a strong response from some participants if correct and respectful terminology is not used. Similarly questions about sex or personal relationships that are framed in stark terms (e.g. male vs female or single vs married) may be off-putting or offensive to some.

f. Do not be overly demanding in what you expect from respondents: Remember that your participants are generally volunteers who are giving their time and efforts. Do not ask unreasonable questions (e.g. 'Rank the following 23 pharmacist services in terms of the frequency with which you utilise them'). The cognitive effort required to complete a task such as this is significant and burdensome.

g. Do not use double-barrelled questions, i.e. asking two questions in one.

For example, a double-barrelled question might be: 'Would you prefer to see your doctor **or** your pharmacist for treatment of athlete's foot?'

h. Avoid use of leading questions that provide clues as to how you want a respondent to respond.

For example: 'How good is your pharmacist at diagnosing athlete's foot?'

i. Avoid making assumptions about your participants: questions such as 'How many university degrees do you have?' may be irritating or offensive to some participants. Rather, ask in two separate questions 'Did you attend university?' [Yes/No] 'What degree did you graduate with?' [MD/PhD/MSc/MPharm].

As individual questions are being written, it is essential that you 'read' them as though you were an average participant in the study and ask yourself these questions:

- Does the question seem reasonable and appropriate?
- Is it too personal and will it look like you are infringing on the participant's privacy?
- Will a question cause distress?
- Will the participant be willing to answer the question?
- Are they able to answer the question?
- Is it written in a way that is clear and interpreted the same way by all respondents, regardless of their background or level of education? Researchers may be more comfortable with jargon and sophisticated vocabulary than the average

person but ask yourself if the terms and language used make sense to your average respondent? Are confusing or ambiguous words like 'nice', 'fine', 'good' explained or defined – or best of all, avoided altogether?

There are many different ways of asking a question; the choices made by the researcher in terms of question design and construction may influence the way participants interpret and respond, and consequently may affect data collection and analysis.

The quality of the questionnaire will directly influence the value of the results. As described in Chapter 5, and in Section 6.7 below, scientific properties of reliability and validity must be carefully considered.

6.5. CHOOSING YOUR FORMAT

The decision of questionnaire format must be closely aligned with a clear understanding of the research goals, timelines, and objectives. It will be influenced by the characteristics, desires, abilities, and resources of potential respondents, including their ease of access to and experience with, for example, web-based applications. Of course, budgetary issues and practical/logistical constraints will also be important to consider.

6.5.1 Pen and Paper

Questionnaires come in a variety of different formats, including traditional pen-and-paper, electronic/web-based, and face-to-face interview style. Pen-and-paper questionnaires can be distributed and collected in person or by mail. The tangible nature of such surveys and (for mail surveys) the perception of anonymity in responding may enhance the authenticity of answers provided by respondents. The cost associated with distribution of mail-based surveys can be high. Beyond the price of photocopying, envelopes, stamps and postage-paid return envelopes required, there is a considerable amount of work involved in opening completed surveys, data-inputting, management, and storage of the completed survey questionnaires. However, once the initial setting up has been done the survey is still the most cost-effective means of collecting large amounts of data.

6.5.2 Web-Based Surveys

Fewer paper-based surveys are being conducted as other alternatives emerge. As web-based technologies become more sophisticated and more widely accessible, electronic surveys using web-based platforms are gaining in popularity. Electronic questionnaires have the significant advantage of permitting instantaneous and accurate uploading into statistical analysis software packages. Some commercial programmes include their own analytics packages which are remarkably sophisticated and allow researchers to observe responses

TABLE 6.1	**Pros and Cons of Different Survey Methods**	
Type of Survey	**Pros**	**Cons**
Paper-based	Can be completed by people who do not have access to a computer. Response rates easier to calculate. Can reach large numbers of people.	Expensive to distribute (e.g. cost of paper, envelopes and post both out to potential respondent and back from them). You need names and addresses. Questionnaires can go missing in the post or be spoiled or damaged. Questionnaires can be completed anonymously.
Web-based survey	Relatively cheap to run and just require a subscription that can be used by a whole department. Responses easy to manage, e.g. most web-based survey providers use software that can export data to your own database. Can reach large numbers of people.	Potential respondents must have access to a computer and be computer literate. More difficult to calculate response rates. May be security issues involving confidentiality.
Face-to-face	Can obtain answers to every question. Can tell if a respondent feels uncomfortable with a question.	Time consuming. Difficult to get large numbers of responses.
Telephone	Can reach greater numbers of people. Less costly as just involves telephone calls.	Respondents must have access to a telephone. Time consuming. Cannot see body language.

and trends in real time. A disadvantage of web-based surveys is that only those with access to computers and familiarity with email, attachments, opening of links and other similar activities can or choose to participate. Elderly individuals in particular may not feel comfortable with this format. Others may be concerned about their privacy and anonymity. Despite assurances of server security and blinding of researchers to individual respondents, well-publicised cases of hacking and information leaks may discourage some individuals from participating or from providing honest responses. The cost of electronic surveys is considerably less than with paper surveys. In the past, response rates from electronic surveys was generally considerably lower than with paper versions but as familiarity with and access to technology increases, this gap has reduced.

6.5.3   Face-to-Face or Over the Phone

In some cases, researchers may wish to administer a survey using interpersonal techniques (e.g. telephone calls or face-to-face interviews). This approach may be particularly helpful for those who are resistant to internet-based or paper surveys, and in situations where open-ended questions are used which may benefit from clarification or follow-up (which will not be possible using internet-based or paper surveys). Of all survey types, this will be the most expensive as it requires personnel, telephone infrastructure and a system for training

researchers to ensure consistency and reliability in questioning approaches and interpretation. This type of approach is frequently used in the lead-up to high-stakes elections, or in consumer marketing research.

6.6   WORKING OUT THE LOGISTICS

Working out what to do, in what order, how and when can be quite confusing especially when you are under pressure to meet a deadline. The answer is to stay calm and write out the steps involved in the design of your survey. You can then talk this through with colleagues and tutors to make sure this part of your study design is as good as you can get it. Using a **Gantt chart**, or other form of table/spreadsheet can help to refine ideas and show where some tasks overlap so extra effort is needed. It certainly helps to be able to multitask! Let's have a look at some of the specific tasks that need to be considered.

6.6.1   Contacting Potential Respondents

It is possible to contact many more individuals through email than through personal approaches. However, many more people will ignore or disregard email invitations than a personal invitation. The cost/logistics of personal invitations (such as telephone calls or mail-outs using traditional mail) will be significantly higher than with email, including the need to 'remind' individuals who have not responded to your invitation to consider your request and agree to participate in the study.

6.6.2 Presenting Your Questionnaire

Whether electronic or paper based, written formats of questionnaire presentation ensure standardisation in the way in which each participant receives the survey. This should enhance overall reliability in most cases but if the questionnaire is poorly designed, and in a written format there are no opportunities for respondents to clarify ambiguities or ask questions, this may actually compromise the quality of responses. If using interviewers to deliver questions and gather data, it is essential that interviewers are well trained and understand the need to standardise so as not to lead or unduly influence respondents. This can be time consuming and expensive and as a result reduce the number of respondents you can feasibly recruit. There are advantages to using interviewers who can clarify answers and ask follow-up questions and probes from both interviewer and participant, but this could result in reliability issues if not all interviewers ask the same questions. The use of face-to-face interviews is more often used in qualitative research which is the subject of Part III of this book.

6.6.3 Recording Your Responses and Answers

Paper-based surveys require individuals to use handwriting and cursive script to respond which may result in transcription errors or misinterpretation. A significant limitation of paper-based surveys (including those in which an interviewer completes a paper-based survey) is the need to export data from the paper into an electronic data management system (such as a spreadsheet). Not only is this time-consuming, there are significant risks for transcription errors during the process which may compromise quality of findings. Electronic questionnaires that connect directly to analytics software packages or databases have the distinct advantage of not requiring additional transcription/inputting. This allows researchers real-time access to data and findings to allow for on-going monitoring of the project.

6.7 VALIDITY AND RELIABILITY REVISITED

As we have said before in Chapter 5, reliability and validity are the foundation stones of measurement and thus of survey design. There are a number of ways we can ensure that what we propose to do is going to work in practice and in this section we consider some of these.

6.7.1. Pilot Testing

Prior to use, questionnaires should undergo a process of validation to ensure that they are indeed reliable and valid.

A useful tool for validation is pilot testing, the process of administering the questionnaire to a subset of the sample and actively eliciting feedback from them about the experience. Part of the pilot testing is also carefully reviewing the actual results to determine whether they conformed to expectations, had reasonable and appropriate data distributions, and yielded useful information aligned with research objectives.

There is no specific formula for validation of a survey, but certain key aspects should be considered:

a. Readability: Asking the pilot-test group to confirm their understanding of each item on the questionnaire is part of the validation process. It allows you to ensure your intention was understood, and that ambiguities do not affect participants' responses.

b. Viability: Can the questionnaire be completed in a reasonable amount of time (that volunteers would be willing to spend) without being unnecessarily burdensome? In general, questionnaires should not take more than 15 minutes to complete; anything longer than this and many participants will simply lose interest and provide inaccurate responses.

c. Member-checking: Presenting the actual data and results back to the pilot test group is a helpful validation technique. Having the actual participants respond to their own responses provides you with confidence that you are indeed measuring what you intend to measure.

d. Open-ended discussion: Pilot test participants should be considered co-creators of a questionnaire – once they have completed the first draft of a questionnaire, it can be helpful to keep them engaged during the questionnaire refinement and editing process. Since they can no longer be used as part of your sample, they can play a valuable role in helping to improve the quality of the questionnaire.

e. Research team members: We often overlook the logistical issues associated with questionnaire distribution and collection. Part of the pilot testing process should also include an opportunity to test-drive your processes for gathering, inputting and analysing data. If you have designed spreadsheets to help manage your data do they actually work as expected? Pilot testing not just the instrument itself but the entire survey design is an important part of the validation process. In Section 6.8 we will outline the process of setting up a database and how this can help you to write the questions for your questionnaire.

6.7.2. Using Previously Validated Questionnaires

As can be seen, the design and construction of questionnaires is an important but complex task with important consequences. Poorly constructed questions will yield poor responses and meaningless data, rendering the survey pointless. The time, energy, cost and expertise required to construct good surveys and questions is considerable: in virtually all cases, researchers (whether they are novices or experienced) are strongly encouraged to consider the use of previously validated questionnaires, rather than attempting to create new ones for specific circumstances.

As part of the survey process, it is essential to undertake a systematic literature review and **'environmental scan'** to understand what is already known about the topic of interest. As part of this process, other researchers' work – including the questionnaires they will have used or developed to address their specific research objectives – will be identified. It is good research practice to familiarise oneself with the details of these previous instruments/questionnaires to determine whether and how they may be utilised or applied for your specific research context and need.

In making this determination, several issues need to be considered:

a. How similar – or dissimilar – is the context? If the research objective of the material you are reviewing is aligned with and similar to your interests and needs, there may be a possibility that the questionnaire that was used could be applied in your context.

b. How similar – or dissimilar – is the research objective? In order to use a previously validated instrument for your research it must be clear that your research objectives are substantially similar to those of the work you may be using.

c. How was the questionnaire/instrument actually validated – if indeed it was validated? In some cases, questionnaires are published in journal articles or posted online with no reference made to their provenance. Simply because something has been published or posted does not automatically mean it has been validated for use. Doing a literature search to find out if questionnaires or other survey instruments have been used in different settings and comparing the results can help you to decide which ones have been well-validated.

d. Do you have permission to use another person's/group's instrument? Once you are satisfied that the context, research objectives, and validation are aligned, and it is appropriate to use another instrument for your research purposes, it is essential you solicit and receive permission to use the instrument. Failure to ask for and receive permission is a serious breach of research ethics and may be seen as fraud or plagiarism.

6.8.   SETTING UP A DATABASE

In the final section of this chapter we will briefly outline some of the essential information about setting up a database.

More detail about setting up and using a database is given in Chapters 9 to 12 but the setting up of the database can help you to word the questions for your questionnaire. For this reason we have included some information here about setting up your database that will give you an idea of how this task should be considered early on in the survey design process. A database is a place where the information collected by questionnaire can be stored and analysed and where the tables and charts for your research report can be generated. Computer software is generally used to set up research databases and this is usually available from university computer services departments. There are also likely to be courses that you can attend that will help you understand the principles of database creation. Software such as Excel and SPSS are especially designed to manage large amounts of information and are set up to provide users with most of the statistics they will need to analyse their data. In Chapter 7 and Chapters 9 to 12 you will find more information about analysing data, and interpreting and reporting on the information you will generate in the course of your data collection.

The database you create will contain information about the characteristics of your sample (demographics) and the answers to every question on your questionnaire. As we have described earlier in this chapter and in Chapter 3, there are ways of asking questions to provide us with the answers in a format that is suitable for data management, and for conducting descriptive and inferential statistics. Thus, the way data are entered into the database will determine the way our results are produced and presented.

All data that are entered onto your database will be anonymous insofar as individual respondents will not be named. However, you will need to be able to identify the different category of respondent in terms of, for example, sex, level of education and place of work. Each of these variables will be measured in a different way. For example, you may decide to offer respondents three choices of answer to the question about whether they are male or female with the third choice being *'prefer not to answer'*. This is because we want to give the respondents the opportunity to keep that information private, but it will be helpful to know whether they ticked that option rather than overlooked the question. When you set up your database there will be space for you to give the question itself and the options for each answer. The information you place on the database will be in numeric form but you will need to know what each number means. So, 1=female, 2=male and 3=prefer not to answer. If you have set up your database with all the questions and options for answers then when you come to analysing your data the software will give you all of this information. If you do not tell the software what '1' means it cannot possibly know – computers are good but they can't read our minds!

The other thing that computer software programmes cannot do is cope with ambiguity and this is our final point (for now) about setting up your database. If you set up your database as you are writing the first draft of your questionnaire you will find out whether you have asked the questions in the best way for your software. This in turn means that there will be no ambiguity in your questions that would make it difficult for your respondents to answer. We will return to this principle in Chapter 7.

6.9. BACK TO DOROTHY

The best way to illustrate the points that need to be considered in the design of any research is to look at an example of research design in progress. To do this we will go back to Dorothy and look at the decisions she needs to make about the design of her research into antimicrobial stewardship. Let's take this one step at a time:

- Step 1: A survey will provide Dorothy with **quantitative results** and she needs to have most of her data in this format to be able to compare answers from different health care professionals involved in the prescribing of antibiotics in her hospital.
- Step 2: A survey will be **cost-effective**. As Dorothy already works at the hospital she will be able to recruit respondents more easily. Hopefully people will trust her more than they would a stranger and might also have more of an interest in the project.
- Step 3: Dorothy believes that the survey **costs** can be kept to a minimum by distributing the questionnaire herself and by asking respondents to return their completed questionnaires to her in the internal post. This means the **logistics** will be simple too as most of her potential respondents are in the hospital itself.
- Step 4: Dorothy needs to make some decisions about who she invites to complete her questionnaire and needs to gather more information before she can make a final decision about **recruitment** of respondents. We will return to this issue in Chapter 7 when Dorothy has all the information she needs.
- Step 5: Dorothy decides that her survey needs to be **cross-sectional**. She will send out her questionnaire to all those who are involved in antibiotic stewardship and will just need to ask her questions once.
- Step 6: Dorothy thinks through her **questions** and how they should be asked in order to get the answers she needs. Dorothy knows that she will use a mixture of formats from **dichotomous** through to **open-ended** questions.
- Step 7: The **format** for the questionnaire will be pen and paper because not everyone will have access to a computer to take part in a web-based survey.
- Step 8: Dorothy decides that she definitely needs to pilot her questionnaire to make sure it makes sense and to find out how long it takes to complete. She can then use the responses from her **pilot study** to inform the design of her final questionnaire and recruitment information.
- Step 9: If Dorothy words her questions carefully she will be able to **draw conclusions** about how her respondents feel about antibiotic stewardship.

CHAPTER SUMMARY

- In this chapter we have outlined some of the key principles survey design quantitative research.
- It has outlined some of the different types of questionnaire design that can be used to conduct a survey and illustrated how they might be used in Dorothy's research.
- It summarises the pros and cons of different types of survey.
- Finally, it outlines how you might begin to set up a database to facilitate analysis of your results.

RESEARCH RESOURCES

A number of academic institutions/departments produce resources for research design that are readily available online. For example, this one from Leeds University is on questionnaire design: http://iss.leeds.ac.uk/downloads/top2.pdf

7

Participants in Your Research

LEARNING OBJECTIVES

After reading this chapter you should be able to:
- understand the importance of identifying a target population
- describe the terms 'inclusion' and 'exclusion' criteria
- explain what 'sampling' is and describe some commonly used sampling techniques
- understand the importance of having a sound and appropriate recruitment technique and the ethics issues involved in these
- understand the need to think ahead about the analysis of the data produced in research

7.1. INTRODUCTION

In most cases, pharmacy practice research will involve people – patients, family and carers, customers, colleagues, pharmacy technicians or other health care professionals. While, in some cases, pharmacy practice research questions can be answered through use of administrative databases or other impersonal sources of information, for the most part working directly with other people tends to be what motivates many pharmacists to undertake research in the first place.

Research involving human subjects must always be considered carefully. Notions of risk and benefit must be negotiated, balanced and communicated effectively to each participant. Issues such as confidentiality, informed consent and the ability to withdraw from a study or withhold data based on the participant's wishes must be carefully worked through prior to initiating any research. Safeguarding participants is a most crucial aspect of health services research, and an absolute requirement for the research ethics review boards that will be overseeing and approving research involving human beings.

Beyond these issues, careful selection of research participants is also a very important consideration. Setting a sample frame, recruiting participants, gaining informed consent, protecting data and confidentiality, and ensuring representativeness when that is required, are just some of the important considerations researchers need to build into their development process. Researchers need to carefully balance idealistic aspirations with pragmatic realism when designing a study, to ensure they can actually recruit the kind and number of participants they need in order to achieve their objectives.

7.2. CHOOSING PARTICIPANTS

Pharmacy practice research generally focusses on things that pharmacists, pharmacies and others involved in the prescription and use of medicines, do that affects those processes. To learn about how people involved in these processes are affected by them we need to elicit information from them. To do this it is important that we choose people who are, for example, either giving or receiving pharmaceutical care. This could be finding out about the side effects of a new medicine or asking pharmacists about job satisfaction. In this section we will look at some of the ways we can choose the appropriate participants for our research. In Chapter 2 we described the importance of involving patients and carers in research. This can greatly enhance the quality of the research and if they are included at the research design stage it can ensure that the results of your research have real-life value. More about involving patients and carers can be found here http://www.invo.org.uk/

7.2.1. Target Population

In Chapter 2 (Section 2.3) we introduced the '**Research Protocol**' and mentioned it again in Chapter 6 when we were telling you how Dorothy might use a survey design to gather her data. When developing a research protocol, it is essential to stay focussed on the research question (Chapter 2, Section 2.6) and research aims and objectives (Chapter

6, Section 6.3.1). When well considered and constructed, these should help guide the researcher in identifying the '**target population**' of interest in the study. The target population is the entire group of individuals the researcher is interested in and is usually a subset of the entire population. For example, our pharmacist Sandy who works in a GP practice, is interested in diabetes management, but is not currently focussed on all patients with diabetes. His interests are centred on younger patients between the ages of 16 and 25, who will have a lifetime of health-related risks and issues ahead of them if their diabetes is not well managed. For Sandy, the target population involves two components:

1. A diagnostic component (diabetes)
2. An age component (between 16 and 25 years of age).

The younger patients with diabetes would be a subset of the practice's overall population of patients with diabetes whatever age.

Carefully defining a target population early on in research planning is necessary as it helps to establish the **inclusion** and **exclusion criteria** that will be used to guide participant recruitment and selection. If the target population is defined too narrowly (e.g. young people with diabetes age 16 years) it may be impossible to recruit sufficient numbers of participants to power the study appropriately. Alternatively, by defining the target population too broadly (anyone with diabetes), there is a risk of drifting away from the original objectives and intent of the research.

Let's see how **Sandy** might make his decisions about his target population.

For Sandy's research, he has a clear objective which has allowed him to define a target population. This is '*male and female patients between the ages of 16 and 25 with a diagnosis of type II diabetes*'. This provides the starting point for defining his inclusion and exclusion criteria. To this, he may consider adding certain characteristics:

a. **English language literacy**: if Sandy is going to be interviewing or surveying people as part of his study he may want to consider listing English language literacy as an inclusion criterion. This would narrow selection so it may be possible to include people who do not speak English by offering the help of an interpreter. This can be a difficult decision to make but any decision must be balanced against the practical reality of how Sandy could recruit, interview, survey or involve people with whom communication might be difficult.

b. **Comorbidities**: Patients with diabetes may also experience other health problems or challenges, and Sandy will need to carefully consider whether comorbidities have any influence on his core research objectives. On the one hand, comorbidities are common and if he wishes to ensure or enhance the validity of his work,

disregarding other health problems may be unwise and unrealistic. Conversely, including comorbidities may make it difficult for Sandy to address his research objectives which are specifically related to diabetes. It may be that people with comorbidities are the ones that have the most difficulty in controlling their blood glucose, so Sandy might decide that a simple question about this is sensible.

c. **Disease progression**: Chronic conditions such as diabetes introduce unique challenges for pharmacy practice researchers. Should an individual who was just diagnosed with diabetes yesterday be in the same study as someone who has successfully managed diabetes for 5 or more years? Sandy will need to consider whether it is advisable or necessary to include some inclusion/exclusion criteria related to duration of diagnosis, and how successfully (or not) the condition is being managed to align with his objectives and research question.

These are just some examples of questions researchers need to consider as they define their target population. There is no pre-developed checklist that will work in all cases. Instead, researchers need to carefully consider their objectives and ensure the identified target population aligns with the research question.

7.2.2. Sampling Research Participants

Choosing the people who will take part in our research is known as '**sampling**' because we are taking a *sample* of the population to explore our research objectives. Once a target population has been defined, and inclusion and exclusion criteria have been identified, researchers need to consider whether sampling is necessary. In some cases, if the target population is reasonably small and readily accessible, it is possible to involve the entire target population in the study. In most cases, however, the target population may be too large, live in different parts of the country, and may not be interested in taking part in research. For Sandy's study, he is interested in all patients with diabetes between the ages of 16 and 25 and how they compare to all patients with type II diabetes. He happens to have the possibility of accessing only some of them (those who are associated with his practice). Even from this sub-group, not everyone is going to want to participate, be available, or be easily contacted. As a result, Sandy will need to consider ways of inviting his potential participants to take part.

There are a number of ways of doing this, known as **sampling methods**, and some of these are defined below:

a. **Random sampling**: This is a technique in which individuals are chosen for participation in a study entirely by chance. By using random sampling, we reduce the likelihood of bias interfering with the study. Simple random sampling is the most basic version of this approach, in which each member of the target population has an equal likelihood of being chosen to participate. Random number generators (available on many commercially available spreadsheet programs such as Excel) can be used to assign each member of the target population a number; the researcher then applies a pre-determined formula (e.g. multiples of four or odd numbers only) to the selection and these are the people chosen to take part in the research (read more about this in Chapter 8). In Chapter 4 Sandy had identified 298 people in his practice with type II diabetes. If he used random sampling each one of those would be assigned a number and then the above formula would be used to select the potential participants.

b. **Stratified sampling**: This recognises that, even within a target population, there may be different groups (or strata) that have different experiences that need to be tracked separately. For example, Sandy may hypothesise that the experience of boys and young men with diabetes may be different from the experience of girls and young women, owing to peer-group influences around diet, exercise, and other lifestyle choices. In order to address this issue, Sandy may wish to stratify (or divide) his sample in such a way as to ensure these sex-based subgroups are adequately represented across the study. Stratified sampling is generally used when the target population is **heterogeneous** or dissimilar, but where certain **homogeneous** (or similar) subgroups can be identified and isolated. If the target population is generally homogeneous, then random sampling is more appropriate. The purpose of stratifying by sex is not simply to ensure equal representation but also to enable Sandy to compare blood glucose control in males and females.

c. **Cluster sampling**: Here, the entire target population is divided into groups of people in whom we are interested (or clusters) and a random sample of clusters is then selected for participation. This can be used when it is not possible to find all of the people in a target population but it is possible to identify clusters. It is often more practical and economical than simple random sampling or stratified sampling when dealing with complex health services research questions. For Sandy, he may hypothesize that family socio-economic status is an important variable in explaining diabetes in young people, e.g. those from poorer families or more deprived backgrounds may be at higher risk of having poorly managed diabetes. Further, he hypothesizes that poorer families and those with deprived backgrounds may 'cluster' geographically in the same neighbourhoods and areas – and that this can be tracked through, for example, UK postal codes. Rather than try to stratify his sample entirely based on individuals (which would be difficult, time consuming and costly), he could cluster sample based on postal codes as a way of determining what, if any, influence family socioeconomic status had on diabetes progression.

d. **Matched sampling**: Sometimes researchers are interested in isolating specific variables to determine their influence on an outcome of interest. For example, if Sandy were interested in determining whether socioeconomic status or deprivation had an impact on diabetes and general health, he may find a group of identical twins separated at birth, with one twin being adopted by a wealthy family, and the other by a less-well off family, and determine what, if any, differences existed between them. The importance of identical twins is that they would have the same genetic make-up and so it would be possible to say that the way in which they were raised made a difference to their health. However, finding sets of identical twins willing and able to take part in research can be logistically challenging and so this type of sampling is not used very often.

e. **Repeated measures design**: In some cases, it may be of importance to take the same measure at different points in time on the same participant to determine if an intervention has been successful or not. For example, Sandy may design an educational programme to motivate young people to take medications as they are prescribed. Prior to delivery of this programme, Sandy may measure their adherence to prescription medications through examination of repeat prescriptions in the community pharmacy. Six months after delivery of the educational programme he may repeat this measure again to help him to determine whether the intervention worked or not. Such 'pre-and-post' testing can be helpful to determine the impact and outcome of a specific intervention on a sample group of interest.

f. **Quota sampling**: Most frequently used in market research and opinion polling, quota sampling is a strategy that is less applicable in practice research, but may be of importance within a business context. For example, if a pharmacist were interested in offering a new cosmetics service to drive customer volume in the shop, it may be valuable to implement a quota sample in which high-value target groups (e.g. women between 18 and 59) are oversampled, given that they may spend more on these products than other subgroups. Quota sampling is not a random sample and therefore it is difficult to generalise from the findings of research using this method of sampling. However, in some cases, it may be relevant and valuable information for a specific context.

g. **Purposive sample**: In purposive sampling researchers decide which people they are going to include in their research. Like quota sampling, it is also a non-representative subset of the target population, designed to fulfil a specific need or purpose. Most frequently, purposive sampling is used when it is not possible to actually specify a target population, or when the target population is not readily accessible. Purposive sampling may be undertaken through the '**snowballing technique**', so labelled because the researcher 'picks up' participants along the way, similar to the manner in which a snowball is built up. In snowballing, the researcher asks a participant to name or nominate someone they know who might be willing to be involved in the study – through such networking, the sample group can be constructed. The snowballing technique is frequently used with hard-to-find or hard-to-track target populations (for example prescription drug abusers) or high-profile very busy individuals (such as senior health executives) who may not come forward when traditional sampling and recruitment methods are used.

h. **Convenience sample**: In a convenience sample, the researcher takes participants whenever she/he can find them. Sometimes called an 'accidental' sample, convenience samples are frequently used in health services research to overcome logistical issues. For example, if a researcher is relying on volunteers to take part in their research this is a type of convenience sample. Like a quota, purposive, or snowball sample, convenience samples are not random and consequently cannot be assumed to be representative of the target population. This causes problems when trying to generalise research findings but there are occasions when there is no alternative. If this is the case, it is important to acknowledge the limitations that this may introduce into inferences made based on findings of the study.

A final thing to note about sampling is that in some types of research it takes place after participants have been recruited. This is particularly so when conducting qualitative studies when people agree to take part and researchers then select participants based on factors such as location, health condition, satisfaction/dissatisfaction with a service. We will be looking at this type of sampling in Part III, which is devoted to qualitative methods.

7.3. RECRUITMENT OF PARTICIPANTS

Experienced researchers doing research that involves human beings will tell you that the most important and challenging aspects of pharmacy practice research involve recruitment.

Recruitment is the process by which potential participants – those who have been identified as meeting inclusion and exclusion requirements in the sample frame – are identified, located, contacted, and invited to participate in the study. Identifying potential participants is described above through the process of sampling. Once identified they need to be located, which is not always easy. In some cases, you may have a patient profile that provides an address, telephone number or email connection. While it may seem straightforward to use this information, unless the potential participant had previously explicitly consented to being contacted for participation in research projects, it is considered unethical to use this information you already have, for this new activity. This sometimes can be frustrating for researchers. You know who you want to contact and even have a way to connect with them but under current research practices, it is considered an invasion of the patient's privacy to use this information for a purpose other than what had been previously agreed upon. This is one of those times when you have to think about how you would feel if your doctor allowed your pharmacist access to your notes and they contacted you.

To address this issue, some pharmacy and medical practices may choose to ask patients when they first register with the practice if they are interested and willing to be contacted for potential research projects. If in our pharmacist Sandy's practice this had been done when patients first enrolled there, Sandy would be able to contact those patients directly. If this had not been done as part of initial enrollment, Sandy would need to consider alternative strategies including the following:

a. **Printed advertising/recruitment flyers**: One of the easiest and most popular recruitment methods is to print up recruitment flyers as a marketing tool to interest participants in contacting the researcher. Typically such flyers are posted within practices, health care settings, clinics and other places where those in the target population and sample frame are likely to go. Information on such flyers usually includes the title of the study, a one- to two-sentence brief description, a listing of inclusion and exclusion criteria, contact information so that those interested can connect with the researcher, and a statement regarding which ethics board has approved this study and who is funding this work. Success with this type of recruitment is highly variable and, in general, researchers do not rely solely upon this technique. Figure X is an example of what a flyer for Sandy's research might look like.

b. **Patient support groups**: When recruiting participants for studies with a specific disease focus (such as diabetes), it may be valuable to target peer support groups. Peer support groups are patient run quasi social gatherings in which individuals with common medical issues have an opportunity to meet and exchange stories and information. Such groups will often welcome approaches from researchers because they are generally passionate about their cause. They will usually ask for written information about the project and then invite you to attend a meeting to tell their members more about it.

c. **National support groups**: Patient support groups may be part of larger, nationwide charities or other organisations that will often help researchers to find participants. They can also provide valuable information about the disease or condition of interest.

d. **Practice-based recruitment**: Pharmacy practice research involving patients can be facilitated by direct requests to patients who are part of the sample frame and this can be done during routine pharmacist–patient interactions. For example, if one of Sandy's patients who meets the requirements for his study was collecting their medicine at a local community pharmacy, Sandy could work with that pharmacist to help recruit participants for the study.

e. **Electronic (web-based recruitment)**: Facebook, Twitter and other social media are increasingly being used as a vehicle for recruitment. Many patient peer support groups maintain web presences, and this can be used for recruitment purposes. This can be particularly helpful if the research itself involves a web-based data collection component (e.g. an on-line survey).

f. **Word-of-mouth**: As discussed previously, snowball sampling can be a useful strategy for recruitment. Similarly asking colleagues, neighbours, friends and others in one's social network to "spread the word" about a study can in some cases be a useful way of alerting potential participants to the research opportunity. In the UK, the Royal Pharmaceutical Society has local forums where members meet to share pharmacy practice issues. These can be good places to start recruitment of pharmacists.

It is important to note that all of the recruitment methods above are variants of purposive or convenience sampling, relying upon interested and motivated volunteers to support research. As such, this may result in a non-representative sample being assembled which may affect the researchers' ability to make inferences from the data and generalize to the target population. Pragmatically and logistically, this is a necessary compromise in most pharmacy practice research projects, to allow sufficient numbers of participants to be identified in a reasonable period of time.

7.3.1.   Data Protection and Confidentiality

A critical part of the recruitment and informed consent procedure involves clearly communicating the processes that will be used to safeguard data that are collected during the study. This safeguarding usually involves two separate issues: (1) ensuring data collected are kept confidential so that personal details/information will not be accessed by anyone not directly involved with the research, and (2) ensuring that any data collected are stored in a secure, retrievable manner for a period of time to allow for audit, review or other requirements.

Confidentiality is an important consideration for most participants. If someone is going to participate in your research and share their perspectives on potentially sensitive or controversial topics, they need to be assured that these opinions will not be broadcast widely. Without confidentiality provisions built into the research method and communicated clearly to the participant, there is a strong likelihood that participants will not be as honest, open and forthright as you might wish them to be. In any and all presentation of data (e.g. manuscripts, theses, research reports, presentations and posters) mechanisms for anonymising and/or aggregating data are required. For quantitative research methods (such as surveys) this can usually be accomplished simply by reporting descriptive statistics such as means, medians, modes and ranges for the entire sample or stratified cohort, rather than results on an individual-by-individual basis. Researchers must carefully plan for an account for this possibility and vigorously ensure all possible (not simply reasonable) attempts are taken to protect identity, or ensure participants fully understand this may not be possible prior to consenting to be involved in the research.

7.3.2.   Ethics of Recruitment

As discussed in Chapter 2, all research involving human beings must have a full and objective review from a relevant ethics research board. Most large institutions (including hospitals, universities and NHS Trusts) have such boards and provide information on the requirements for researchers. Typically, a standardized form is completed outlining the research objectives, methods, data collection tools, and analytic methods that will be used. Their focus is on safeguarding patients' interests and rights throughout the research process and it is through this lens that they will consider your work. Ethics review boards will consider the scientific or scholarly merit of the research itself and the strengths or limitations of the method used if they directly impact on patients' interests.

Key ethical issues related to recruitment include the right to privacy, the right for patients to decline to be involved in research and not suffer any consequence or harm, and the right to have full informed consent prior to involvement in the research.

It is important to remember that ethics review boards are there to protect the researcher too. They do this by making sure that the way research is conducted safeguards participants and thus ensures that researchers do not put themselves in a position whereby they might not treat research participants appropriately.

Informed consent is considered the cornerstone of health services research, and is based on the belief that everyone has a right to know what is being done to them (not just their bodies, but also their words and thoughts) and to have the option to participate or not. Depending upon the nature of the research, informed consent provisions may be more or less detailed and extensive. For example, in a clinical trial for a new medication, where side effects and risks may not be fully known and where periodic blood samples are required to monitor therapeutic levels, the nature of informed consent will be detailed and extensive. There will be an expectation that a researcher will personally talk the potential participant through the details, answer questions and respond to concerns. While this is expensive, time consuming and logistically challenging, it is an essential safeguard because of the risks involved if the participant does not fully understand what they are agreeing to. Simply asking patients with varying levels of education and scientific expertise to read a document and sign a form is considered insufficient for this purpose.

In contrast, some forms of health services and pharmacy practice research are much less invasive. Sandy's role is as a pharmacist working in a GP practice where he has responsibility for (amongst other things) caring for patients with diabetes.

Let's leave Sandy for now and take a look at some of the issues our MSc student, Dorothy, might face – her challenges are different to Sandy's. If Dorothy is interested in better understanding physicians' perspectives on Antimicrobial Stewardship, and wants them to complete a survey, she is dealing with a highly educated and sophisticated target population. There is unlikely to be any risk of physical or psychological harm to the participants through enrolment in this kind of a study. Consequently, a written recruitment flyer and basic informed consent process will be sufficient in this case, so long as participants can access Dorothy to ask questions should they have any.

Most ethics review boards provide examples and models for researchers to consider as they determine the appropriate level and amount of information necessary for recruitment and informed consent based on the specific characteristics of their research. Familiarizing yourself in advance with your ethics boards' requirements and expectations, and in particular with the requirements for expedited review (which will allow for an abbreviated review process due to minimal or no risk to participants) is essential.

At the end of this chapter we will return to Dorothy and look at how she might find participants for her study.

7.3.3. Reminders

Recruitment of participants and finalization of informed consent is a process requiring both patience and vigilance. Participants need to be provided with sufficient time to reflect and consider whether or not to participate, and researchers need to recognise that, in some cases, no response actually means 'No thank you' (but the participant is simply too polite or too shy to say this directly). Researchers must make it very clear to potential participants that it is OK to say 'No'. On the other hand, sometimes interested participants simply forget or lose track of requirements and need to be gently reminded to complete informed consent or other procedures prior to enrolment in a study.

Reminders are a useful tool to structure into any research protocol to enhance the success of recruitment and facilitate more complete data collection. Reminders can be provided electronically (e.g. via email), by phone, in person, or by mail. As part of a research protocol, it is useful to consider and try to anticipate recruitment challenges and data collection needs and schedule reminder notices to be automatically triggered. Wherever possible, a sorting mechanism should be developed so that those who have responded or returned data to the research team are not bothered by a reminder notice that does not apply to them. Ethics review boards will want to ensure that the reminder process is neither unnecessarily meddlesome/irritating nor coercive. Respectful wording, ensuring participants are reminded of their rights and protections around declining to participate, withdrawal from the study, and withholding of data, etc., should be included in the reminder if applicable. In general, no more than two reminders should ever be used in a study. This is because more than this may be regarded as putting undue pressure on potential participants. If, after two reminders, there is no response or no return of data, the researcher must conclude the individual is not interested in participating and consequently simply leave them alone.

7.3.4. Participant Withdrawal From a Research Project

A critical ethical requirement for all research involving human subjects is the notion that participants are free to withdraw from a study at any time without being forced to provide reasons and without fearing consequences. This must be directly and explicitly explained as part of the informed consent process, and participants should be reminded of this option throughout the study. Once informed by the participant that they are withdrawing from the study, no coercion, force or threat may be used to convince them to change their mind. As discussed above, non-responsiveness to reminders may also be interpreted as dropping out. If data has been collected anonymously, e.g. if people have completed a questionnaire and did not have to provide their personal details, they cannot withdraw their response. Participants who have given their personal details may choose to withdraw from the study and they may be asked during the consent process if they will still allow any data they have already contributed to be used in the study. At the end of this hyperlink you will find more information about the design of consent forms in England: http://www.hra.nhs.uk/resources/

before-you-apply/consent-and-participation/consent-and-participant-information/. Please refer to your own country's Research Ethics Service if you are working/studying outside England. An example of wording is given below:

> Please indicate below how you would like any information you have given to be treated should you decide to withdraw from the study:
>   'If I withdraw from the study I wish any data I have already given to be destroyed' [ ]
>   'If I withdraw from the study I give my permission for any information I have already given to be used in the study'   [ ]

Researchers must carefully keep track of all participants and account for dropouts as part of their data analysis. In some cases there may be a sufficient number of dropouts from a study to threaten the on-going viability of the research, or the sample size ('**power**' see text box below) required to allow statistical inferences to be drawn. In such cases, contingency plans must be developed around the feasibility or desirability of reinstituting a recruitment plan if that is possible.

> ## POWER
>
> This refers to the likelihood that a statistical test will allow a researcher to correctly reject their null hypothesis that no difference will be found between the groups being tested. The power of a statistical test is influenced by the size of your sample (number of participants), the level of statistical significance and the size of the treatment effect. Power analysis can be used to ascertain the sample size you will need to detect a reasonable treatment effect. There are a number of free to use power calculators available online. For more information about power please see the 'Further Reading' section of this chapter.

Accounting for dropouts is a mathematical exercise. In data analysis and reporting of findings, it is essential that all participants who started in the study are accounted for at the end of the study. While participants are not required to explain reasons for dropping out, in many cases they may freely volunteer this information, in which case it should be reported to allow consumers of the research an opportunity to understand the circumstances more clearly.

There is no magic number of dropouts that will render a study impossible to complete; each study is considered on its own merits. Nevertheless, researchers need to be concerned about any number of dropouts and how this may be affecting the overall health and feasibility of the study, and why individuals who had previously agreed to be involved are now withdrawing. In some cases, this may require modification of the original research protocol, or re-examination of the questions, processes and methods used in the research which may inadvertently alienate or disturb participants.

7.3.5. Recognition for Participants

Motivating members of your target population and sample to participate in a study can be challenging. In some cases, researchers have the advantage of being able to offer incentives to recognise the time and effort required to participate in research. For example, in some projects potential participants are offered the opportunity to take part in a prize draw. This offers some recognition that return of a completed questionnaire is valuable to the researchers but can also act as an incentive to do so. In this situation, participants are encouraged to enrol in a study in order to gain an opportunity to 'win' some object of interest (e.g. an iPad, a gift card, or something else of some value). Researchers must make it clear that only a limited number of prizes are available, and describe the process by which the winner may be selected (e.g. usually a random draw of all participants). This is generally a less successful method of recognising participants' contributions to research, but pragmatically may be the only method available if budgets are constrained.

In some cases, it is possible to provide a flat honorarium to each participant, as a token of appreciation for participating but where sample sizes are large this will be a costly option. Researchers need to work with financial officers involved in managing research funds to identify the most cost-effective and meaningful form of recognising participants.

In other cases, research participants may actually receive more formal compensation for their participation. It is very rare (and in many cases considered unethical) for a participant to receive a 'salary' or 'wage' for participating, but higher levels of compensation may be used in certain situations. For example, clinical trials for new medications that require overnight stays, blood testing and many repeat visits to the study centre.

Regardless of whether financial forms of compensation are available or not, it is still important that researchers consider means to effectively acknowledge and thank participants for their contributions. Simple follow-up thank you notes or emails may be suitable. Public acknowledgement in the form of suitably anonymised notes at the beginning or end of the research report saying 'Thank you to all those who participated in this research', may also be considered. Above all, treating participants politely and professionally throughout the recruitment, informed consent and research processes is essential.

Before completing this chapter with some initial thoughts on data analysis, let's return to our case study pharmacist, Dorothy, and explore some of the challenges she may face when recruiting participants for her research.

CASE STUDY: DOROTHY'S RECRUITMENT

When we left Dorothy in Chapter 6 she had decided she needed to gather more information about her target population prior to writing her **recruitment strategy**. The purpose of this additional work was to identify everyone in the hospital who is involved in antimicrobial prescribing and decision-making. Dorothy has made a list of those people who are involved. There may be others and she can add these to her recruitment strategy as she identifies them. So far, on the list Dorothy has staff involved with:

- prescribing and administering, e.g. doctors, pharmacists, nurses
- infection prevention, e.g. patient safety and quality assurance team
- higher level decision-making, e.g. department heads
- pharmaco/epidemiology, e.g. staff involved in auditing, analysing and reporting data
- laboratory services, e.g. staff involved in the use of tests and the flow of results
- information technology, e.g. staff involved in integrating protocols at the point of care

Sampling

As can be seen from the list above Dorothy has a variety of potential participants and each group of staff may have different experiences that need to be captured in the questionnaire. Dorothy has decided that she will use stratified sampling to take into account not only the different people involved in the prescribing and administration of antimicrobial drugs but those involved in all of the other categories she has identified.

Recruitment of Participants

Dorothy has the advantage that all of the people she would like to recruit work in the hospital she works in, so she decides to have three different ways of recruiting: (1) printed advertising of her research that can be placed in different departments in the hospital and in rest/eating areas, (2) word of mouth – Dorothy will ask her colleagues to tell their colleagues about the research, and (3) electronic recruitment through the hospital intranet system. This is where all staff go to find out what is going on in the hospital and will be a good place to place her advertising.

7.4. DATA ANALYSIS

Although we will not be dealing with data analysis in detail in this chapter, there are aspects of data analysis that should be considered alongside the recruitment of participants. Giving thought to the answers we want from our research and how these will help us to meet our research objectives can save time later on. For this reason, we will introduce some key aspects of data analysis now and these will be expanded on in Chapters 9, 10 and 11.

7.4.1. Data Types

In Chapter 3 we looked at the different levels of measurement that are available to us, why, when and how they might be used. We also discussed the importance of choosing the level of measurement that is most appropriate to provide us with the answers we want in a format that can be readily interpreted. Each level of measurement introduced in Chapter 3 can be used in quantitative research to measure variables that correspond with participant characteristics such as age or place of work, and to measure participants' attitudes and beliefs (see Chapter 6).

The reason we are introducing data analysis at this point in the book is that the type of data collected will determine how we describe or compare the responses of our participants. For example, **Dorothy** has done her further background work and realised that in order to understand the barriers and facilitators to the development of an antimicrobial stewardship programme, she needs to collect data from everyone who might be involved in that programme – or have an opinion about it. If you look back at Dorothy's list of the staff that she believes should be included in her study it is extensive. Now she needs to think about those staff – the health care professionals and other human beings in her study and ask herself what she needs to know about them and from them that will help answer her research question. Dorothy's questionnaire design will be based on her participants and how she can best capture the information she needs. The responses to her questionnaire will be collected in different ways and translate into different **data types**. Ideally Dorothy needs to make a plan in the form of an explanatory framework (see Chapter 2) that shows the organisational relationships of the participants she has decided to recruit. She must always keep in her mind that whatever numbers she collects and enters numerically into her database, they represent the characteristics or thoughts and feelings of her participants.

Let's look at a possible framework for the relationships between Dorothy's participants. Prescribing decisions are made about the medicines that should be administered to patients to help make them better so that might be a good place to start (Fig. 7.1).

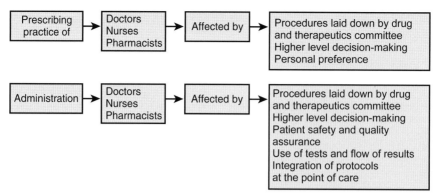

FIGURE 7.1 Diagram showing the relationships.

TABLE 7.1	**Information About Dorothy's Participants**			
Profession	**Sex** **1=female** **2=male** **3=prefer not to say**	**Age**	**Number of Years** **in Practice**	**Clinical Specialty**
Pharmacist	1	34	10	Paediatrics
Doctor	3	32	8	Orthopaedics
Nurse	2	51	25	Oncology

As can be seen from the Fig. 7.1, there are a number of relationships that Dorothy can explore in her research. She has chosen to use the stratified sampling technique which is structured to represent particular groups within her target population (people involved in the prescribing and delivery of antimicrobial therapy). The next step is to work out how these relationships can be described and compared.

7.4.2. Describing Our Research Population

One of the first things that Dorothy will want to do is thoroughly describe her study population. Some of the variables included in this description will be the demographics of our population. Table 7.1 shows some of the data Dorothy might collect.

As you will see from the table the answers to the questions 'What sex are you?' have been assigned a number that represents each participant's answer. Remember from Chapter 6 that this is because our database can only work in numbers.

Dorothy has decided that the length of time a participant has been practicing might make a difference to their level of knowledge about antimicrobials and their experience of using them in different contexts. Clinical specialty will also be important because prescribing decisions are made on the basis of clinical need and that need will vary depending on, say, the age and condition of the patient.

This is just a brief example of the information Dorothy will be collecting during her survey and these are based on her initial thoughts. By thinking about data analysis now, Dorothy can ensure that she includes all of the relevant people in her study. Being structured in her thinking and planning in advance will contribute to a recruitment strategy that will be fit for purpose.

7.4.3. Comparing Groups Within Our Research Population

This is where things get a bit more complicated and at this point in the book we will just outline some of the issues that must be considered when seeking to quantify relationships between research participants. To be able to draw assumptions from her data Dorothy must ensure that the groups and sub-groups she wants to compare have roughly equal numbers in them. There would be no point in trying to compare the responses of two pharmacists with those of 22 nurses and the same will apply when Dorothy comes to compare the means of, for example, age, across her groups. In the final four chapters of Part II of this book we will describe data analysis in more detail, but for now you might have gathered that Dorothy's sampling technique is going to be crucial in her study, if the key stakeholders in her research are to be adequately represented. She still has to rely on her potential participants volunteering to take part and will need to win the hearts and minds of her colleagues if she is to succeed. Antimicrobial resistance is a major health issue around the world so it is hoped that most clinicians will feel they have a responsibility to contribute to the safe and appropriate use of such drugs. Dorothy works in the same hospital as most of the major stakeholders and can use her personal connections to promote her work.

7.5.   CLOSING THE LOOP WITH PARTICIPANTS

Many participants volunteer for research studies because they are genuinely interested in the topic being studied and want to contribute in some way. In such cases, some participants may be very interested in the research findings. In most cases, participants should be offered the opportunity to receive summary reports, publications, abstracts and other forms of scholarly dissemination associated with the research if they would like to do so. Usually researchers will ask participants at the beginning of the research process if they would like to receive such reports. The time and expense required to facilitate this needs to be built into the research protocol itself to ensure this is possible.

Another important aspect to consider is the role of 'member-checking' which is a mechanism for 'closing the loop' with research participants. This means that participants have been fully involved from the beginning of the research to the publication of findings. By involving participants in the whole process the researcher can confirm and validate analysis and understanding of data gathered in the course of the study. In member-checking, the researcher presents his/her findings, data analysis and conclusions to the very participants (or a sample of these individuals) who were involved in the research in the first place. They are invited to reflect upon, comment, disagree, contextualise, or dissect this work as a way of helping the researcher better understand what has occurred through the research process, through the eyes of the actual participants. Going back to participants in this way allows the researcher to make sense of data gathered, to test models that may have been generated through the study, and to confirm analyses and conclusions. It also gives participants the opportunity to raise issues around the interpretation of results that they may not agree with. Researchers must respect this important aspect of research and acknowledge the contribution the research participants make to increasing knowledge about pharmacy practice and health care research. If our research is to have genuine, real-life value, then we must be able to implement it in practice. We cannot do that without our research participants.

CHAPTER SUMMARY

- In this chapter we have looked in some detail at how we choose the participants in our research.
- It has highlighted the value of including patients and carers in health care research.
- It sets out some of the most commonly used sampling procedures and uses Sandy's research to illustrate some of these.

- It outlines recruitment strategies including data protection and ethical considerations using Dorothy's research as an example.
- Finally, it looks at some data types and relationships that Dorothy might explore in her research.

FURTHER READING

Power Calculation
Ellis, P. D. (2010). *The essential guide to effect sizes: statistical power, meta-analysis and the interpretation of research results.* Cambridge, UK: Cambridge University Press.

8

Experimental Design and Randomised Controlled Trials: Deciding What Treatment Works

After reading this chapter you should be able to:
- understand what clinical trials are, including their advantages and disadvantages
- describe the critical features of a clinical trial
- understand the process of randomisation
- identify how participants in a trial are recruited
- describe how to define the outcomes of your clinical trial
- understand the difference between clinical and statistical significance

8.1. INTRODUCTION

Of all forms of research, pharmacists are likely most familiar with – and reliant upon – clinical trials. While there are many different ways of understanding this term, for the purposes of this chapter, we will use the traditional notion of a clinical trial as a double-blinded, randomised, placebo-controlled study. While some clinical trials are neither randomised, nor placebo controlled, nor double-blinded, many of the salient characteristics of this form of study that will be described in this chapter will still be relevant. Specific reasons for using a double-blinded, randomised, placebo-controlled clinical trial are described in Section 8.3. When designed and implemented well, clinical trials are a uniquely powerful type of study design that can not only facilitate individual clinician-patient decision-making, but can also be useful in guiding health care policy formulation. While traditionally, clinical trial study designs have been used to conduct specific types of research (e.g. medication or treatment comparisons), the actual design of a clinical trial can be used for a diverse array of interventions *not* specifically related to medication, medical procedures or treatment devices and there is now interest in using clinical trial study designs to test other types of interventions such as risk-factor modifications, lifestyle changes or health education provided by clinicians.

Some of the concepts found in this chapter have been introduced elsewhere in this book. However, in this chapter they are discussed specifically in relation to clinical trials.

8.2. ADVANTAGES AND DISADVANTAGES OF CLINICAL TRIALS

Amongst health professionals (and perhaps especially pharmacists), there is great respect for the findings that flow from rigorously designed and well-conducted clinical trials, and a general acceptance that this research method often provides the strongest evidence in support of cause–effect relationships between interventions and outcomes. As a result, individual clinicians, institutional and governmental policy makers, and patients tend to emphasise findings from clinical trials as part of decision-making processes. There are, however, advantages and disadvantages in undertaking a clinical trial and relying on its findings. These will be outlined in the following sections.

8.2.1. Advantages

A critical advantage of clinical trial study design is its purported ability to eliminate the bias, and **confounding** that influences data collection, analysis, and reporting.

Another significant advantage of clinical trials is the rigorous system that has evolved to standardise their implementation. This is a relatively recent occurrence, and in large part evolved due to perceived shortcomings, errors, and procedural biases in the past. The Consolidated Standards of Reporting Trials (CONSORT) initiative which relates specifically to Randomised Controlled Trials (RCTs) has had a significant positive influence on the structuring and implementation of clinical trials and provides an algorithm-driven method for researchers using clinical trials study designs to ensure critical and expected components of a quality trial have been utilised. The structure of the CONSORT recommendations also provides readers of clinical trials with an opportunity to cross-check researchers' work, to ensure that they have actually adhered to requirements for high-quality clinical research. Requirements include evidence of sample size calculations to establish **power** of a study (the likelihood that a statistical test will distinguish an effect that has occurred because of an intervention, rather than the results occurring by chance) appropriate randomisation systems to minimise procedural biases, clear guidelines for blinding of investigators and/or patients to minimise potential Hawthorne effects (see Chapter 5), accounting for participants and participant withdrawals, and ethics approval mechanisms to protect potentially vulnerable participants. Further details of these CONSORT recommendations will be discussed later in this chapter. See the end of this chapter for some Further Reading that gives examples of how to calculate sample size to establish the power of your study.

8.2.2. Disadvantages

Many of you may recognise and value the many and important advantages of clinical trials study design. However, there are a number of logistical, scientific and other challenges that are inherent in the process, which may put many researchers off from actually using this type of study design. First and foremost, it is important to acknowledge that many important research questions cannot be tested and answered through a clinical trials study design. For example, if we were interested in knowing whether a drug may potentially cause harmful or **teratogenic** effects in a fetus, it would be ethically indefensible to undertake a clinical trial in which you knowingly administered a medication to a woman that may (or may not) cause fetal harm. Unfortunately, the history of medical and health services research is littered with examples of unethical types of clinical trial research which may have yielded interesting and valuable scientific information, but only at a horrendous and unacceptable cost to uninformed participants. One of the most notorious and infamous of such studies is the Tuskegee Syphilis Experiment undertaken between 1932 and 1972 by the United States Public Health Service: its objective was to study the natural progression of untreated syphilis in rural African-American men in the south of the United States. Participants, who

were mostly poor and often demonstrated health literacy challenges, were recruited for this study by being told they would be provided with 'free' medical care and meals. Despite the knowledge that penicillin was a viable and available treatment for syphilis, the researchers deliberately withheld care for those enrolled in the study to meet the study objective of observing the natural progression of untreated syphilis. As a result, many of the participants suffered unnecessary harm simply because they were tricked into participating in the study with promises of free medical care. This sobering example should serve as an important reminder to all researchers of the critical importance of maintaining the highest ethical standards in all research, and especially in clinical trials research.

Beyond ethical considerations, there are other issues associated with the use of clinical trials as a study design. Not all health or medical questions can be answered using this method due to the nature of the condition itself. For example, there can never be a clinical trial that could prove smoking causes lung cancer, or that vitamin D supplementation prevents multiple sclerosis (MS). Conditions like lung cancer and MS evolve over a decades-long time frame, and are influenced by literally thousands of confounding variables that simply can never be controlled through a clinical trial. While clinical trials may be useful at answering very specific sub-questions within a broad domain such as lung cancer or MS, it is rarely possible to answer the most important 'big' questions as to causes, prevention and cures, solely through use of clinical trials.

A significant advantage of clinical trials is the methodological rigour and systematic attempts to minimise bias that are built into the process itself. These, unfortunately, introduce significant time, resource, and logistical complexities into the process. Clinical trials are expensive, require extensive and detailed documentation, and take time and resources to complete. This is not the type of research that individual clinicians, on their own and without support, are able to implement without an experienced and well-qualified team of diverse individuals behind them.

Finally, in some cases, certain conditions or diseases may be rare or evolve so rapidly in a clinical setting that it is simply impractical to go through all the CONSORT-required steps for a clinical trial. Further, in some cases, foundational scientific knowledge and treatments are evolving so rapidly that it makes no sense to 'stop' this progress to undertake a clinical trial knowing that in a few months' time other treatments may have appeared as well.

While it is important to acknowledge and carefully consider these disadvantages and limitations, it is equally important to not overemphasise them. Though challenging and complex, clinical trials study designs have been an invaluable tool for generating the evidence base in pharmacy, medicine and other clinical professions that we now rely upon to guide treatment decisions. Recognising that it is very unlikely that individual pharmacists will ever run their own clinical trials, and that in almost all circumstances pharmacists will be important members of any team of skilled professionals running such trials, we must still understand the basic features of trial design and understand how to optimise value from clinical trials.

8.3. CRITICAL FEATURES OF CLINICAL TRIALS

The term 'clinical trial' is frequently a shorthand description of the term 'double-blinded, randomised, placebo-controlled study', (often shortened to Randomised Controlled Trial (RCT)) which perhaps more accurately summarises the intent of the CONSORT recommendations. The objective is to minimise opportunities (inadvertent or deliberate) for investigator bias, enthusiasm or expectation to influence the outcome of a study, whilst simultaneously providing participants (patients) in the study with the utmost confidence that they and their interests are protected at all times.

8.3.1. Parallel Arms

The most common type of clinical trial study design involves parallel-arm trials involving two or more groups. Comparison between existing and possible new treatments/ interventions, or comparisons between interventions and doing nothing at all ('placebo') are of great interest to clinicians and policy makers; clinical trials facilitate the kind of head-to-head comparison of outcomes that can greatly inform decision-making.

In a basic parallel-arms trial, there is a comparison between the intervention (or treatment) group of participants and a control group which either receives no treatment/ intervention or a current standard one. In this design, participants once allocated to the intervention or the control group, will stay with that group for the duration of the study. An important feature of a clinical trial is the randomisation of participants to these groups: the decision as to whether an individual is in one group or the other is neither made nor known by the participant or the researcher, so it is said to be 'double blinded'. This is a crucial design characteristic for minimising any bias: since neither the participant nor the researcher know whether a participant is in the treatment group or the control group, it becomes less likely that observational bias or the Hawthorne effect (see Chapter 5) will influence outcomes.

8.3.2. Randomisation

The idea of randomised *sampling* was introduced in Chapter 7. In clinical trials a system called randomisation is used once participants have been identified and agreed to take part in the trial. The process by which randomisation in an intervention or control group occurs must be rigorous, reproducible and transparent. Examples of such methods include using a random number generator to assign each participant a unique identification number, then allocating even-numbered participants to one arm and odd-numbered participants to another arm. The use of the random number generator (generally available through most spreadsheet software programs such as Microsoft Excel) to make this allocation removes the necessity for decision-making from any individual involved in the study itself. Some forms of randomisation may appear 'random' but inadvertently will introduce bias. For example, allocating participants into groups based on surnames (e.g. A-L in one group, M-Z in another group) may not take into account the fact that within certain ethno-cultural communities there may be a large number of surnames beginning with certain letters (e.g. Chang/Chung/Chan/Chong) which in turn may mean randomisation is not as effective or true as required.

The cardinal virtue of randomisation is its ability to distribute as evenly as possible the factors and confounding variables (both known and unknown) that may influence trial outcomes. Even with the most effective randomisation methods, however, it is important to note that (by chance alone), it is still possible to end up with groups within each parallel arm that in fact do differ on some particularly important predictive factor. This is a problem that can occur in studies of all sizes, but it is one that is particularly important to consider in clinical trials with a small number of participants. One mechanism that can be used to address this potential issue is **stratification** based upon an important sub-variable. How might this work? Consider the example of our primary care pharmacist **Sandy**, who is interested in the growing numbers of young people with type II diabetes in his community. In his literature review, Sandy notes that many experts believe this trend is occurring because younger people lack appropriate knowledge around the influence of lifestyle factors (e.g. diet, exercise, alcohol consumption and smoking) on diabetic risk factors. Based on this, Sandy wishes to design a new intervention: an educational programme aimed at teenagers in his community to alert them to such risks. If Sandy wanted to structure his research as a clinical trial, he would randomise participants into two parallel arms: participants in one arm would receive the educational intervention while those in the other arm would not. Sandy would then follow-up and measure some relevant outcomes (for example, self-reports of diet or whether any participants increased the amount of daily exercise) of interest to determine whether his programme had any influence in changing the behaviours of the participants.

However, Sandy would also be aware that, amongst teenagers, there may be different learning styles. For example, young women may be more likely to be quiet, attentive and focussed in a classroom setting than young men or it might be the other way round. If Sandy is concerned that he has a relatively small number of participants in his study, simple randomisation using a random number generator could mathematically still result in more boys being in one group than in the other. If this is a concern, and mindful of the importance of sex in learning styles differences, Sandy may elect to stratify his randomisation. In this case, he may randomise all the girls separately from all the boys into two different groups, then compose an intervention and control group by simply adding these stratified randomised groups together. In this way, Sandy can control for the unlikely, but mathematically possible, situation where simple randomisation of the entire set of boys plus girls results in a situation where boys are under- or over-represented in one of the groups.

For practical reasons, it is usually difficult to stratify on more than one or two sub-variables within one study. In the example above, if Sandy felt ethnic background, as well as sex, was an important factor for him to consider, it would be possible for him to stratify based on those two different factors. If, however, he also felt family income, or academic performance in school, or some other variable were also important, attempting to stratify on three or more different variables may mean Sandy needs to rethink the entire design of this study. The more variables upon which one stratifies, the smaller the number of potential participants within that pool becomes, and as a result, it becomes very complex beyond a certain point to actually assemble viable intervention and control groups.

Within the literature on clinical trials, a variety of different alternatives to randomisation and stratification have been proposed, though none of these appear to be as effective. For example, allocation based on the month of a person's birth, or odd–even allocation based on the last digit of a person's national identification number or passport may be sufficient. Ultimately the research team must be satisfied that they have controlled for – as best as possible – the factors that may influence the outcome of a clinical trial, whether those factors are currently known or not.

To help clarify the concept of stratification, please see Fig. 8.1.

8.3.3. Superiority or Equivalence?

In many cases, clinical trials are traditionally used to evaluate whether a new treatment or intervention is better than, or superior to a control or placebo group, or the traditional standard of care provided. This design is referred to as a superiority trial, and is generally most appropriate when

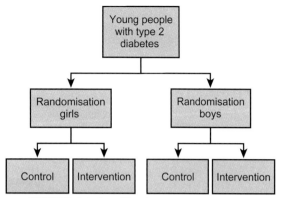

FIGURE 8.1 Stratification according to sex.

there is no current effective therapy/intervention and/or when the new intervention may potentially be more effective than conventional/traditional therapy. It is also possible to design a clinical trial to show that an intervention is not inferior to standard/conventional treatment in terms of outcome, but may be preferable anyway due to lower cost, greater convenience, or some other important factor. These are equivalence trials (sometimes called non-inferiority trials).

It is critical for researchers to honestly and accurately frame whether their research is about superiority or equivalence. In general, the challenge with equivalence trials relates to the sample size, and ensuring it is large enough and appropriately representative of the target population to adequately rule out any small differences that may be clinically relevant.

8.4. FINDING YOUR PARTICIPANTS

Chapter 7 of this book was devoted to how we go about choosing participants for our research, and many of the principles discussed in that chapter apply to clinical trials. However, there are some features of participants in clinical trials that make recruitment to a research study challenging. In this section we outline some of the principles of recruiting patients to clinical trials.

8.4.1. Establishing a Target Population

The set of individuals or participants to whom the results of a clinical trial may be relevant or applied to constitutes the target population. This is, in essence, the 'type' of people (e.g. demographically, medically or socio-economically) who may benefit from the findings of the study (see Chapter 7 for more information about participant characteristics). For clinical trials to be meaningful, it is important that those who are actually enrolled in the study are representative of those who will ultimately receive the intervention should findings be positive.

Historically, this has been a challenge in some clinical trials involving medications. For safety and ethics reasons, in the past, many clinical trials for new medications have enrolled relatively young, healthy male participants. The rationale for this being that, should there be any unanticipated problems with the medications, young, healthy participants would be more likely to 'bounce back' and recover. Male participants were preferred to prevent any questions or concerns about women of childbearing age unknowingly or inadvertently receiving a clinical trial medication while being pregnant, thereby exposing the fetus to unknown risks. Of course, the challenge with this approach is that most medications studied using clinical trials are eventually prescribed for older, less healthy men and women, not young healthy men. Thus, the clinical trial sample set is unrepresentative of the target population itself, which raises issues regarding how transferable findings may be between the clinical trial and the real-world practice setting.

Where possible (and in some circumstances, it may actually NOT be possible, in which case an unavoidable methodological limitation has occurred), those enrolled in the study should represent those who will ultimately be using the intervention itself, and this is frequently defined through use of inclusion and exclusion criteria. Inclusion criteria are typically framed using positive terms and phrases while exclusion criteria provide researchers with a list of specific factors or criteria to consider disqualifying potential and interested participants from involvement in the trial. To maximise generalisability of results, there is frequently an effort to minimise the number and nature of exclusion criteria, so that only those that are truly and legitimately related to participant safety and project viability are used.

If, for example, our pharmacist Sandy were interested in defining inclusion and exclusion criteria for his study involving implementation of an education programme to help young people in his community manage diabetes, he would first need to identify the target population for his intervention. If he has specifically designed an intervention aimed at 14–25 year olds, it would be legitimate to include this age range as an inclusion criteria (noting of course that in this instance an 'inclusion criteria' of 14–25 years of age is simultaneously an exclusion criteria for those <14 and >25). A unique challenge for Sandy may be the issue of health literacy: how literate, or how much English do potential participants need to know in order to participate in his trial? If Sandy has an exclusion criteria related to 'fluency in spoken English and ability to read documents at a 6th form level', this may make perfect sense to him. There is some written material participants will need to

read, and Sandy will be presenting his programme in English so in order for it to be understood, clearly his participants will need to speak English, right?

While there may be common sense to this, such exclusion criteria may inadvertently reduce the generalisability of Sandy's study, particularly if he considers that those in most need of help and support to prevent diabetes are perhaps those with the lowest health literacy and English language fluency levels. As can be seen there is an important but delicate balancing act to consider here: if we set inclusion/exclusion criteria too broadly, we may end up with unrepresentative samples and unworkable trials. If we set them too specifically, we may delude ourselves into thinking our intervention works well, even if the reality is that it only works in a very specific and narrow group within our target population.

8.4.2. Calculation of Sample Size

For both novice and experienced researchers, one of the most difficult challenges within a clinical trial is identifying the number of participants necessary to produce defensible conclusions. As we have already seen, clinical trials are inherently complicated. Having more participants involved than are really needed is expensive and cumbersome. It is also ethically questionable as it can be seen as 'wasting the time' of participants whose data will not actually contribute meaningfully to any conclusions. On the other hand, given the time, effort and resources invested in clinical trials, having too few participants may in the end result in meaningless results; which is both disheartening and a waste of effort.

Ultimately, sample sizes are merely estimations or educated guesses – however, the implications are significant if these estimations are incorrect. There have been numerous mechanisms proposed to calculate sample size requirements for clinical trials. While there may be multiple formulae and mathematical operations to perform in this calculation, which may give the appearance of confidence and certainty, ultimately they are still only estimates.

Most approaches to sample size calculation require the researcher to:

a. estimate the number of participants in the control group who will experience the outcome of interest (in some cases, a literature review or consultation with experts in the field may provide a useful starting point to make this estimation)

b. estimate a reasonable, plausible and defensible change in the outcome of interest that one might expect to occur as a result of the intervention (again, in some cases, previous literature/experience or consultation with experts in the field may provide a useful starting point to make this estimation)

c. establish the type 1 error (also known as the alpha-level) which represents the statistical probability of falsely rejecting the null hypothesis. Most frequently, this level is arbitrarily set at 0.05, meaning that the null hypothesis will be falsely rejected 5% of the time

d. establish the type 2 error which is the statistical probability of falsely NOT rejecting the null hypothesis (i.e. when the alternative hypothesis is true). Most frequently, this is arbitrarily set at 0.2, which is equivalent to falsely not rejecting the null hypothesis 20% of the time when the alternative hypothesis is true. The way to control a type 2 error is to make sure that you have a large enough sample size to make sure that any differences found are true. It is always sad when researchers do a great piece of work but finish it off by saying that 'if the sample size had been larger or if more people had taken part in the study…'.

We will talk more about type 1 and type 2 errors in Chapter 9, but for now we will focus on the people who take part in the clinical trial – the participants.

8.4.3. Recruitment of Participants

Experienced researchers who use clinical trial study designs frequently note that the most challenging aspects of this work involve recruitment of participants. First, this involves identifying an accessible population – a subgroup of the target population whom the researchers believe have both the capacity and interest to participate in a trial. This can be a challenge – many clinical trials rely heavily on the goodwill of participants to give of their time and energy to support research. Even when clinical trials involve an incentive (such as a small monetary honorarium, the chance to win an iPad in a draw, parking and transportation costs subsidised), such incentives rarely truly compensate participants for the time, trouble and risk involved in their participation. An important limitation of clinical trials is that this recruitment issue generally means the sample group is not truly representative of the target population, or of the accessible sample. Those who agree to participate in a clinical trial are likely to be more literate, more interested, more motivated and more curious than those who do not, and these underlying individual differences may in some way influence the outcome of the study itself in ways we do not quite understand.

Common recruitment strategies for clinical trials include mass mailings (snail- and/or e-mail), referrals from physicians, advertisements in newspapers, or preliminary screening of medical charts/hospital records. In most cases the number of people who agree to be involved in the study is much smaller than the number contacted or accessed. Study recruiters must be prepared for disappointment and constant revision of their recruitment strategy in order to achieve the sample size required.

In some cases snowballing-recruitment may be helpful: in this technique, the recruiter will ask an individual who has agreed to be involved in a study to nominate, name or direct the research team towards a friend or other potential participant (see Chapter 7, Section 7.2.2.g). Snowballing tends to be somewhat more successful than simply advertising; however, snowball samples run the risk of being less representative of both the target population and accessible sample as those who refer friends will likely share demographic similarities.

Ultimately, recruitment of participants requires a delicate balance between pragmatic realism and research idealism. Mindful of the importance of representativeness, appropriate sampling and other characteristics of good clinical trials, researchers must also be practical and recognise the challenges inherent in the process. Careful documentation of the compromises made throughout the process will help the researcher – and readers of the study – to better contextualise how these necessary deviations from an ideal clinical trial ultimately impact on the final results.

8.5. CONSIDERING THE OUTPUT: WHAT ARE WE MEASURING?

As discussed previously, the main intent of running a clinical trial is usually to determine the general or overall effects of a particular intervention across a representative sample of a target population. Results of clinical trials, however, are frequently used by clinicians to make individual treatment decisions for specific patients. These specific patients may have similarities or differences to the sample group that had been studied, based on demographic characteristics such as sex, age, race, genotype, stage of disease or comorbid conditions.

8.5.1. From Large Samples to Individuals: Practical Implications

The fact that all patients are different may result in interesting issues related to analysis and interpretation of data from trials and application to real world decision-making at the individual patient level. For example, some interventions may produce benefits for some groups of patients while actually causing harm to other groups. Simple descriptive statistics (see Chapter 10) that treat all participants within a clinical trial as being equivalent may end up masking real sub-group differences. For example, men may respond differently from women to a medication, or individuals from different ethnic groups may have different clinical responses based on genotypic differences. Failure to analyse data in a manner that allows you to use such demographic characteristics effectively may result in problems of interpretation. For example, some individuals of East Asian genetic heritage may lack a certain metabolic enzyme (acetaldheyde dehydrogenase) more common in the Caucasian population. A medication that relies upon acetaldehyde dehydrogenase for its metabolism will therefore be processed quite differently in a Caucasian population than in an East Asian population; failure to account for this difference within the clinical trial may result in problems if the medication is used by a subgroup that wasn't adequately or actually studied during the clinical trial. As this example illustrates it is becoming more important, and increasingly more common practice, to provide subgroup analyses where possible, in which data from clusters of study participants with similar characteristics or demographic features may be dealt with separately to ensure no significant harm or non-beneficial effects have been masked or blended in and therefore lost through data analysis. In most cases, these differences emerge during the data analysis stage and are dealt with through demographic stratification or use of other characteristics. In situations where the researcher is aware of a demographic or other reason to expect different response in advance, it can also be incorporated in the study design and recruitment stage (i.e. stratifying your sample and recruitment based on particular demographic characteristics in anticipation of differential results).

8.5.2.   Surrogate Outcomes

The reason we do research in the first place is to find something out that we didn't know before, or we knew it about one group of people and wanted to find out if the same held true for another population. In Chapters 1 and 2 we used the example of antibiotic therapy with the question '*Do patients with a bacterial infection get better more quickly if they are treated with antibiotics than those who are not?*' Whether or not patients recovered, how well and in what time frame would be some of the outcomes of the study. However, there is another type of outcome, a '**surrogate outcome**', which we need to highlight here because they are often used in clinical trials because they are cheaper and in many cases a smaller number of patients is exposed to the risks of trialling a new treatment.

In many cases, researchers face an almost insurmountable obstacle when studying certain processes or diseases: the time lag between interventions and effects can take decades to manifest. For example, if our pharmacist **Sandy** believes an educational programme can ultimately help reduce incidences of development of diabetes amongst young people in his community, he will need to be mindful of the multiple steps between intervention and outcome that are implicit in his hypothesis. 'Education' per se does not automatically 'prevent' a disease like diabetes from developing. The assumption here is that education produces a change in thinking, which in turn produces a change in behaviour, which over time will result in better lifestyle choices around eating, drinking, exercise, smoking, etc., which ultimately after decades will improve overall health (including a reduction in risk for diabetes). There is no direct straight line cause–effect relationship between education and health improvement. Instead, education is simply the first of many steps that may over time lead to positive health outcomes.

Similarly, when studying diseases like diabetes, it is difficult to actually 'observe' the condition itself. Instead, medical practice has evolved in such a way that markers (such as **HbA1c**, or fasting blood glucose levels, or other laboratory test parameters) provide us with an indirect method of describing, classifying, defining and monitoring a disease. These laboratory parameters are NOT the disease itself; they are simply accepted numerical standards or proxies that health professionals use to describe an unobservable health process and are known as surrogate outcomes.

KEY TERM

HbA1c: If you have diabetes you will usually have a blood test once a year to measure your HbA1c, which is your glycated haemoglobin. This test enables your clinician to find out how much glucose is being carried in your red blood cells over the previous 2 or 3 months. This gives a far better picture of how well controlled your diabetes is as it does not just rely on a few measurements.

Surrogate outcomes like blood glucose levels and body mass index (BMI) can be a useful answer to the complex question, 'Am I healthy'? However, the issues around BMI are a useful reminder that such proxies come with significant problems: a BMI between 18.5 kg/m2 and 25 kg/m2 is considered normal and healthy, while anything outside this range is considered unhealthy. First, by this definition, well over 60% of individuals in most developed countries may be categorised as unhealthy. Second, the emphasis on weight placed by BMI fails to consider other aspects of health, including genetic makeup, cardiovascular responsiveness, flexibility, etc. Third, this weight emphasis may actually be misleading. Many of us in our day-to-day lives know of people who may appear visually to be slim or slender but may have other health-related issues, while others who may visually appear to be on the larger side may be strong, flexible and athletic.

As the examples of BMI and diabetes illustrates, surrogate outcomes may be required out of necessity: complex constructs such as 'healthy' or 'diabetes' defy simplistic measurement, definition and assessment, and as a result, clinicians and patients must find viable, practical alternatives to facilitate decision-making. However, when surrogate outcomes actually become the outcome itself, not simply an indirect reflection of that outcome, we may make poor decisions. Do we treat laboratory test values and numbers, or do we treat patients? Outcome measurement is central to the value of clinical trials. In many cases, this outcome will be a surrogate outcome, given the limitations described previously. Acknowledging and recognising that we are dealing with surrogate, not real outcomes, is important. Even the most qualified researchers and clinicians may understand this reality but forget to actually apply it in their day-to-day work. Clinical trials researchers in particular need to be constantly vigilant that they understand and respect the differences between real outcomes of interest and the surrogate outcomes that are practical to measure, and ensure this is contextualised appropriately in research questions, methods, analyses, and reporting of findings.

So, recognising and appreciating this reality, our pharmacist Sandy has a new way of looking at his work. He now understands that 'learning' (or the result of education) is simply a proxy or surrogate outcome of interest with respect to diabetes management and disease prevention. If, as part of his study design, Sandy had focussed his research and measurement efforts on tracking his participants' change in knowledge about causes and consequences of diabetes (with the assumption that a person who now knows what causes diabetes and why it is unhealthy will then naturally take steps necessary to change his/her behaviour), he has used education and learning as a proxy outcome for behavioural change. Education does not cure or prevent diabetes: it is simply one tool among several that may be helpful to some people in some contexts. While education and learning are important in the behavioural change process, there are of course other factors that are important; Sandy must consider how to measure and study these factors (such as increasing exercise, improving diet, adherence to medications, etc.). As these behaviours change, Sandy could then study effects on biomarkers of diabetes (e.g. blood sugar levels, HbA1c, etc.), which are, from a medical perspective, the findings of greatest importance.

When designing a clinical trial to establish the value and impact of an educational intervention on prevention of diabetes amongst young adults in his community, Sandy needs to put this particular intervention in the broader context of health and disease progression. This does not diminish the importance of Sandy's intervention or work, or the value of using a clinical trials method to answer the question of whether an educational intervention 'works'. Instead it helps Sandy to better understand the meaning of the word 'works' in this context. Raising awareness and interest in one's health, providing access to resources that may be accessed in the future, giving individuals a new vocabulary to describe medical conditions like diabetes are

TABLE 8.1	**Surrogate and Real Outcomes**
Surrogate Outcome	**Real Outcome**
Education and learning	Cure or prevention of diabetes
Wellbeing	Cure or reduction of mental health symptoms
Cholesterol levels	Prevention of death from heart disease

all legitimate, valuable and helpful outcomes. They are not necessarily the grandiose and lofty outcome of 'preventing diabetes' but they are still important and worthy of study.

To clarify the concepts of 'surrogate' and 'real' outcomes we have provided some examples in Table 8.1.

8.6. OUTCOMES AND WHAT WE DO WITH THEM

An important criticism of many clinical trials is the otherworldly, unrealistic way in which such research may be operationalised. In an important twist on the Hawthorne Effect or Heisenberg Principle (see Chapter 5), critics of clinical trials methods maintain that the design and implementation of such studies fundamentally skews results, despite attempts to control bias through double blinding, randomisation or placebo controls. Why? Because the simple fact of participating in a clinical trial means individual participants are 'different' to average people (more motivated, interested, engaged, mobile) and that, during the clinical trial itself, they are more closely watched, monitored and scrutinised than average people.

This criticism is important to contextualise, and has been used as the foundation for differentiating trials based on effectiveness vs efficacy. **Efficacy** refers to the positive effects of an intervention under the optimal (or near-optimal) conditions of a clinical trial, which likely will exceed the quality of care routinely available to individuals. While enrolled in a trial, researchers and clinicians are very interested and closely monitor patients, even if they do not know (due to double blinding) whether the patient is in an intervention or control arm of the trial. In contrast, **effectiveness** relates to the effects of an intervention under more typical, routine conditions – the kinds of conditions that more accurately reflect the real-world of medical or pharmacy practice.

This can be particularly relevant in the context of adherence. During a clinical trial (whether for a medication, a medical procedure or an intervention such as an educational programme), there are strong efforts made by researchers and clinicians to encourage participants to do what they are told. Participants themselves have a strong incentive to comply with instructions and may be more psychologically open to adherence given their interest in volunteering to enrol in the trial in the first place. During the trial period, participants may have greater access to study nurses or medical care; they may have their parking and transportation costs paid for (which in the real world may actually prevent some people from attending medical appointments) and in some cases will even receive monetary compensation to follow instructions. While it may be argued such incentives are essential to motivate patients to want to participate in trials in the first place, the reality of course is that such incentives also make clinical trial conditions different to real-world conditions.

It is critical that researchers clearly and accurately state when they are running efficacy trials or effectiveness trials. A common criticism of clinical trials is that efficacy trials do not conform to real-world practice and consequently the outcomes achieved in such trials cannot be expected in routine practice. A strong counterargument to this may be that efficacy trials must precede effectiveness trials so as to understand what target or maximum benefits can reasonably be expected.

Even though those running clinical trials are typically running efficacy trials it is important for researchers to clearly state their intentions to allow stakeholders in the research findings to better contextualise findings. An important component of this contextualisation may include clarity around the difference between an intervention 'working' under the idealised, highly controlled and well-supported circumstances of the trial and what barriers exist to this intervention achieving similar outcomes in the real world - which is much less idealised, controlled and well-supported. For example, if **Sandy** were to find that his educational intervention resulted in participants learning more about their diabetes and translating this learning into positive behavioural change, he would equally need to consider what environmental gaps exist between the study conditions and the real-world conditions of someone else who may implement a similar programme. Explicitly acknowledging and describing this within the context of the efficacy trial provides readers with greater understanding as well as providing them with more practical tools for implementing clinical trial findings in their own practice.

Finally in this section we must mention '**intention to treat (ITT) analysis**'. The CONSORT guidelines describe this as 'A strategy for analyzing data in which all participants are included in the group to which they were assigned, whether or not they completed the intervention given to the group. Intention-to-treat analysis prevents bias caused by the loss of participants, which may disrupt the baseline equivalence established by random assignment and which may reflect non-adherence to the protocol.' The reason for this analysis

> ### EXAMPLE: THE DASH TRIAL
>
> One of the best known examples of this important distinction relates to the findings of the DASH trial. The Dietary Approaches to Stop Hypertension clinical trial run by the US National Heart, Lung and Blood Institute (part of the National Institutes of Health), explored the role of diet as a tool to prevent and control hypertension. Building upon observations of different rates or prevalence of high blood pressure in different parts of the world, the researchers were interested in whether diet could play a role in reducing blood pressure or risk of developing high blood pressure (note here the way in which the researchers focussed on surrogate outcomes (see section above)). This large, well-designed, and widely reported trial demonstrated a link between dietary intake and blood pressure in the high-normal blood pressure and moderately hypertensive adult populations. The so-called DASH diet was described as one rich in fruits, vegetables, whole grains, and includes meat, fish, nuts, and legumes, but limits sugar-sweetened foods, red meats, and added fats. Critics of this study noted that the trial itself was well-designed and implemented – almost too well-designed and implemented because, as it was a study, participants had much more support, monitoring and encouragement to comply with the DASH requirements than would those trying this dietary approach on their own in the real world. As an efficacy trial, DASH demonstrated diet can positively influence outcomes related to blood pressure: it was not an effectiveness trial and needs to be contextualised appropriately. Changing one's diet on one's own (without the support of clinical trials staff) is extraordinarily difficult – DASH did not make the claim this would be easy. Instead, as an efficacy trial, it simply helped confirm that indeed there is a connection between diet and blood pressure.

is to ensure that the positive effects of a drug that is the subject of the clinical trial are not overestimated due to the removal of people who drop out or who do not comply with the trial regimen. These are things that happen in real life and so should be taken into account in a clinical trial.

For more information you can find the CONSORT web site at the end of this link: http://www.consort-statement.org/.

8.6.1. Clinical vs Statistical Significance

One of the most overused words in research is 'significance'. Most researchers want and expect their work to be important and valuable, and for it to 'matter' to a broad and diverse audience. The threshold for defining value and importance is vague, and will generally depend upon context and application. One important tool for clarifying this importance is the distinction between statistical and clinical significance.

You will have heard researchers use the term '**statistical significance**'. This refers to the probability that the observed result occurred by chance alone. It is normally expressed through the p-value statistic and the rule of thumb is that a p-value of less than 0.05 would be a good result. This would mean that the probability of the results we have obtained happening by chance in our target population is less than 1 out of every 20 people. That is good, because we don't want the results to occur by chance – we want them to be because of the intervention we have used in our research. Statistical significance is a function of both the size of a difference/benefit, and the size of the sample in which it was studied and observed. For example, a clinical trial with a very large sample size is powered sufficiently to detect statistically significant but very small differences or benefits. Conversely, a clinical trial with a smaller sample size may not detect such a small difference. When making decisions about the implications of results of clinical trials those small differences are crucial because for some patients, they may mean the difference between life and death if the drug is approved for use.

In contrast to statistical significance, and of generally far more relevance to readers, clinicians and patients, is the concept of clinical relevance. Clinical relevance describes the threshold of difference or benefit required to change individual practice or general health policy. It is not a fixed number or concept and will vary based on context and application. An example of this might be the decision to treat a patient suffering from atrial fibrillation and at risk of having a stroke (**cerebro-vascular accident (CVA)**) with either warfarin or aspirin, which will depend on the individual's relative risk of having a stroke in the future. The calculation of this risk includes taking into account age, previous medical history and other conditions such as diabetes. It also includes taking into account the side effects of warfarin and aspirin and whether it is worth the risk of severe bleeding from warfarin, to prevent stroke. This is the clinical relevance of treatment with warfarin vs aspirin and it relates to the individual rather than a whole population.

Confusingly, the term 'significance' is sometimes used in clinical trials without the modifier 'clinical' or 'statistical' to help readers differentiate one from the other. While statistical significance may be of academic or intellectual interest, clinical significance is what most readers will be interested in. Therefore it is general convention now to refer to 'clinical relevance' and 'statistical significance' to ensure clarity in communication.

Not all things that are statistically significant may be clinically relevant. On the other hand some clinically relevant study findings may not achieve the threshold of statistical significance within a specific study (particularly if the study has a relatively small sample size or is underpowered). For example, a new medication for treatment of blood pressure may demonstrate a statistically significant decrease in **systolic** readings of 3 mmHg. Is this clinically relevant? Is it important? Does this finding matter to the individual clinician or patient? We cannot answer these questions without knowing the context within which they are being asked – in some cases the answers might be yes, in other cases the answers might be no. The important issue here is to clearly contrast between the concepts of statistical significance and clinical relevance in a way that is transparent, meaningful and respectful of the reader.

In this chapter we have outlined in some depth the way that clinical trials are designed and managed, and how important issues like outcomes are established. In pharmacy practice research these principles can be applied to any proposed intervention where the purpose of the research is to find out if changes in practice 'work' for patients. After all it is the individual patients that matter.

CHAPTER SUMMARY

- In this chapter the term clinical trial has been described along with some of the key features of this type of research.
- It also outlines procedures of randomisation and stratification using Sandy's research into diabetes control as an example.
- It describes the CONSORT guidelines and Intention to Treat.
- It highlights the use of the principles of a clinical trial in various forms of research.

FURTHER READING

Power Calculation

Röhrig, B., du Prel, J.-B., Wachtlin, D., Kwiecien, R., & Blettner, M. (2010). Sample size calculation in clinical trials. *Deutsches Ärzteblatt International*, *107*(31–32), 552–556.

9

Managing Your Results: A Step-by-Step Guide to the Principles Underpinning Your Choice of the Right Statistics to Use

LEARNING OBJECTIVES

After reading this chapter you should be able to:
- understand what statistics are and how they might be used
- understand what a database is and the tools available to help create one

- describe what 'data treatment' means
- understand the difference between statistical and clinical significance

9.1. INTRODUCTION

The word 'statistics' is concerned with the way in which researchers collect, organise, analyse, interpret and report data they have accumulated during the course of their research. Quantitative data lends itself to mathematical description and analysis, and statistics provide us with a common language and approach for understanding the numbers that are generated through research. A wide range of software tools is available to help organise, manage and analyse data – and do the statistical tests for you. In most cases (particularly in relatively small-scale pharmacy practice or practice improvement research projects) the data analysis is done by the researchers with support from a supervisor, but if additional help is needed then, we give you some advice on finding this at the end of the Chapter 11. This textbook is not all about quantitative methods. In Part III of the book the chapters are all devoted to qualitative research methods, so you will be able to understand which methods best suit your research question. At the end of this chapter you will find a reference to a published case study that provides you with examples of how to manage quantitative data. We will refer you to this at different points along the way.

9.1.1. Thinking Ahead

In almost all cases, you are well advised to develop some frameworks and data management plans before actually implementing or undertaking any research or data collection. A clear understanding of the research question (see Chapter 2) should help you to clarify what specific data must be collected in order to address your objectives. As a general principle, you should aim to collect only that data which are actually required to answer research questions and meet project objectives. Although a topic might be 'interesting' or 'may lead to further insights', if all our interesting and insightful ideas were explored, data collection would become an endless enterprise. Establishing from the outset what the remit of your research project is, and collecting only that data which are relevant and essential to fulfilling this remit, will keep your data down to manageable levels and keep you focussed.

9.1.2. Support From Others

Having clarified, refined and narrowed the scope of a research interest into a specific research question it is a good idea to talk your ideas through with your supervisor or other members of your research team. Working as a team and hearing what other people say about your ideas can be very rewarding, and they can be an invaluable sounding board in refining your research question to the point where it becomes feasible, answerable and appropriate for quantitative research.

The pre-planning of your data collection, management, analysis and interpretation is essential. Whether you are using surveys to gather opinions, frequency counts to establish behavioural patterns, laboratory results, audits to track progression/evolution of a medical condition, demographic data to better understand a population or sample, or pre- and post-knowledge tests to define participants' understanding of an issue, it is essential that data are collected in a manner that will support both answering of the research question and management of all the data that will be encountered. If you are working on a research project as part of your MPharm programme then you will have the support of your other team members and your supervisor(s).

9.1.3.   More About Statistics

A word about statistics: many health care professionals (including pharmacists) have a great deal of respect for the quantitative, and a general faith in the power of numbers. While quantitative research projects – and the statistics we use to analyse and describe the phenomena we are researching – can be powerful tools to enhance understanding, it is imperative that we never blindly accept without question numerical 'answers'. Whether a consumer of health research or a producer of health research, it is essential that pharmacists recognise and work within their comfort zone with respect to statistics. Ultimately, statistics are simply mathematical formulations – there is nothing magical about them. It is easy to allow yourself to feel daunted by the numbers, the formulae and the options for analysis that are available. Rather than simply give up, you are strongly encouraged to spend some time not only learning, but trying to truly understand the statistical foundations of the work you are consuming and the work you are producing. The chapters in this book that focus on statistical analysis will not provide all the answers, but it is our hope that in reviewing this material you will feel less intimidated by the mathematics and more confident in your ability to knowledgeably apply, use, consume and produce statistical information.

9.2   SETTING UP A DATABASE

Paradoxically, a critical first step in research involves consideration of the end point. What are you going to do with the data you have collected in the course of your research, and how are you going to organise and manage all this information? The different options and the costs and benefits of various data management tools and systems need to be considered at the outset to ensure well-intentioned research plans are not spoilt by the reality of being inundated by data.

When you first start to do research it is tempting to rush into the development of questionnaires, audit forms or other data-collection instruments because you are in a hurry to get started. Sometimes, though, a slower, more methodical and careful approach to planning results in greater success. For example, as discussed in Chapter 6 (Survey Design), careful selection of survey items is essential to ensure only relevant and meaningful questions are asked of participants.

In designing a survey or other data collection instrument, it is important to clearly understand the research objective. There are two main methodologies used in statistical analysis: descriptive and inferential. **Descriptive statistics** (see Chapter 10) are used to summarise data and present it as a snapshot in time. **Inferential statistics** (see Chapter 11) are used to draw conclusions (or inferences) from the data about the population or sample of interest. Before proceeding with data collection (or even design of a data collection tool), you must ensure you are clear in your own mind as to the true objectives of the research. The time to decide about statistical tests used to analyse data is when you are actually designing the data collection instruments themselves … not in the weeks after data have already been collected. See the case study in the Further Reading section.

9.2.1.   Thinking About Your Database

In designing a data collection instrument, the operational efficiency of your research will be significantly enhanced if a database is set up at the same time. A database is simply a repository (usually but not always computer-based) into which data points from a study may be entered, stored, retrieved, manipulated and analysed. The database you establish at the outset of your study will have tremendous importance as the research progresses. A poorly constructed database that is illogical in its construction, opaque in its design, and overly complicated to access will hinder your ability to actually do anything useful with the data you are collecting. There are many different software tools and systems that can be used for data collection. **Spreadsheet programmes** such as Microsoft Excel can be perfectly appropriate for some kinds of research, while in other cases, more complex database programmes such as Microsoft Access may be better. As the complexity of the research increases (including the numbers of participants, the nature of data collected, and the desire to shift more strongly towards inferential statistical analysis occurs), research-specific software programs, such as SPSS, SAS, or R may be needed. (Please see references at the end of this chapter for more information about this type of software.)

So the key message here is, before you start your project reflect on your study design and make sure you have the right support for the statistics you want to use.

9.2.2.   Importing and Exporting Data: Some Tips

No matter what software program is being used, it will be important for you to construct a template, form, database or some kind of tool to allow for the transferring of data from individual collection tools into a central repository. Mindful of the fact that transcription errors may occur during the movement of data from one tool to another, many researchers prefer to use systems that simultaneously and automatically tabulate quantitative results in real time without the need for human involvement. For example, those using survey methodologies may be interested in purchasing subscriptions to services such as Survey Monkey™ or FluidSurveys™. While there is often a cost associated with use of these commercial packages they have the advantage of coupling data collection, management and analysis all in one service, saving time and virtually eliminating risk of transcription error. Free versions of these programs are available but they sometimes limit you to the extent of the features you can use. You should be able to get advice about the right software to use from your supervisor or your computing services department.

9.2.3.   Characteristics of Databases

What are some characteristics and attributes of a good or fit-for-purpose database? In large part this will depend on the actual nature of your research (e.g. the amount of data you expect to collect, the method by which you will collect and input it, your need for descriptive and/or inferential statistics, etc.). A few key points to consider include the following:

a. **Minimising data replication**: A spreadsheet or database should be constructed in a way that captures all critical data once and once only. Constructing your database in a way that ensures minimal redundancy will reduce risks of transcription or data inputting errors (see Further Reading for more about capturing data on your database).

b. **Minimising manual data inputting and transcription**: Databases are only as powerful as the data they contain. Inputting and transcription errors (particularly when data is transferred manually) are the most frequent source of error. If you are using paper-based surveys or other methods of data collection that require transcription, it is essential to establish an audit or review practice for random second-checks of data inputting, as a way to mitigate errors. If at all possible, consider using a data collection system that allows you to simultaneously collect data and populate your database electronically, as a way

to guard against transcription errors.

c. **Using your database correctly**: You might have some experience of using commercially available software such as Excel for some other purpose but this may not be sufficient for research purposes. Explore the software you are going to use and make sure you understand the different functions and symbols and know what these mean. It can be mind-boggling at first but most software comes with an online handbook that you can use for support.

d. **Protecting the safety, integrity and confidentiality of your database**: As a researcher, your database represents the culmination of a significant amount of your time, energy and work. Back-ups and double-back-ups of critical databases are essential (and of course, do not keep your back-up copies on the same computer or on a USB stick adjacent to your computer – physical separation of back-up and original copies is safer). It is also important that your database is managed and stored securely as required by your ethics approval. For example if you have identifying information in your database (e.g. a patient's name or address), you will need to ensure two levels of password protection: one to open your computer and one to access the specific spreadsheet/database. Managing the integrity of your database is also important: particular challenges may occur when, for example, software upgrades occur and you are migrating data from one version of software to another. Random spot checks to ensure successful migration (particularly when formulae are part of your database) should be undertaken.

e. **Managing the paperwork**: In some cases, your primary data collection tool will be a paper-based survey, form or document that will ultimately be transferred to an electronic database. While most of your work in data analysis will likely occur using a computer, the question of what to do with all the paper copies can be tricky. For most researchers, storing large numbers of paper surveys in a way that facilitates any sort of reasonable retrieval is irritating or impossible, yet most research ethics boards require you to find a mechanism to do just that for a period of several years (as a way of ensuring back-up and possible audit of data inputting). Some researchers have developed systems where paper copies are scanned and stored electronically, allowing the original paper copies to be shredded and disposed of in a confidential manner. If this is permitted by your local research ethics board, it can be a valuable tool to manage the paper that your research may generate. Most academic institutions have a way of disposing of confidential papers, and your supervisor will be able to tell you what this is.

9.3. BEFORE YOU START

One of the most challenging issues for researchers involved in quantitative studies is determining the 'right' statistical test to use for the research objective of interest. The number of options appears overwhelming and matching the kind of data collected (e.g. nominal, ordinal, interval, ratio) (see Chapter 3) to the correct kind of statistical test can be difficult. On top of that, you have got to find a way of understanding what all your data means and also present your findings in a way other people can understand. Before you begin to look at your data and the ways you might use statistics to analyse them, there are some terms that you will come across that it might be useful to understand. We explain some of these below.

9.3.1. Data Treatment

The collection of data (e.g. from a survey, observations, chart audits, or other sources) is only the first step of the process – so called 'raw data' must be statistically treated to facilitate analysis and interpretation. The way in which data are organised and mathematically manipulated is referred to as **data treatment**, and it allows raw data to 'come to life' and become meaningful information. In data treatment it is important to use certain terminology accurately. Here are some common terms:

- Data point

One particular number or item from a broader collection of data (e.g. one participant's response to a specific question would be considered a data point).

- Data set

Simply a group of data points, but the way in which data sets are organised is critical in data treatment. For example, forming data sets based on age of the participant (i.e. clustering data into groupings based on a demographic characteristic (see Chapter 3, Section 3.7)) may result in masking of certain features of the data such as socio-economic effects (i.e. if those of similar chronological age but with widely divergent incomes are all put into the same data set, then the effects of wealth or poverty on an outcome of interest may be harder to detect).

- Raw data

All of the data you have entered onto your database before you have done anything with it. This is almost never reported as-is, since the sheer volume of data points would be overwhelming to anyone other than the researcher. Equally, raw data without treatment has little meaning – it is literally numbers on a page without patterns or significance. Statistics are the primary vehicle by which data points can be treated and formed into data sets that can be further treated, analysed, described and used to make meaningful inferences.

9.3.2. Significance

Most researchers are interested in ensuring their work has meaning and impact. For example, practitioner-researchers frequently undertake research as a way to improve a system or process, or to determine how to optimise care for patients. The term 'significance' has many meanings and interpretations. On a personal level, researchers want their work to 'matter', to have significance to someone other than the researcher him/herself. The desire for this kind of significance can sometimes lead researchers to downplay or ignore negative findings (i.e. findings that are not statistically significant or run contrary to an initial hypothesis). It is essential that researchers remain open to all possibilities of outcomes, including ones that do not achieve a level of statistical significance: these findings are real, important and meaningful, and should be reported in just the same manner as any other kind of research:

a. Statistical significance

In a statistical sense, significance has a precise meaning associated with a diverse array of tests and measures that will be described in Chapter 10. In any research involving a sample (rather than a population), there is always a risk that the observed outcomes were a result of some kind of sampling bias or error (see Chapter 7), rather than a true result. The p-value is the outcome of a statistical test that helps researchers and readers understand the extent to which the observed outcomes actually reflect characteristics of the population that was sampled, rather than a random or biased sampling error (see Chapter 9). Importantly, statistical significance is no guarantee of clinical, practical or real-world significance.

b. Clinical significance

Clinical significance can be thought of as the practical, real-world importance of a finding. Does it actually produce a meaningful, observable difference or change, in a way that a patient or health care provider would notice? Some changes may be measurable (in terms of a clinical laboratory value), but not necessarily noticeable by a patient – for example, a change in 4 mm Hg for systolic blood pressure may be statistically significant, but may not be noticed by a patient, or affect their health care outcome or trajectory, or their day-to-day life.

Within the health professions, most practitioners are generally interested in the real-world application of research, and, consequently, clinical significance is of greater importance than statistical significance (see Chapter 8). An outcome may be of statistical significance, but for a specific practitioner and his/her patients this may not translate into clinical significance. Since clinical significance is highly dependent on the unique characteristics of patients, contexts, and practitioners, it is sometimes difficult to define in a general way: what is clinically significant for Sandy the pharmacist in his context, may not be clinically significant at his colleague's GP practice down the road. As a result, the best we can do in most cases is simply report statistical significance and outline features or characteristics for readers to consider that may allow them to draw their own inferences about clinical significance in their context. See the case study in the Further Reading section.

9.3.3.   Causality

The final term to mention in this section is 'causality'. This refers to the attempts to find out whether one thing causes another, and in health care this is a very important issue. If researchers can establish what causes illnesses they may be able to develop new treatments that can prevent the illness happening in the first place. An interesting example of causality is the issue of cigarette smoking. We know that there is a link between smoking and a number of life-threatening conditions, such as lung cancer. But if smoking was the one thing that caused lung cancer, everyone who smoked would get lung cancer, and they don't. The best we can say is that research has shown a strong association between smoking and lung cancer.

9.4.   LOOKING FOR RELATIONSHIPS BETWEEN VARIABLES

When looking for relationships between variables, sometimes it is best to begin with the two main statistical methodologies described previously: descriptive statistics and inferential statistics (see Section 9.2). While it is tempting to always aim to be able to generalise the conclusions and inferences from your research, the reality is that in most cases this may be beyond the scope of most practitioner-researchers. The statistical requirements for defensible, inferential conclusions are many, and relate as much to issues of sample sizes and powering (see Chapter 11) of the study as they do to the choice of statistical test. The value and importance of descriptive statistics may sometimes be overlooked. Descriptive statistics provide a wealth of information about a topic of interest and can form the solid foundation of future work more appropriately scaled for inferential analytical methods. For this reason it is important to think about what statistics you might use right at the beginning of the research design process. In framing a research question, it is usually helpful to determine how data collection and analysis will inform the project. In some cases, we are interested in determining whether different processes are related, linked or associated with each other in some way. Such **correlational** research aims to uncover the extent to which changes in one variable may impact another.

So, the design of your research will have an impact on what statistics you can use, but it may not always be possible to draw conclusions about a population or process of interest using only descriptive statistics. Indeed, it might be necessary to use qualitative analyses to help answer your research questions.

EXAMPLE

Rosi's project focusses on whether there is need and demand for a pharmacy on campus at her university. A question on her questionnaire might be:

'Should there be a pharmacy on campus?'
Yes [ ] No [ ]

Using descriptive statistics to count the numbers of people who said 'Yes' and the number who said 'No' might reveal that *'75% of those polled said there should be a pharmacy on campus'*. However, it would be premature to then conclude that a pharmacy should be built on campus. This is because Rosi would need more information before drawing such a conclusion. For example:

- Was there a statistically significant difference between the number of people who said 'Yes' and 'No' compared to all of the people that work and visit the university campus?
- Does Rosi need more information? For this question she forced respondents into a dichotomous response (i.e. 'Yes' or 'No' only) when in reality their preference may have been to say 'Yes, with the following exceptions' or 'No, unless these things change'. Throughout the research process, it is essential to remember (and constantly remind oneself) that the data must lead to the conclusion, rather than having a preconceived conclusion looking for data to support it.
- Does Rosi need to talk to some of the people who run the university about the practicalities and costs of building the pharmacy?

In Part III of this textbook we will look at qualitative research methods and how Rosi might use these to gather more information for her project.

Another example comes from Sandy's research project. He may be interested in determining whether a change in baseline understanding of how and why type II diabetes occurs in young people may lead to a change in behaviour (e.g. improvement in diet, increase in exercise, weight loss) which may in turn lead to a change in outcome (e.g. improved diabetes control). In this situation there are three distinct variables of interest that might be considered:

1. Understanding of the disease
2. Lifestyle choices and behaviours
3. Control of type II diabetes.

Understanding of type II diabetes ➡ Lifestyle choices ➡ Control of type II diabetes

In this model, there is a one-way association between these variables. Sandy is hypothesising that how much people understand about their condition will bring about (or cause) a change in behaviour, which in turn will bring about (or cause) a decrease in the diagnosis of diabetes. This kind of association – a causal connection between variables – is particularly challenging to demonstrate statistically, as it means we must also rule out or allow for other possible reasons for the observed change.

For example, Sandy might decide to run a class on diabetes for young people and some people may attend every session. One or more might demonstrate an increase in understanding of the causes of diabetes through pre- and post-testing (e.g. Sandy might create a questionnaire that tests their understanding). Six months later these regular attendees might return to Sandy having lost 15 kg of weight and their next blood test shows that their diabetes is better controlled than it was before they lost weight. Can Sandy rightfully claim it was his education session and his intervention that caused this outcome?

It may be tempting to do so, but statistically it will be difficult to prove one way or another. Without further study, it is hard to know if individuals' levels of understanding about type II diabetes actually caused them to behave in a certain way (e.g. lose weight) and that this caused the improvement in blood sugar control. There might have been other things that happened to some of those young people. For example, perhaps at the same time a peer might have been made fun of the weight of one of the young people and that was the driver for the behaviour change. Or perhaps the young person caught sight of him/herself in a mirror and that was the real cause of the weight loss, not the knowledge and understanding acquired through Sandy's course.

9.4.1. Designing an Intervention

What Sandy set out to do in his research was to find out if the level of understanding of the young people with diabetes of their condition might lead to better outcomes. In the example in the previous section Sandy thinks about designing a study to see if what he thinks might actually be true. The running of a class for young people with diabetes with the purpose of finding some answers is called an **intervention**.

When trying to establish associations or relationships between different variables, it is tempting to assume that

our interventions are the reason. We all hope that our research can contribute to health care in some way; that's why we do it. It is important to remember, however, that just because there may be a relationship between two things, it does not necessarily mean that one has caused the other (see Section 9.3.3).

9.4.2. Statistical Tests

When trying to establish relationships or associations, a certain kind of inferential statistic is required. There are a series of **tests** for correlation (such as Spearman Rho or Pearson r) that can be used to establish the strength of relationships between different variables such as those in the example of Sandy's research. In Chapter 11, we will explore these types of tests in greater detail, recognising that they are useful for establishing correlation, not causation.

In some cases, we may be more interested in exploring differences between groups because these can be revealing and lead us to conduct further studies to find out why those differences are seen. In some cases we can use qualitative research (see Part III) to help us answer the 'why?' questions, and we will give examples of this in those chapters. For now we are going to concentrate on how we can explore differences between variables using quantitative methods, and to do this we shall go back and see how Dorothy's research might progress.

Let's go back to the theory and have a look at how we might do this.

9.4.3. Statistical Significance

Testing for significant differences is an inferential statistical method used to answer this question: 'What is the probability that the observed change occurred because of the intervention, and what is the probability that this change would have occurred in any case, simply by chance?' The statistical methods used to answer these questions result in a '**level of probability**' – a number that must then be interpreted by the researcher to establish whether or not it is actually significant or meaningful. The inferential statistical tests most frequently used when comparing two groups on one variable only are the **Pearson's chi-square test** and the **t-test**, both of which will be described in more detail in Chapter 11. In health services research similar to Dorothy's project, the usual convention is that up to five occurrences in 100

CASE STUDY EXAMPLE

You may remember (see Chapter 6) that Dorothy, our hospital pharmacist doing an MSc, wants to find out about the feasibility of beginning an antimicrobial stewardship programme in her hospital. This is an inter-professional collaboration designed to encourage optimal prescribing which can have the added benefit of reducing overall health care (including drug) expenditures.

When we left Dorothy in Chapter 6 she had decided on some of her research objectives which included to:

1. describe the attitudes of the interprofessional team towards antimicrobial stewardship
2. compare the views of doctors, nurses, pharmacists, microbiologists and others involved in the antimicrobial prescribing decisions made at XX hospital
3. identify barriers to implementation of an antimicrobial stewardship programme
4. identify the enablers to implementation of an antimicrobial stewardship programme
5. develop a draft programme

In Chapter 7 we left Dorothy trying to figure out who her participants should be and how she could compare the responses to her questionnaire from different groups of prescribers, e.g. doctors, nurses, pharmacists (see Section 7.5.3). If Dorothy were to design a checklist or form that all prescribers were required to complete prior to initiating a patient on a new antimicrobial, she would want to know what value it had (if any) in promoting better quality prescribing and use of these medicines. The checklist she designs must help prompt critical self-reflection on the part of the prescribers to consider:

a. whether an antimicrobial is indeed required in this situation
b. whether the specific choice of antimicrobial has been carefully thought through (for example, based on actual culture-and-sensitivity laboratory results)
c. if the most appropriate duration has been identified (including specification of monitoring parameters to ensure expected response to therapy).

Using a checklist-/form-based approach to stewardship issues would allow Dorothy to consider a **quasi-experimental design** for her research. Quasi-experimental studies fall somewhere between correlational studies, where we are trying to establish a link between variables, and experimental design studies, where we are trying to establish causality. It is not always possible, for example, to randomly allocate our participants into two distinct groups and an example of a quasi-experimental design is where there is only one group of participants but measurements are taken of the variables of interest at different points in time. This is called a 'Time Series Design' and more about this and other quasi-experimental designs can be found in the 'Further Reading' section at the end of this chapter. The reason we include this type of design here is because in real-life things don't always fall into neat patterns where peoples' health behaviours can be measured by an experimental design. Therefore we need other ways of finding out what we need to know about our participants, and quasi-experimental designs can be a valuable step in the research design process that can help inform future research.

How Might Dorothy Approach Her Study?

Dorothy might design an intervention where one group of clinicians may be asked to use the form, in addition to their traditional/routine practices around antimicrobial prescribing, while another group of practitioners may be asked simply to continue their traditional/routine practices (see Chapters 6 and 7 for details regarding sampling, sample size and participant recruitment for further important logistical details). Dorothy now has two distinct **cohorts** or groups in her study – one group using the new intervention and one group continuing without the intervention. After a month, let's say that the group using the new tool prescribed, on average, 15% fewer antimicrobials than the group using its traditional/routine practices. Can Dorothy claim credit for this change or improvement in practice?

To establish this, she would first need to apply inferential statistics to determine whether observed differences in average prescribing rates between the two groups were a result of the intervention (the new form/checklist) or were simply the result of chance or random events (they might have just happened anyway for reasons other than Dorothy's checklist). Further, she may want to establish to what extent chance or random events, in addition to the actual success of her intervention, resulted in the outcome she observed.

of the observed change being caused by random events or chance is a reasonable enough level to accept, and that any number less than this becomes meaningful, or 'statistically significant'. So, if only 1 out of the 100 was found to have occurred by chance then we would know that we were on to something. Flipping this around into more everyday language, this means that Dorothy can be 95% certain that the change she observed in prescribing behaviours was caused by her intervention. Of course, in some situations, 95% certainty may be too low – or too high. Further details of how significance is determined and tested will be discussed in Chapter 11.

To finish up this chapter let's look at the step-by-step principles underpinning your choice of the statistics to analyse your research data.

9.5. SOME GENERAL GUIDELINES FOR USING (AND AVOIDING MISUSING) STATISTICS

Statistics can be powerful tools to help us better understand our world. Unfortunately there have been a sufficient number of instances where statistics have been improperly used to warrant coining of the phrase 'there are three kinds of lies: lies, damned lies and statistics' (popularised by the writer Mark Twain), reflecting the wariness of the general public with the role of statistics in decision-making. What follows is a series of guidelines that all researchers – regardless of their experience or expertise – should consider prior to using statistics in their work:

Principle 1: Always remember the real audience for your work. While the mathematics of significance may be important, it is more important to remember that the real end-user of most research is not an academic journal or a fellow researcher, but the general public who hopes for better things in life through the work of researchers. Try to make the statistics you use clear, transparent, understandable and usable so that your research can truly inform public discourse about an issue.

Principle 2: Do not use statistics you actually do not understand. While this may appear to be a self-evident piece of advice, you may be surprised by the frequency with which even experienced researchers feel the need to go beyond their actual statistical skill set as a way of impressing others or appearing to 'know' more than they actually might. All research must be defensible, and researchers must be prepared to engage in active discussion with others regarding their study question, design, methods, and analyses. Using complex statistical tests you do not actually understand does not make your work appear more scholarly or important … it simply makes you more vulnerable to those who will legitimately ask questions.

Principle 3: Do not attempt to interpret statistical results if you do not fully understand the statistical tests themselves. In some cases, it is tempting to comment upon the work of others, or to interpret the results of a statistical test. In both cases, it is essential you actually understand the mathematical and probabilistic underpinnings of the statistical test upon which you are commenting. This is particularly important with respect to inferential statistics which require significant contextual interpretation. In many cases there are multiple simultaneously valid interpretations of a given statistic and defining which one is 'better' in a particular context takes more than mathematical knowledge: it requires judgment and wisdom.

Principle 4: When in doubt, consult someone who knows more about statistics. Health professionals such as pharmacists often believe that they must be jacks-of-all-trades – independent workers who can confidently solve problems and make decisions by themselves. Indeed there is a great premium placed within the health professions' culture on decisiveness and being a 'quick study'. While this may be applicable within a clinical context where time is of the essence in decision-making, in most cases, a more thoughtful, collaborative approach is warranted in a research context. In most cases, pharmacists (or other health care professionals) who do research are not specially trained in statistics. To enhance both the quality and credibility of your work consider including a biostatistician in your research as early in the process as possible, to optimally benefit from this support.

Principle 5: Try to provide readers of your work with as much information as needed so they can make their own interpretations of your data. Most statistics (whether they are inferential or descriptive) are used to persuade readers – simply providing them with a conclusion without the ability to take your data and reconstitute your conclusions themselves diminishes the strength of your work. Further, if you do not provide readers with sufficient information and details about your data, the statistical treatments used and why, and how these results lead to your conclusions, it may give readers the impression you are being at best lazy or careless and at worst deceptive. In general people are convinced by a logical argument built up systematically with premises clearly presented. Your data and statistics should be similarly systematic and clearly presented for readers to understand how you arrived at the conclusions you did.

Principle 6: Be aware of how statistical data are presented. Depending upon the size and scale of your study, you may generate a large amount of data that are difficult to condense into a traditional manuscript or paper. As a result, you may rightly choose to present data in a graphic or tabular format as a way of converting numbers into a more appealing and intuitive visual depiction. Caution must be exercised when converting raw data into visual representations. Pay particular attention to the scales used, recognising measurement units on an axis may have profound influence on the slope of a curve, which in turn may shape the interpretation of data by the reader.

As can be seen, it is relatively easy to subconsciously shape a reader's perception of the importance or impact of data and statistical analysis simply by presenting it in a visual form. In general, steeper slopes on curves appear more dramatic and meaningful, even though the slope itself is a function of the units used on each axis. Selecting the correct unit and scale for your graphical presentations of data is important for establishing the credibility of your work.

Principle 7: When using descriptive statistics, always present the range or variability, not simply the central tendency. As you will see in Chapter 10, both characteristics are important to accurately understand a data set. Simply presenting the central tendency (e.g. mean, mode or median) without the dispersion, range or variability of the data set described does not allow the reader to understand the magnitude of this central tendency.

Principle 8: When using other researchers' work cite clearly and appropriately. In many cases, your research will be building upon the work of others. At the very least, you may be presenting others' work as part of a literature review or environmental scan to provide readers with a context within which to understand your work. When citing the work of others, it is prudent to (i) wherever possible, rely more heavily upon peer-reviewed literature; and (ii) provide details so the reader understands where these data came from and how it connects to your work. Peer-reviewed literature has a higher degree of credibility than other forms of so-called 'grey' literature. Through the peer review process, there is some greater assurance that issues of research design, statistical treatment, and inferences drawn are defensible. While a peer-reviewed citation is not necessarily fool-proof, and the peer review process cannot detect all irregularities or problems with research, it is generally considered to be of higher quality than other forms of publication and consequently should, wherever possible, be the source for your citations. When citing others' work, avoid giving the impression that a fact is simply appearing out of nowhere. Providing a citation or footnote is of course required, but in the text of your work it is a good idea to give the reader some context within which to interpret what they are reading. Consider this final example:

Bad Example: 75% of patients trust pharmacists to prescribe, renew, adapt or modify prescriptions.

Better Example: A study commissioned by the NHS in 1995 indicated that 75% of patients agreed or strongly agreed with the statement 'I would trust my pharmacist to prescribe, renew, adapt or modify prescriptions for me'.

As can be seen through this example, the better example contains:

a. the date of the work, which helps the informed reader put into context the fact that at the time of this study pharmacist-prescribing was new and unfamiliar to most patients in the UK. This will affect the reader's interpretation of the statistic presented

b. the specific question asked of participants, highlighting the notion of 'my' pharmacist rather than pharmacists in general (which again will affect interpretation of the finding)

c. the strength of the response (agree and strongly agree), albeit collapsed into one category. In the better example, the reader is provided with more information to help contextualise the statement for him/herself.

These principles are by no means comprehensive. Our intention is to provide some guidance in the appropriate use and presentation of statistics to enhance the credibility and quality of your work. It is important for researchers to consider issues of credibility and not believe that 'the numbers speak for themselves'. If this were true, there would be no need for researchers to actually be involved in analysis and interpretation of data. So remember, it is your name and your credibility that are at stake. Within the research community, there is a strong premium placed on the credibility of researchers. The culture of the scientific community recognises the central importance of trust. We trust researchers to work with integrity, to report findings honestly, and to manage and disclose any personal biases that may interfere with the production of high-quality research. Even as a novice researcher, your name will be associated with the work you do. Particularly at the start of your research career, it is imperative that your name be associated with high-quality, trustworthy work.

Statistics are frequently the cause of misunderstanding and contention, which may be surprising to you given the seeming certainty of numbers and mathematical formulae. As you shall see in Chapters 10 and 11, the selection of statistical treatments, the way in which data are presented, and the context within which analyses occur all will be scrutinised by readers. Not fully understanding the statistics you use, accidentally or deliberately presenting data in a way that skews interpretation by the reader, or misuse of statistics that suggests your personal bias or lack of knowledge interfere with the quality of the work and will be detected. There are ALWAYS more experienced individuals with greater expertise who will review your work and will ask legitimate questions. Having the knowledge, skill and confidence to answer these questions and to defend your choices and decisions along the research pathway – particularly with respect to statistical treatments – will in many ways govern whether your work is considered important and successful or meaningless and unhelpful.

So let's get started. For some pharmacists, the simple thought of having to learn or apply statistics is the most significant barrier to undertaking research. Remember, statistics are merely tools to help support us in better understanding the things we observe – they are your friend, not your enemy. Learning statistics for the purposes of applying them for research should not be an exercise in memory and anxiety. Instead you should be focussed on thinking through the questions you are asking, the methods you are using, the data you have collected and how all of this taken together can help us to better understand a process or system. There is no need to memorise a formula or recite by rote in an unthinking manner the circumstances under which one statistical test should be used vs another. Instead, statistics should be seen as simply a vehicle to help you to understand what you have seen and communicate it more effectively and accurately to diverse audiences who may be interested in your work. In Chapters 10 and 11 that follow, we will focus in greater depth on first descriptive then inferential statistics.

CHAPTER SUMMARY

- In this chapter the examples of our case study pharmacists Sandy and Dorothy and our student, Rosi, have been used to show how they might establish whether or not their results are significant.
- It defines statistical tests.
- It explains a quasi-experimental research design.
- The chapter ends with the principles of using statistics.

FURTHER READING

Statistics

https://www.discoveringstatistics.com/.
This is a link to Andy Field's website that accompanies his book.
Field, A.: *An Adventure in Statistics: the reality enigma.* London: Sage.
Statistics Software, 2016.
Field, A. (2013). *Discovering Statistics Using IBM SPSS Statistics.* London: Sage.

The R Project for Statistical Computing. https:// www.r-project.org/.
Statistical Analysis Software. http://www.sas.com/en_us/ software/analytics/stat.html.

Case Study Example Using Statistics

Unne, A., & Rosengren, K. (2014). Using numbers creates value for health professionals: a quantitative study of pain management in palliative care. *Pharmacy*, *2*, 205–211.

10

Descriptive Statistics: How Many People Said What and Who Were They?

LEARNING OBJECTIVES

After reading this chapter you should be able to:
- explain central tendency and dispersion
- understand some of the more commonly used analyses
- describe, mean, median, mode and range
- decide on the best way to depict the results of your own descriptive statistics

10.1. INTRODUCTION

As described in Chapter 9, statistics involves the collection, management, analysis, interpretation and presentation of data. This can be data collected using both quantitative and qualitative methods, but in this chapter we will be concentrating on quantitative data. We will explore how to describe qualitative data in Part III.

Frequently, it is not possible to collect data from every single person or participant who is eligible to take part in our research interest because it would be costly. The logistics of doing so would also be very difficult to manage. When such a population-wide census is not possible, most researchers collect data by developing targeted interventions and specific tools involving samples of their population of interest (see Chapter 7). As described in Chapter 7 representative sampling is a technique that is frequently used to support researchers in generalising their findings from the sample group to the population as a whole.

Regardless of whether a sample or census is used, or whether an experimental/interventional or observational approach is taken, there is always a need to manage and analyse the data which has been collected. As we said in the previous chapter two main methods are used in analysis of quantitative data: descriptive statistics (involving a summary of the data gathered using mathematical formulae) and inferential statistics (involving the drawing of conclusions and generalisations to a broader population).

This chapter is focussed on descriptive statistics and Chapter 11 is devoted to inferential statistics. Descriptive statistics most frequently focus on two particular properties of a data set:

1. The **central tendency** of the distribution (sometimes referred to as its location, which seeks to define the central or most typical value of the data)
2. The **dispersion** (or variability) which seeks to characterise the extent to which individual data points depart from the most central/typical value and from one another.

Unlike inferential statistics, descriptive statistics are not developed on the basis of any kind of probability theory. Instead they are a form of data accounting that can be presented either mathematically/numerically or visually (for example in the form of a graph). Descriptive statistics are essential for understanding a group that has been studied, and form the foundation for initially describing data that have been collected. In some cases, descriptive statistics by themselves may be sufficient for understanding what is going on in our population. In other cases, descriptive statistics are first undertaken in order to help researchers move to inferential statistics.

Some people might assume that descriptive statistics can be used for making inferences and generalisable conclusions that will lead to decision-making. This is a misuse of descriptive statistics that can be problematic. Summarising data and presenting central tendencies and distributions by themselves does not allow us to draw inferences and conclusions. For example, stock market investors may be tempted to believe that the performance of a favourite stock over the past decade should somehow predict its future performance. A stock that has, on average, gained 15% in value over the previous decade may sound like a sure-fire way of building wealth. A slightly more sophisticated investor may recognise that 'on average' is somewhat vague and learn that the range of growth over that decade was somewhat broad; in its best year, the stock gained 30%, but in its worst year the stock lost 85% of its value. Simply reporting an average (gained 15%) does not provide the investor with as much information as they would get if the dispersion were also noted.

An even more sophisticated investor would recognise that even knowing both the average and the best/worst year gains and losses does not provide sufficient data to make forward projections (or inferences) about how the stock will perform in the future. Researchers – and investors – need to beware of the tendency to want descriptive statistics to say more than they are actually capable of saying. Experienced investors – and researchers – both recognise and appreciate the value and importance of descriptive statistics as one important (albeit limited) source of information that, when blended with other types of analysis, can facilitate further understanding of a process or system.

10.2. CALCULATING DESCRIPTIVE STATISTICS

As discussed above in Section 10.1, descriptive statistics tend to be most focussed on describing mathematically two critical features or characteristics of a data set: its central tendency and its dispersion. Why are these characteristics of such importance? As noted in Chapter 3, most research involves the collection of data from diverse individuals, settings, or processes. Except in rare circumstances, research typically involves multiple participants. With this diversity, there is a challenge to better understand and interpret data that have been collected, and, as a first pass, central tendency and dispersion provide a useful vehicle for summarising or encapsulating these data.

In calculating descriptive statistics it is important to first consider the kind of analysis that is most appropriate in a given circumstance. This is generally based upon the number of variables involved in the research and is important because some statistics are more robust than others when trying to mathematically describe our sample. **Univariate** analysis involves research focussed on a single variable. For example, if during an election campaign we were interested in knowing which political party would receive the greatest number of votes, we might simply ask those of voting age '*For which political party are you most likely to vote?*' The single variable of interest in this case would be the political party and data would be reported based on the number of respondents who indicated their support for a specific party (or no party at all).

In contrast, **bi-** or **multivariate** analysis is useful when the sample being studied consists of more than one variable. In this context, descriptive statistics can be useful for describing the relationships between and amongst different variables. For example, if during an election campaign we were interested in a better understanding of WHO actually supports a specific political party, we may ask other questions in addition to '*For which political party are you most likely to vote?*' We may want to ask about the respondents' age, sex, marital status, income level, postal code (as a **proxy** for income levels) or other respondent characteristics of interest. With these data it becomes possible to develop a statistical 'portrait' of the typical political party supporter. For example, it may be possible through descriptive statistics to establish that only 12% of single female voters under the age of 35 support a specific political party. This might provide that political party with some evidence indicating that they need to work harder in their election campaign to attract single female voters under the age of 35. Multivariate statistical analysis allows us to more thoroughly and deeply describe the sample of interest which can provide useful information for further consideration. Importantly, multivariate analysis helps us to describe relationships between and among different variables through use of cross-tabulations, and (in some cases) the degree to which dependence exists between certain variables of interest. Though not quite at the level of inferential statistics, such analyses can provide researchers with valuable insights into how our participants might be thinking or the characteristics of a system.

10.3. CENTRAL TENDENCY AND OTHER DESCRIPTIVE STATISTICS

A descriptive statistic of particular importance is **central tendency**. We introduced this term in Chapters 4 and 9 and the central tendency is a mathematical way of describing the 'typical' data point within a set of data points. There are three descriptive statistics that are most useful in describing central tendency. They are mean, median and mode, and more detail about these is given in the next three sections.

In most cases researchers are gathering and compiling multiple data points from multiple participants around a research question of interest. The following example illustrates an important point regarding the collection of data points for our descriptive statistics. What questions we ask and how we ask them can make a difference to the results we obtain.

Our hospital pharmacist Dorothy may be interested in knowing how frequently prescribers in her practice use a specific antimicrobial drug. This may inform her effort to support an antimicrobial stewardship programme in her institution to encourage optimal prescribing of costly medications. Let's say Dorothy undertakes a **retrospective** chart audit of eight key prescribers in her practice. Using historical records from the previous 30-day period, she is able to tally up the frequency with which an antibiotic of interest is being used. For this example, let's consider the antibiotic **vancomycin,** which is relatively expensive to use, has certain side effects that warrant concern, and has an antibiotic resistance pattern (vancomycin-resistant enterococcus, or VRE) that means it should not be used indiscriminately. Dorothy consults her dispensing records and identifies the following pattern:

EXAMPLE

Prescriber #	Frequency of Prescribing Vancomycin in Last 30 Days
1	6 times
2	8 times
3	7 times
4	8 times
5	7 times
6	6 times
7	7 times
8	42 times

Her simple study immediately points to some intriguing patterns. First, without any descriptive analysis at all, she is able to identify there is an '**outlier**'. Prescriber number 8 has used vancomycin in a manner that is entirely inconsistent with his or her peers, and this may be a **red flag** for Dorothy to think about talking to that person to find out why they have used vancomycin more often than the other prescribers in her sample. Simply glancing at (or 'eyeballing') the data without actually mathematically or statistically analysing it, she can see that seven of the eight prescribers are all in a narrow range in terms of frequency of prescribing.

10.3.1. Beware of Drawing Premature Conclusions

At this point, it may be tempting for Dorothy to immediately conclude something is 'wrong' with Prescriber 8 and that everyone else is 'fine'. Drawing these kinds of inferences or conclusions from this kind of data may lead to errors. These data in isolation tell us nothing about the nature of the patients for whom vancomycin was prescribed. Perhaps Prescriber 8 has a unique type of practice with specific patients who in fact do need vancomycin. Perhaps Prescriber 8 is an infectious diseases specialist, while prescribers 1–7 are generalists with few cases of infectious disease in their practice.

You see, at this point we have no other information about the patients receiving vancomycin. Specifically, we have no idea what percentage of patients within that prescriber's regular practice received vancomycin. Perhaps prescribers 1–4 only work clinically part time and see relatively few patients. For them 6, 7, or 8 incidences of prescribing vancomycin, when they have only seen 10–12 patients over the course of the study period represents a very high percentage of their patients receiving this medication. On the other hand, perhaps Prescriber 8 has an exceptionally busy practice and, over this same time period saw hundreds of patients: in this case, his/her frequency of prescribing vancomycin is actually relatively lower than the rest of the peer group.

10.3.2. Setting Descriptive Statistics in Context

Clearly, the numbers by themselves cannot allow Dorothy to draw any inferences or conclusions about the appropriateness of vancomycin prescribing. She will need other pieces of information to put these numbers into context; for example, the number of patients seen during the time period, and the nature of the prescriber's practice. Recognising that simply adding up the numbers without this information helps Dorothy realise her initial question may not have been the clearest or most helpful one to pursue if her goal is to assess appropriateness of vancomycin prescribing. As a result she reframes her question and this time undertakes a **retrospective chart audit** to identify the percentage of patients receiving an antibiotic prescription who were prescribed vancomycin. In other words she looks back over patients' medicines charts and records the number of patients who (a) were treated with an antimicrobial drug and (b) were prescribed vancomycin. The results of this audit are shown in the text box below.

RETROSPECTIVE CHART AUDIT

Prescriber #	% Of Patients Receiving Antibiotic Prescription Who Received Vancomycin
1	10
2	50
3	15
4	75
5	20
6	25
7	35
8	25

This revised research question is significantly more complicated to answer, but is also significantly more valuable from a research perspective. To answer this question, Dorothy's chart audit will become far more complicated than her first attempt. She will need to locate and identify all occurrences of antibiotic prescriptions for each prescriber, then from this subset of all prescriptions reviewed, will have to create another subset (or sub-subset) of vancomycin prescriptions.

Because she has specified percentage frequency as her measurement Dorothy is dealing with a ratio; as a result, she needs to also calculate the total number of all prescriptions written for antibiotics during the study period for each prescriber. This can be a time-consuming task but fortunately for Dorothy, her hospital uses computerised prescriber order entry (or CPOE) so these data can be readily retrieved.

10.3.3. Re-Examine Your Data

As Dorothy examines her data this time, it is clear that Prescriber 8 is no longer the outlier, and the range (or 'spread') is much broader than in her first attempt. If Dorothy had satisfied herself after her first attempt, her antimicrobial stewardship efforts may have focussed on the wrong target (Prescriber 8). Now, she has much more work to do to determine what – if any – problem actually exists with vancomycin prescribing.

With her new data set, Dorothy's first task is to generate descriptive statistics that are focussed on central tendency. In everyday conversation, we often use the word 'average' when we discuss central tendency involving multiple data points. Importantly, 'averages' are not always or necessarily the same thing as central tendency. Understanding the different conceptions of central tendency allows you to select

the most appropriate one to use when analysing your data. Now is a good time to have a look at the three most useful descriptive statistics that we mentioned earlier.

10.3.3.1. Mean

The mean is the most frequently used form of central tendency calculation, and is (in most cases) what we mean when we say 'average'. It is calculated as the total sum of all numbers in the data set, divided by the total number of data points. For example, in Dorothy's first study, the mean is 11.38; in her second study the mean is 31.88. Note that the unit measurement that is reported in the mean is the same as the unit measurement of the numerator.

10.3.3.2. Median

The median is the middle value of a data set. To find the median, we simply re-order the table that was produced in the study, from lowest-to-highest and select the middle value. If there is an odd number of values in the data set, it is a straightforward matter to identify the median as there is (literally) a mid-point in the table between the lowest and the highest values. It is somewhat more complex if there is an even number of values in the data set. While statisticians continue to debate this point, most researchers agree that in the event of an even number of observations or data points, the two middle numbers are selected and a mathematical average (or mean) of those numbers is used to calculate the median.

10.3.3.3. Mode

The mode is the most frequently occurring number in the data set, that is, the number that is repeated most often in the measurement or observation. Unlike the mean and (in the event of an even number of data points, the median), the mode is not mathematically calculated; instead, it is simply derived from an observation of the data set in its entirety.

Why are there so many ways of describing central tendency, and why can't the commonly understood concept of 'average' be used instead? Measures of central tendency have evolved in this way to recognise that data can be complex and overly simplistic interpretations can lead to errors in judgment and decision-making.

10.3.4. When to Use Means or Medians, and Understanding Bimodality

A key issue with respect to data relates to the influence of outliers. In both of Dorothy's studies, there were participants whose data were misaligned with the rest of the group. How do we know they were misaligned? A superficial review of the numbers from her first study illustrates that Prescriber

8 reported prescribing vancomycin roughly six times as frequently as anyone else in the study. In a situation like this, even a statistically untrained eye can identify this discrepancy. In less conspicuous cases, it is necessary to use descriptive statistical tests of variability to help us to establish the magnitude and importance of such discrepancies.

Because the mean is simply a mathematical operation involving addition of all data, it will be pulled in the direction of an exceptionally high – or low – data point. A positively **skewed** distribution (Fig. 10.1) is one in which the value of the mean is larger than the median. For this reason the median would be more commonly used when data are skewed, and we will explain this using the examples below. The term 'positive' here does not imply any sort of ethical value or moral judgment placed on this finding. It is simply an indication of the direction of the skew and could just as easily be described as a 'rightward' skew.

A 'negative' or leftward skew (Fig. 10.2) is one in which the value of the mean is less than the median, again reflecting how one extreme case can have a disproportionate effect on the mean.

Consider, for example, the situation if Bill Gates were to move into your neighbourhood. The legendary business man is renowned for living a very modest lifestyle, driving his own very average car and owning a typical suburban home, despite being one of the five wealthiest people on the planet. If he were to move into a typical suburban neighbourhood and a statistician wanted to calculate average household wealth … there would most definitely be a strong positive or rightward skew to the data. The combined household wealth of you and all your neighbours would come nowhere near to a fraction of his wealth, so the 'mean' calculated from such a study would be quite meaningless. Determining whether mean or median is the most appropriate measure of central tendency is essential, and requires you to actually understand the subtle qualitative dynamics of the phenomenon you are examining.

In other circumstances, neither mean nor median may actually be an appropriate way of describing central tendency. Consider the plight of politicians trying to make decisions on highly controversial or contentious social issues such as assisted suicide or abortion-on-demand. Such issues are typically quite polarising: most people already have a well-formed opinion on the issue and in most cases this opinion is quite strong. If you were to do a survey and asked the question '*Do you support health-professional assisted suicide for those with incurable diseases who are mentally competent and have chosen to end their own lives?*' and used a scale of Strongly Agree/Agree/Neutral/Disagree/Strongly Disagree (or a 1–10 scale in which 10 = strongly agree) there is a strong likelihood you would end up with a mean that suggested the study group was 'neutral' on the issue. This is because the majority of responders would either strongly agree OR strongly disagree and consequently counterweight one another in any mathematical calculation of an average. This is called a '**bimodal**' distribution.

Bimodal distributions create unique problems for our politicians as this means there is no societal consensus for how to proceed AND there are strong opinions on both sides which means there is no clear, easy 'win' in terms of a solution: a classic 'damned if you do, damned if you don't' situation. Fortunately, for statisticians, it is a bit easier to manage: bimodal distributions are simply a representation of data in which two non-adjacent categories (e.g. Agree and Disagree) have roughly the same number of responses. Where data splits bi-modally, it is generally best practice to present central tendencies of each mode separately, and not try to lump all the data together in a meaningless 'average' (Fig. 10.3).

10.3.5.   Measures of Variance

As described previously, central tendency is only one aspect of descriptive statistics, and consequently only one piece of a jigsaw puzzle. Measuring and reporting variation within the study group is as important to understanding the big picture. There are a variety of different techniques used, each of which conveys a certain kind of information.

10.3.5.1.   Standard Deviation

The most commonly used measure of variability is the standard deviation: the standard deviation is, in essence, a

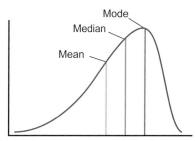

FIGURE 10.1 Positively skewed distribution.

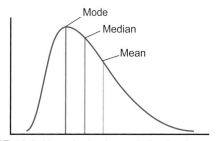

FIGURE 10.2 Negatively skewed distribution.

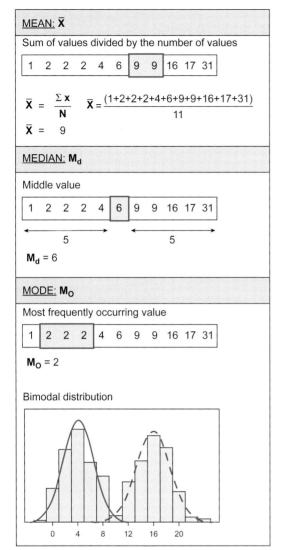

FIGURE 10.3 Calculation of central tendencies: mean, median, mode.

This provides a mechanism for understanding the spread or dispersion of data away from the mean. Why does this matter? Understanding the relative or relational position of your data points in comparison to one another can provide insights into the group as a whole, and can help us to consider the impact of outliers on our calculation of means. Simply reporting a mean value without reporting a standard deviation does not allow readers to understand the spread of values and how this may impact upon interpretation of results.

10.3.5.2. Range

Closely aligned with the notion of standard deviation is the importance of reporting the range. The range is a descriptive statistic that isolates the highest and the lowest (top and bottom) numbers within a data set, and provides another mechanism for understanding the spread of data. A tightly clustered range in which there is little difference between the top and bottom numbers suggests uniformity or **homogeneity**, while a broad spread of data suggests much greater **heterogeneity**. Strictly speaking, the range is calculated as range = highest value – lowest value +1. Since the range can be altered drastically by outliers or one exceptionally high/low value, it is not by itself a good summary measure for most purposes. Increasingly there is a tendency in health services research to move away from the statistical calculation of range described above and instead simply present the highest value AND the lowest value as two different numbers and call this presentation 'range'.

> There is some debate as to how this is calculated. Taking the high score minus the low score, plus one (1) this is an inclusive measure of range, rather than a measure of the difference between two scores. For example: the inclusive range for data ranging from 6 to 10 would be 5. Exclusive range would be just the different between high point and low point. Inclusive is used for whole numbers as it gives the size of the range – inclusive of the high and low points. 'Inclusive' is the most common method of calculating range but different statistics texts vary.

mathematical representation of the mean distance of individual data points from the mean.

> The Standard Deviation is a measure of how spread out our numbers are and is calculated by taking the square root of the variance. If you follow this link you will find more information about this: http://www.mathsisfun.com/data/standard-deviation.html

One way of addressing the problems created by outliers is to calculate **interquartile** ranges, which help us to understand the range within which most of the measurements lie. Quartiles are points in the distribution that correspond to the first 25%, 50%, 75% and 100% of measurements. The 2nd quartile (50%) is another name for the median. Presenting data in quartiles is a way of ensuring that outliers do not disproportionately influence reporting, particularly in observations where a high degree of variance exists. For example, in the reporting of annual income for a country, a few high-wealth individuals would clearly skew the mean; there may not be enough of them to warrant a bimodal distribution analysis, and yet there is a distributive justice issue in knowing how much the top quartile (or decile, or percentile) makes compared to the rest. Interquartile (or interdecile or interpercentile) range reporting can help address this issue.

Within descriptive statistics, there is an adage that 'a statistician once drowned in a river that was – on average – 2 feet deep'. As the example above illustrates, an average

(be it mean, median or mode) cannot tell us the whole story: we need to consider the range of values and the standard deviation of results to get a true picture (or description) of what we are looking at. Had that mythical statistician known that the mean depth of the river was 2 feet, with a range of 1 inch to 100 feet and a standard deviation of 10.2 feet, perhaps he/she would have reconsidered such a perilous journey! Similarly, if you are considering implementation of a new clinical service for pharmacists (like initial prescribing of antibiotics for strep throat) and are building your case for it on a foundation that includes previous positive

---

PRACTICE EXAMPLE

Let's say you were interested in understanding GPs' readiness to accept pharmacists in the role of primary independent prescribers of antibiotics for **strep throat** infections. You may believe that this is a relatively routine task that can be undertaken using a protocol or algorithm. A possible algorithm is shown below:

- Interview with a patient to obtain a careful medical and medication history
- Identification and assessment of current signs and symptoms
- The pharmacist may take a throat swab and assess whether initial empiric therapy is warranted or not
- If a swab is taken then follow-up based on the results of the swab itself, without involvement of or approval from a physician

You also acknowledge that this role for pharmacists may be controversial, particularly amongst GPs who may believe pharmacists are not qualified or ready for this kind of role on a routine basis without some sort of advanced credential or education. You are also astute enough to recognise that physician resistance may delay or prevent implementation of this new service, so you are interested in gauging what they think.

A simple survey could be developed and distributed to GPs to gather information about:

- medical practices
- experiences of working with pharmacists
- opinions and beliefs about pharmacists' expanding scope of practice.

Let's say that one of the questions asked GPs to report '*how often in a typical week do you seek advice from a pharmacist about a prescribing decision related to one of your patients?*' If 100 GPs responded, and a **descriptive statistical analysis** was undertaken, the response may be 'the mean weekly **frequency** was 8.5 consultations.' Further, if you calculated the median and the mode, and

they were 8 and 9 respectively, you may be tempted to conclude that this represents a reasonable amount of interaction amongst physicians and pharmacists to establish mutual respect for roles and capabilities.

However, if you were to report the **range** of responses, and discovered it ran from 0 times/week to 41 times/week, you may then assume that there are some GPs who clearly are very or almost entirely dependent on pharmacists, and some who have no contact or interaction with them and, as a result, your understanding of the situation may change. Rather than concluding that GPs (as a group) have a reasonable amount of weekly interaction with pharmacists (as a group), the range statistics helps to highlight that the group averages do not necessarily accurately reflect individual GPs' and pharmacists' experiences. Further, if you were to calculate the **standard deviation** from these data and discover that it was 7.5, that would further cloud your understanding of the issue. If mean weekly frequency of consultation was 8.5 +/- 7.5, with a range of 0–41, it would suggest that the **mean**, **median** and **mode** by themselves do not tell the full story. It would suggest instead that there is an extraordinarily wide spread of experiences within the study group; even though mathematically it 'averaged' out to a specific number, the dispersion of data points in this study would suggest you would need to exercise extreme caution in assuming that your data meant GPs have regular interactions with pharmacists. Instead, all you may be able to conclude from these data is that some do and some don't. Here is a good example of not taking the numbers on face value and finding different ways of looking at them until you are sure you have the whole picture. This would also be a good time to start asking yourself why some GPs work together with pharmacists and some don't. In Part III of this textbook we will look at how qualitative methods can help us answer some of the '**why**?' questions.

GP-pharmacist interactions, getting the whole picture (not just an average result) will be important.

10.4. VISUAL REPRESENTATIONS OF DATA AND HOW TO USE THEM

One of the most important ways researchers have of communicating with their diverse audiences is through the reporting of findings. While readers of your work will have legitimate interests in your questions and methods, they are initially drawn to your research because they want to know what you have discovered or learned in your study. The way in which data are presented is a crucial choice for researchers so outputs should be presented in a way that is clear, accurate, and concise. Overly wordy paragraphs or tables unnecessarily cluttered with raw data can cause your readers to become disinterested in your work. The presentation of your data can be as important as the data themselves. Visual formats for data presentation can display a lot of information that can be quickly understood by readers, and should be used wherever possible. In the Further Reading section of this chapter you will find some examples of research reports and how the data have been represented.

10.4.1. Tables

Tables are simply structured formats that allow you to present summarised information in a clear manner. Rather than presenting blocks of explanatory text, tables allow 'the numbers to speak for themselves'. Consider the following example, building upon the case discussed above around implementation of a new pharmacy service. This focussed on independent prescribing of antibiotics for suspected or confirmed strep throat infections. If you had asked survey questions about previous collaborative experiences with pharmacists, and **stratified** your responders based on frequency of interaction into three separate cohorts ('no interaction', 'low interaction' and 'high interaction') you may find a different pattern of results than simply reporting the overall respondent pool mean/mode/median.

You may have defined 'no interaction' as literally 0 consultations/week, 'low interaction' as 1–4 interactions/week, and 'high interactions' as 5+/interactions/week. Based on this categorisation, you could then calculate that, of the 100 respondents, 40% were in the 'no interaction' group, 25% were in the 'low interaction' group, and 35% were in the 'high interaction' group. Within each of those groups, you could calculate and report means, ranges and standard deviations, to allow the reader to then better understand how different types of pharmacist–GP interaction are occurring in primary care practice.

Did reading that previous paragraph simply exhaust you? Frankly, it was exhausting to write! It would be far easier to concisely present a table (Table 10.1).

Presenting the data from this study in this format (see Table 10.1) is so much easier to make sense of. Key attributes of an effective table include the following:

a. Sequentially numbering your tables to correspond to a citation in your text. By convention 'Tables' are different from 'Figures' (which are typically graphs or other non-tabular forms of visual depiction)

b. A clear and coherent title that relates to the content of the table as well as the corresponding text

c. An indication of the size of the study sample (in this case 'n=100') to remind readers of the size of the respondent pool

d. Clarification of any bespoke definitions you have created (in this case, the definitions of no/low/high collaboration are included in the table itself)

e. Specification of units of measurement (in this case, indicated by an asterisk (*) to indicate 'times/week' to save having to re-write this each time in each cell of the table)

f. Reporting of all relevant data in one table (in this case, reporting mean, range and standard deviation all together rather than in separate tables or partially in a table and partially in the text)

g. Taking care to not produce an all-in-one table in which all data you collect and report are provided to the reader in one enormous table. While this may be tempting in

TABLE 10.1	Weekly Frequency of Pharmacist–GP Consultation (n=100)		
	No Interaction Cohort (0 Interactions/Week)	Low Interaction Cohort (1-4 Interactions/Week)	High Interaction Cohort (>/=5 Interactions/Week)
Proportion	40%	25%	35%
Mean no. of interactions	0	2.2	8.6
Range*	0	1–4	5–41
Standard Deviation*	0	0.6	3.2

*times/week.

the name of brevity and to allow for convenient cross-tabular comparison, there is a limit to what readers can digest in a tabular format. While there is no specific rule as to how much information should be presented in a single table, use your judgment to decide when a new table is warranted

h. Consider what should be put into a table versus what should be put into another format (charts, graphs, or text). Generally speaking simple lists of frequency and percentage can be effectively presented in a table. Tables are useful for condensing and summarising large amounts of data, and to illustrate findings from descriptive (or inferential) statistics (more in Chapter 11).

10.4.2.   Charts and Graphs

It is sometimes said that a picture is worth a thousand words. In the case of charts and graphs, this can be very true, as they can eliminate the need to write complicated and boring sentences. As with tables, however, exercise caution – too many charts and graphs can also become overwhelming for a reader. Charts and graphs can be a more effective way of communicating to help readers understand 'the big picture'. In the examples below we present the pharmacist–GP data in a different ways:

1. Frequency polygon/line graph

One of the most common types of graph is the frequency polygon or 'line graph' in which a single line joins frequency points of occurrence to provide a 'moving picture' of a process. Most typically, the y-axis will depict the frequency of items or events, while the x-axis indicates the specific item being studied (Fig. 10.4).

2. Histogram/bar graph

The histogram (or bar graph) is somewhat similar to the frequency polygon, except it is formed by drawing vertical bars at each frequency across the entire width of the measurement. With histograms it is also possible to use visual methods to indicate ranges when categories are presented, which can be an advantage over frequency polygons. Strictly speaking, Bar Charts are graphics for qualitative variables (such as 'strongly agree/agree/disagree/strongly disagree') in which the response is displayed with solid bars separated by spaces. A histogram is a graphic for quantitative variables (such as frequency distributions) in which the response is displayed using adjacent bars with no spaces, to emphasise continuity between each variable (Fig. 10.5).

3. Pie charts

The pie chart provides an alternative method for presenting data that is particularly well suited to situations where the reader is interested in proportions or 'shares' Metaphorically, the pie chart is built on the assumption that the size of the 'pie' itself is fixed so we are interested in who or what consumes how much pie.

There are many more ways of depicting data and you will find more examples in the Further Reading list at the end of this chapter.

In general, graphs and charts of the sort noted above should be labelled as 'Figures' rather than 'Tables', 'Graphs' or 'Charts'. In the text that refers your readers to these figures, signpost salient highlights. As with tables, accurate and complete titles, axes labels, explanatory footnotes and clarity in presentation are essential.

10.4.3.   Units and Scaling

While visual depiction of quantitative data can be both powerful and emotionally resonant for readers, it also opens up potential opportunities to introduce researcher bias or inadvertently (or deliberately) mislead readers about the importance of a finding. For example, this can be done through scaling of units on the 'y' axis of a frequency polygon

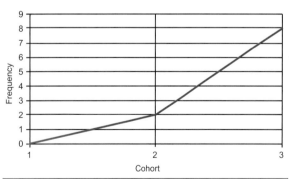

Cohort	No Interaction Cohort	Low Interaction Cohort	High Interaction Cohort
Frequency	0	2	8

FIGURE 10.4 Weekly Frequency of Pharmacist-GP Consultation (n = 100) %

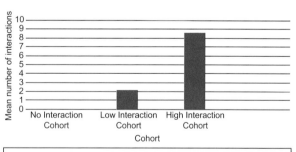

Cohort	No Interaction Cohort	Low Interaction Cohort	High Interaction Cohort
Mean number of interactions	0	2.2	8.6

FIGURE 10.5 Weekly Frequency of Pharmacist-GP Consultation (n = 100)

in such a way as to emphasise the slope of the line (see Chapter 9) and make the findings appear more pronounced. Consider the following example.

Let's say you are interested in understanding the public's perception of pharmacists as you have heard that, in the past at least, pharmacists are the 'most trusted professional' in the view of the public. Here are the data you have retrieved from the last 5 years:

Question:

I trust my pharmacist to look out for my best interests and take care of me   Yes [ ] No [ ] Not Sure [ ]

2010:   85% Yes
2011:   86% Yes
2012:   84% Yes
2013:   83% Yes
2014:   82% Yes
2015:   81% Yes

This year, when you ask that same question, the response is 79% yes. Take a look at the following two frequency polygons visually depicting 7 years of responses to this question.

These are the same data presented using the same reporting mechanism (a line graph), but they visually appear quite different. As you will note the units of measurement on the 'y' axis for each graph is '% saying YES'. But note how different the slope of each of these graphs is when the units of measurement on the y axis are changed. You can create an apparently much steeper slope on the line graph by only focussing on the units of measurement between 75% and 90%. However if you scale the y axis from 0 to 100, the slope decrease is almost imperceptible. A person examining one graph (a) may conclude there has been a precipitous drop in public support of pharmacists. On the other hand a person examining the other graph (b) may conclude there is no meaningful or discernible difference in public opinions about pharmacists over the past 7 years.

As this example illustrates, it is important to pay careful attention to the way in which charts and graphs are drawn so as not to provoke unnecessary or inaccurate emotional responses to the data you are presenting.

10.5.   HOW NOT TO USE DESCRIPTIVE STATISTICS?

Descriptive statistics are a critical way of understanding quantitative data. As the name implies, they help to describe our study group in a way that facilitates further understanding and generation of additional questions. Descriptive statistics can be deceptively easy to calculate and use, but as illustrated above, caution must be exercised in simply reporting means, or overlooking bimodal or skewed distributions. When used in a routine or unthinking way, descriptive

statistics can hide many important and interesting issues and can gloss over major themes requiring further exploration. When using descriptive statistics, it is essential the researcher understands his/her objectives and uses descriptive statistical analysis appropriately. Blindly calculating means, not reporting standard deviations, or distorting the slope of a line graph (frequency polygon) through an inappropriately scaled y-axis are just a few examples of how descriptive statistics can be misused.

In other cases, researchers may overemphasise the importance of their work and try to draw generalisable inferences from descriptive statistics. This is an inappropriate application of statistical analysis because descriptive statistics do not allow us to generalise in this way (see Chapter 11 on inferential statistics for further details about this). Recognising the strengths and limitations of descriptive statistics is important, and not inappropriately amplifying your findings is essential.

Descriptive statistics are an essential part of quantitative research and reporting. They are usually our first opportunity to understand the group or process we are studying. In almost all cases, you will be calculating and reporting descriptive statistical analyses of your work so readers have the foundation for any further inferential statistical analysis you may undertake. A solid understanding of how descriptive statistics work, their limits, and how to apply different analyses in different situations depending upon your research context is critical to further statistical interpretation.

Case Study Example

Throughout Parts I and II of this textbook, to illustrate how quantitative research methods can be used, we have followed some of our case study students and pharmacists. We will now summarise what Sandy has done so far in his research and give you an example of how he might report his descriptive data. At the end of Chapter 11 we will catch up with him again and see what he thinks about using inferential statistics!

In Chapter 1 we introduced Sandy and his role as a pharmacist working in a GP practice. Sandy has a special interest in patients with type II diabetes and had noticed that the blood sugar control of some of his younger patients wasn't as good as it should be. Sandy thought that he needed more information about the blood glucose control of his patients and if he found there was a problem he might be able to design an intervention to help patients have better control over their blood glucose in the future. If, on the other hand, what he had noticed was just by chance then at least he had investigated things properly. For example, Sandy could look at whether the blood sugar of his younger patients is being controlled over time. He could ask his younger patients to keep a record of two blood glucose readings a day over 6 months and find out what percentage of them met their target blood sugar. See Table 10.3 for NIHCE recommended target blood glucose for people with type II diabetes. Before we look at how Sandy might do this, let's continue with our recap.

In Chapter 2, we followed Sandy as he grappled with the research question he should ask in order to get the answers that would help him (and others) in his practice. There we showed you how the theory underpinning how to do research can inform the perspective from which we view our chosen research topic. If Sandy just assumed that the fact that he had noticed poor blood sugar control in a few patients meant that it was true of all patients, then any intervention he made would not necessarily be accurate. Sandy needed some hard evidence that young people are really not controlling their blood glucose and then try to find out why. In Section 2.5.3 we gave you some examples of the different perspectives Sandy might take. In Section 2.7.1 we left Sandy thinking through this research situation not only from his own perspective but from the patients' perspective too and developed the research question: '**How do my patients feel about their diagnosis of diabetes and the need for consistent blood sugar control?**' Sandy feels content with this question as a starting point and can now embark on his own clarifying process to further refine and narrow the question.

In Chapter 3 Sandy explored some of the levels of measurement he might use and in Chapter 4 he focussed on how quantitative methods could be of most use to him at the early stages of his research. He thought through his choice of study sample, how to collect his data (through questionnaires) and what characteristics about his potential participants he might want to look at. In Chapter 6 Sandy looked at the actual measurement of blood sugar and how valid and reliable such measures are and in Chapter 6 he took a break to think all this through.

When we re-joined Sandy in Chapter 7 he had got as far as thinking through some of the sampling issues he needed to consider and choosing his participants. He was particularly keen to have a clear research objective that helped him define his research population. In Chapter 8 Sandy grappled with the whole issue of experimental design including how far he would be able to generalise his research findings across a wider population. In Chapter 9 Sandy did some initial background work on which would be the best statistics to use to analyse and make sense of his data and now in Chapter 10 we join him again as he works through his descriptive data and decides how best to present these in a meaningful and engaging way.

In the box below you will find a summary of the information Sandy has collected.

- Patient Identifier (this is in numeric form in the order Sandy has their details on to the database e.g. patient 1, 2, 3...)
- Age
- Sex
- Work status (School or university or employed)
- Family history of diabetes
- Weight
- Height
- Date of diagnosis
- Blood glucose (there will be more than one entry for each patient)

In reality, Sandy may have collected data on other things about his participants, but we have kept this to the minimum so that we can give examples about how he might make sense of his data.

Remember Sandy's target population is '*male and female patients between the ages of 16 and 25 with a diagnosis of Type 2 diabetes*'. In order to compare this group to others with type II diabetes in his practice, he has identified 298 patients in total who have been diagnosed with the condition and at this point he will concentrate on the ones in his target group. Sandy has sent all of these patients a questionnaire and asked for their age, sex and work status (school or university or employed), he has also asked the patients to enter a record of their daily blood glucose for 1 month. He has asked all of them to complete the questionnaire so that later he will have the opportunity to compare younger patients with those in older age groups to identify any similarities and differences.

From the patients' medical records Sandy has family history of diabetes, weight, height, and date of diagnosis. All of this information has been entered into a spreadsheet that Sandy has designed especially for this study.

Let's say for argument's sake that Sandy has a really high response rate and 250 patients have returned completed questionnaires! This almost never happens in real life but here we can dream! Table 10.2 is an example of what a sample of the data might look like on a database.

We have assumed for argument's sake that each participant has been asked to keep a record of two blood glucose readings a day. The columns on the right are the spaces for the blood glucose readings. Table 10.3 shows the recommended target blood glucose levels for people with type II diabetes.

Diabetes UK suggests that for the majority of healthy individuals, normal blood sugar levels are as follows:

- **Between** 4.0 and 6.0 mmol/L (72 to 108 mg/dL) when fasting
- **Up to** 7.8 mmol/L (140 mg/dL) 2 hours after eating.

TABLE 10.2   Example of the Target Group on Sandy's Database (Without Data)

ID	Age	Sex	Work Status	FH	Weight	Body Mass Index (BMI)	Date of Diagnosis	Day1 BG1	Day1 BG2
1	17	m	school	Yes					
2	16	f	school	No					
3	22	f	uni	No					
4	19	m	work	No					
5	25	m	work	No					
6	19	m	unemp	No					
7	18	m	school	Yes					
8	24	f	school	Yes					
9	21	f	work	Yes					
10	20	f	uni	Yes					
11	18	m	work	No					

TABLE 10.3   NIHCE Recommended Target Blood Glucose Ranges

Target Levels by Type	Before Meals (Pre Prandial)	At Least 90 Minutes After Meals (Post Prandial)
Non-diabetic*	4.0–5.9 mmol/L	under 7.8 mmol/L
Type II diabetes	4–7 mmol/L	under 8.5 mmol/L

*The non-diabetic figures are provided for information but are not part of NIHCE guidelines.

Source: http://www.diabetes.co.uk/diabetes_care/blood-sugar-level-ranges.html

For people with diabetes, blood sugar level targets are as follows:
- **Before meals**: 4 to 7 mmol/L for people with type II diabetes
- **After meals**: under 8.5 mmol/L for people with type II diabetes.

We have used these numbers to 'make up' some readings for our first 11 participants (Table 10.4). This is just for one set of readings. Please remember these are to show you how Sandy might use descriptive statistics to explore the data he has collected and may not be exactly as everyone might expect to see.

In the two columns to the right A = blood glucose before meals and B = blood glucose after meals. All readings indicate mmols of glucose per litre of blood (mmols/L). See Chapter 8 for more about the measurement of blood glucose.

The aim of the first part of Sandy's study is to find out if his initial thoughts that the younger people with type II diabetes seem to be having difficulty controlling their blood glucose are borne out by the evidence.

Let's have a look at this small set of data and see what it might be telling us. In Section 10.3 we talked about 'eyeballing' the data to see if anything leapt out at us from the page. We are sure you have already noticed that there is one set of figures that stands out from the rest. This is participant number 9, whose blood glucose looks a little high and might be regarded as an outlier (a number quite different from the rest). This participant is a 21-year-old female with a family history of type II diabetes; however, let's not jump to any premature conclusions based on the results from just one person (see Section 10.3.1). If we have another look we can see that the blood sugar readings of participants 3 and 4 are a little higher than we might expect and these participants are age 22 and 19 respectively. The final thing to note is the readings for participant number 5, a 13-year-old male, whose blood glucose looks a bit low compared to the others. However, we must be sure of our facts and need to carefully interpret all of our data after thorough examination – maybe more than once. Sandy could also ask colleagues to have a look at his preliminary ideas about what the data are telling him.

You will also notice that we have added some figures for body mass index (BMI). Although there is some controversy over the use of BMI as a proxy measure for a healthy weight, it is widely used. You will find some further reading about BMI compared to other representations of weight at the end of this chapter.

The next steps for Sandy would be as follows:
- Look at means for blood sugar for each participant over the whole 6 months to see if any patterns emerge that might indicate particular times, days or weeks that might reveal changes in blood glucose.
- Look at the standard deviations to try to understand spread or dispersion of data away from the mean. This will help Sandy to see whether the blood glucose levels

TABLE 10.4   Example of Sandy's Database (With Data)

ID	Age	Sex	Work Status	FH	Weight	Body Mass Index (BMI)	Date of Diagnosis	DAY1 BG1 A	DAY1 BG1 B	DAY1 BG2 A	DAY1 BG2 B
1	17	m	school	Yes		25		4.2	7.4		
2	16	f	school	No		28		5.6	8.4		
3	22	f	uni	No		19		7.9	9.2		
4	19	m	work	No		29		6.2	9.3		
5	25	m	work	No		15		3.6	5.4		
6	19	m	unemp	No		33		6.0	8.7		
7	18	m	school	Yes		31		5.4	8.0		
8	24	f	school	Yes		22		4.1	7.1		
9	21	f	work	Yes		35		9.3	11.4		
10	20	f	uni	Yes		19		7.6	9.3		
11	18	m	work	No		26		7.2	9.9		

of his sample deviate from the values that would be expected in the population.

- Look at the range of scores to identify the highest and the lowest – this can help Sandy to see what the pattern of blood glucose levels is amongst his sample and he can compare those too with a wider population of people with diabetes type II in the UK.
- Later on, Sandy might be able to compare BMI with target blood glucose to see if being overweight is related to high blood sugar (see Chapter 11).

Finally, Sandy needs to think about how he might present the data from his study. As an example, Table 10.5 presents the data clearly and provides a column showing the means, standard deviations and range of scores for the set of readings above. We have included a column for the second set of readings so that you can see how Sandy might present these data. Ultimately, Sandy is interested in educating young people about the risks of diabetes, so in Chapter 11 we will explore how inferential statistics might provide him with the evidence to continue with his intervention and develop such a training package.

TABLE 10.5   Means, Standard Deviations, Ranges

	BLOOD GLUCOSE DAY 1 BEFORE AND AFTER BREAKFAST Reading A	Reading B	BLOOD GLUCOSE DAY 1 BEFORE AND AFTER DINNER Reading A	Reading B
Mean	6.1	8.6	XX	XX
Standard Deviation	1.69	1.59	XX	XX
Range	3.6–9.3	5.4–11.4	XX	XX

N.B. Reading A = before meal; reading B = after meal.

CHAPTER SUMMARY

- This chapter focusses on descriptive statistics and how they might be used.
- It describes some of the mostly commonly used calculations.
- It provides detailed information about how to depict descriptive statistics.
- It uses the example of Sandy's research to explain these.

FURTHER READING

Body Weight Calculators
http://www.thecalculatorsite.com/articles/health/alternatives-to-bmi.php.

Descriptive Statistics
Holcombe, Z. C. (2017). *Fundamentals of Descriptive Statistics.* Abingdon, UK: Routledge.

Inferential Statistics

After reading this chapter you should be able to:
- understand the difference between descriptive and inferential statistics
- describe the difference between parametric and non-parametric data
- understand how and when to use specific statistical tests
- call on others for help when you need expert advice

11.1   INTRODUCTION

Arguably, the essence of statistical analysis is use of inferential methods. Descriptive statistics (covered in Chapter 10) are generally straightforward and easy to calculate, present and interpret. While descriptive statistics are the foundation for any statistical analysis, they do not allow us to discover the properties or patterns within the data that are of relevance to researchers or participants trying to draw conclusions or make predictions. Inferential statistics are complicated and in some cases may generate competing interpretations or produce paradoxical outcomes. It is this complexity and the ability to draw conclusions that make inferential statistics so powerful – and an important tool for health services researchers.

As discussed in Chapters 9 and 10, it is important for you as a researcher not to become overwhelmed by the numbers and formulae that will be presented in this chapter. Inferential statistics can be like a new and unfamiliar language, filled with nuances and complexities that can be difficult to interpret. For some, this may result in avoidance, while for others it may result in incorrect or ill-informed application to a specific situation. Indeed, inferential statistics can be mathematically, intellectually, and conceptually challenging, but this is not a reason to ignore or avoid using them. You don't need to be an expert or mathematician to use inferential statistics, but it is essential you reflect upon, acknowledge and accommodate your limitations. Worse than avoiding use of inferential statistics, is pretending to understand them and then misapplying them through your research. This chapter is not intended to turn you into a biostatistician or expert,

but rather to provide you with the context within which to understand the power and potential of inferential statistics in your work. If you are interested in learning more about the detailed mathematical calculations and formulae used for the statistical tests we will discuss below, there are several biostatistics texts in the Further Reading section that may be useful. For this chapter, we assume that you will not need to manually calculate any statistics that are discussed and instead that you will have access to software (such as SPSS) that will perform calculations for you. No software program, however, can make the decision for you as to which statistic is appropriate for your specific need. We hope the content of this chapter will provide you with the skills and confidence necessary to select and apply inferential statistics to support your research objectives.

11.2   WHAT ARE INFERENTIAL STATISTICS?

At their core, inferential statistics are tools for helping us to infer (or discover) some property or characteristic, or general pattern about a large group by first studying a much smaller group so that those results can then be generalised back to the larger group of interest. Inferential statistics help us to assess the strength or magnitude of relationships (associations) between **independent (or causal)** variables and **dependent (or effect)** variables. An example of this might be cigarette smoking as an independent variable, e.g. something that people do, and lung cancer as a dependent variable that is a possible outcome of smoking. See glossary for definitions of independent and dependent variables.

See Chapter 7, Section 5 if you would like to revise what you have learned about relationships between variables.

Why are inferential statistics so powerful and important? In large part it is because they are of incredible practical value, not just to researchers but to those who consume research. Inferential statistics can help us to understand whether our interventions actually work and allow us to determine the probability of success. The ability to generalise findings from a small and manageable subset of your population of interest to the larger population makes inferential statistics a most valuable tool for health services researchers. In short, inferential statistics can help us to determine not simply what could possibly happen, but what actually tends to happen in a situation, by allowing us to generalise more confidently from a sample to a population.

Inferential statistics should only be applied under the following circumstances:

- When you have a complete list of the members of your population of interest
- When you are able to draw a truly random sample from this population of interest
- When you have established that the size of your truly random sample is sufficient to allow you to draw inferences

While biostatisticians are able to manage data that does not, strictly speaking, meet all of the criteria listed above, these methods are complex and beyond the scope of this chapter.

11.3 STATISTICAL INFERENCE

The predictions we make about a sample population can form the basis of real-life practice changes, so we really need to get them right. Inference is a powerful tool, but it is important to recognise its limitations. At its worst and least statistically defensible, inference can be seen as a type of stereotyping. For example, if we were to observe a group of drunken hooligans and note that all those involved had a y-chromosome (most commonly present in males), it may be tempting to conclude that everyone with a y-chromosome behaves badly. Simply extending from your own observation to the general population is NOT statistical inference, it is biased stereotyping that unfortunately happens all too commonly.

What makes statistical inference powerful is the nature and size of the sample upon which the inference is based. When the sample is correctly structured and constituted (i.e. it is representative of the population of interest, it is truly randomised, and it is of sufficient size), statistical methods can be used to generalise to the broader population in a defensible and confident manner.

Individuals who are less well versed in statistical analysis may sometimes attempt to generalise and draw inferences when the sample itself is unrepresentative, non-random, or too small. They may attempt to take a personal experience with a few members of a group/population and assume this extends to all members of that group. This type of stereotyping leads to poor outcomes, biases and prejudices. Without a properly constituted and appropriately scaled sample, inferences are simply not possible.

11.4 PARAMETRIC AND NON-PARAMETRIC DATA

Recall from Chapter 3 that quantitative data collected in your study can be categorised in four different ways: nominal, ordinal, interval and ratio. Let's just recap those. Nominal data provide a way of quantifying non-numerical variables when each category of data is mutually exclusive. An example of nominal data may be 1=diagnosis of pregnancy and 2= no diagnosis of pregnancy. This is considered nominal data because one is either pregnant or not pregnant: there is no 'sort of pregnant' intermediate or hybrid category that is possible. **Nominal data** are sometimes referred to as 'discrete' rather than 'continuous' data. Despite having a number assigned to each category, the numerical value itself is meaningless so you cannot perform any mathematical operations with the numbers (e.g. you could not calculate an 'average' or 'mean' of pregnancy using the example above).

Ordinal data are numbers that are still discrete but they have meaning in a sequence or order. Key to the definition of ordinal data is the notion that the interval between categories or numbers is not actually known and therefore cannot be assumed to be equal. Numbers are still assigned to group, and these numbers can be placed in a meaningful sequence, but the numerical differences (for example) between 1st, 2nd and 3rd place in a contest are not known using ordinal data. Ordinal data are frequently misunderstood and can be presented in a manipulative way. For example, in determining who the 'best' runners at the Olympic Games are, it is conventional to give gold, silver and bronze medals. The absolute differences in time-to-race-completion between these three individuals may be vanishingly or infinitesimally small, and the order may be different tomorrow, or if the crowd had cheered more loudly. Most reasonable people would conclude the gold, silver and bronze winners were substantially interchangeable and all 'the best'. Still, in an ordinal ranking system, there is curious tenacity and power associated with such numerical rankings.

Interval data are also ordered in a logical sequence, with the key difference here (compared with ordinal data) being that the intervals between numbers are considered equal and represent real and quantifiable amounts. Unlike ordinal and nominal data, interval data are considered continuous as they represent a scale or a continuum. Despite their inherent limitations, IQ scores are considered a form of interval data as they represent fixed numerical gradations of increasing intelligence.

Ratio data are also a form of continuous data, with the key difference (compared with interval data) being that there is a meaningful zero point. The zero point in a ratio scale indicates a total absence of whatever is being measured. Ratio data can be conveniently mathematically manipulated. For example, consider a patient experiencing epicondylitis (or 'tennis elbow') who is taking naproxen 500 mg bid. At the start of her treatment, the range of motion in her right arm may have only been 25 degrees from horizontal; after 1 week of medication therapy, her range of motion has extended to 50 degrees from horizontal. Using ratio data, we can say that she now has twice the range of motion since she began therapy, thereby indicating improvement in her condition. Nominal and ordinal data are known as non-parametric data, while interval and ratio data are called parametric data. While descriptive statistics (see Chapter 10) can be used on both parametric and non-parametric data (the exception being that mean and standard deviation cannot be calculated on nominal data), different inferential statistical methods must be used for these different categories of data.

11.4.1 Why Do We Have to Use Different Methods for Different Types of Data?

Specific properties of the data (e.g. whether they are ordered, or the intervals between numbers are equal and meaningful) make it challenging to draw defensible inferences from the data itself. For this reason it is necessary to use different methods for different types of data. Some statistical tests are simply not powerful enough to cope with unordered or unequal data, while others are. Table 11.1 provides a summary of categories of data and which inferential tests are most appropriately applied.

In order to use parametric tests, several criteria must be established:

1. The sample must be representative of the target population, so that the variables being measured actually fall within the **normal distribution** for that population. This is simply a more mathematical way of saying that truly random selection has actually occurred.
2. Variables must have been measured in a way that generates interval or ratio data.
3. Participants in the two or more groups being studied must have the opportunity to actually be similar. This is simply a more mathematical way of saying that truly random assignment of individuals to treatment and control groups has occurred.

TABLE 11.1 Inferential Statistics Used Based on Type of Data Collected

Category of Data Collected	Classification of Data	Examples of Inferential Tests
Nominal data	Non-parametric	Fisher's exact Pearson's chi-square
Ordinal data	Non-parametric	Spearman rho Man–Whitney u Kruskal–Wallis
Interval data	Parametric	t-test Analysis of variance (ANOVA) Analysis of co-variance (ANCOVA)
Ratio data	Parametric	t-test Analysis of variance (ANOVA) Pearson product moment correlation

When any of these three conditions has not been established, then non-parametric statistics must be used:

1. If random selection has not occurred, so that the sample is not actually representative of the population of interest
2. If variables have been measured in a way that generates nominal or ordinal data
3. The number of participants in the sample is too small to have statistical power (see Chapter 7 for discussion of sample size calculations).

Non-parametric statistical tests will generally mean that substantial differences must be found between group scores in order to consider these differences meaningful. This does not mean these tests are less valuable or less important; it is simply the case that one must use the correct type of inferential test for the kind of data that have been collected.

11.5 DIFFERENT TYPES OF INFERENTIAL TESTS

An extensive array of inferential tests exists which are used depending on the nature of the sample and data you have collected. There is no need for or value in simply memorising lists of different tests and cases where they should be applied. Instead, it is more important to understand the principles that guide decision-making around which test to select: everything else can be looked up in a textbook on an as-needed basis. Most books dealing with statistics provide a decision table that guides you through the process (see the Further Reading section of this chapter). At the end of this chapter you will find an example of a decision tree and a description of how Sandy reached his conclusions about which tests to use.

Inferential statistics allow us to take results from a sample and decide whether (and how) likely they are to occur in the population as a whole and these can be broadly divided into three categories:

1. Tests that try to find if the **differences** observed between two sets of scores are significant
2. Tests that examine *two sets* of scores to establish the strength of association or **correlation** between them
3. Tests that compare *more than two sets* of scores to establish the **extent to which they vary** amongst each other.

Let's consider each of these in turn.

11.5.1 Tests for Significant Difference

One of the most common reasons for using inferential statistics is to establish whether a real – or significant – difference exists between two observations. Consider the case of Sandy, our pharmacist who is interested in educating young people about risks of diabetes. To achieve his objective, Sandy has developed a 90-minute interactive educational session. He has worked on this presentation, and to deliver it to his target group he will need to take time out of his busy schedule. Moreover, his audience – young people at risk of diabetes and their families – will also have to take time out of their busy schedules. If the session is useless, a lot of people will have wasted a lot of their time … and a very negative impression of pharmacists and their value may also be generated along the way. Before booking weekly educational sessions, Sandy is rightly concerned about this and wants to ensure there is a real- or significant – impact of his session on his audience.

In such a case, a pre- and post-test research design would be considered appropriate. Sandy would design a questionnaire or survey consisting of 10–15 straightforward multiple choice questions designed to assess a patient or family member's knowledge about diabetes risk factors and complications. It would be administered to each participant on two separate occasions: once, before taking the educational intervention, and once after the educational intervention has been completed. Comparing performance on the pre-test to the post-test for each participant, and for the group as a whole, Sandy can start to understand whether his educational programme actually made a difference.

If everyone scored 15/15 on the pre-test, then clearly there is no need for the session: his participants already know a lot about the subject! However, if the mean on the pre-test was 6.5/15 +/- 2.3, and the mean on the post-test

was 10.8/15 +/- 1.2, how should Sandy interpret these findings?

The first thing to recognise is that test scores such as this represent ratio data: equal intervals between numerical scores with a true zero point. As a result, parametric tests could be applied. Sandy wants to determine whether these test findings are significant. Significance testing is based on the laws of probability, and helps him to answer the question *'What is the likelihood that the change observed in the pre- and post-test scores occurred because of my educational intervention, and what is the likelihood that it may have occurred anyway, simply by chance?'* In any evaluation of the value of an intervention, it is essential to consider whether random chance may have produced the finding, rather than intervention itself. For example, if Sandy's participants took the pre-test several days before his educational session, and prior to the delivery of the session there was an interesting documentary on television about diabetes that many of them watched, this unpredicted or random event could conceivably have produced the improvements he detected in the post-test. Conversely, if some of the participants decided they wanted to cheat the second time around and looked at each other's answers on the post-test, this unpredicted or random event might have contributed to the improved post-test scores.

SUMMARY OF WHAT SANDY IS TRYING TO DO

- Sandy wants to find out if his educational intervention 'works'
- That means he is trying to establish whether education, e.g. knowing more about diabetes, improves blood sugar control
- Specifically his question is *'What is the likelihood that the change observed in the pre- and post-test scores occurred because of my educational intervention, and what is the likelihood that it may have occurred anyway, simply by chance?'*
- If participants' scores for the questionnaire completed after having the educational intervention are higher than the same questionnaire completed before, then it may be that Sandy's educational programme works
- BUT, whether or not the pre- and post-test scores are significantly different will largely depend on Sandy's sample size

---

In most health-services research, an arbitrary but widely accepted threshold of 5% is commonly used to determine the influence of random chance on an observed outcome. This is usually expressed as $p < 0.05$, meaning that one wants to be 95% certain that the improvement in post-test scores that Sandy observed were in fact due to his intervention and not due to random chance. In some cases, more stringent proof may be required, in which case the standard may be $p<0.01$, meaning 99% certainty that the intervention caused the observed outcome.

TYPE I AND TYPE II ERRORS

For most of the quantitative research we do we will have an hypothesis that states what the outcome of our research might be. For Sandy's research question in the text box above he might hypothesise that: 'a difference in the pre- and post-test scores will have occurred because of my educational intervention'. This would be written as shown below and we would indicate that this is our first hypothesis by putting the number 1 in superscript after the 'H' for hypothesis:

H^1 is that there will be a significant difference between the pre- and post-test scores.

Sandy could make a specific prediction that the difference in the scores will be greater post-test than pre-test. Saying that there will just be a difference leaves his options open to explore which way the difference goes, e.g. there may be a difference but the scores might be higher pre-test. This would be disappointing for Sandy because it would mean his educational programme had not increased his participants' knowledge – in fact it had decreased it!

We also have something called a null hypothesis, and this is more important in some respects than the hypothesis. This would be written like this:

H^0 is that there will be no significant difference between the two tests.

This means that Sandy would not be able to say with any confidence that the results might not have occurred by chance. The aim of all researchers is to be able to reject the null hypothesis.

A **Type I Error** happens when the null hypothesis is true but you reject it. Being able to reject the null hypothesis hinges on the level of significance you set for the hypothesis test. If you set a probability of 0.05 that means you are happy to accept a 5% chance that you are wrong when you reject your null hypothesis. You can lower this risk by lowering your probability but beware because lowering the probability means you may not detect a real difference if there is one.

A **Type II Error** happens when your null hypothesis is false but you do not reject it. The probability of making a type II error is dependent on the power of your statistical test (see Chapter 9). To avoid this you should make sure that you have a large enough sample size.

One of the most critical decisions researchers face is to establish this threshold. How 'certain' must we be of our results in a world where 100% certainty is not possible? If we set the p value too high (e.g. $p<0.1$) we may too easily and generously accept everything as significant. Conversely if we set the p value too low (e.g. $p<0.001$) we may make it virtually impossible to ever demonstrate significance, thereby dismissing findings that actually are meaningful.

The tests most frequently used to determine significance levels are the t-test for parametric data and Pearson's chi-square test for non-parametric data. Both of these tests can be used to compare two groups on only one variable at a time:

a. t-tests

There are three different kinds of t-tests that are commonly used. While all three compare mean scores of two groups, each is applied within a different study design context. **Paired-group (or dependent) t-tests** are used when each subject acts as his/her own control group, or when groups of individuals who are being compared have been matched on some demographic characteristic. For Sandy's study, he has collected two data points for each participant in his study: a pre-test score and a post-test score. Since the post-test score represents knowledge following delivery of his educational programme (the intervention), each participant in Sandy's study is acting as his/her own control group. If Sandy had hypothesised that his educational intervention would produce a positive upward score on the post-test results, he would use a **one-tailed t-test** to determine the significance of his results. If, in another circumstance, a **non-directional hypothesis** had been used instead, a **two-tailed t-test** could be employed to determine the direction of significance, if any.

A key attribute of t-tests is that they can help us to understand whether observed differences were 'real' or 'random'. Further, they can be used on relatively small groups of participants (i.e. <30). Let's look at some more statistical tests:

i. **Mann–Whitney test**: this is an alternative to the t-test that can be used with non-parametric data. It tests for differences between means on two independent groups.

ii. **Wilcoxon Signed Rank Test**: this test can be used on non-parametric data, and can be used to determine the significance of differences between pre-test and post-test scores for individuals.

iii. **Wilcoxon Rank Sum Test**: similar to (i) and (ii), this test can be used for independent groups and with non-parametric data.

b. Pearson's Chi-square test

This test is used when data are non-parametric (e.g. nominal or ordinal). For example, if in Sandy's study there was

SUMMARY OF HOW SANDY WOULD USE A T-TEST

- There are two types of t-test: t-test (related) and t-test (unrelated).
- The related test is used for experimental designs where two things are happening; we call these '**experimental conditions**'. For Sandy these are the scores for the questionnaire completed before and after the educational intervention.
- The two conditions are testing one independent variable which for Sandy are the scores on the educational programme.
- The same participants do both conditions and therefore the participants are *related*.
- The t-test (unrelated) would be used if Sandy had two different sets of participants completing the one condition each (one set completing the pre-test and one completing the post-test). This would not make sense for Sandy because it wouldn't tell him if the educational programme made any difference to his young people with diabetes.

SUMMARY OF HOW SANDY WOULD USE PEARSON'S CHI-SQUARE TEST

- The chi-squared test is the only test that is suitable if your data are nominal.
- This means that instead of being able to measure your participants' scores you can only allocate them to one or more category.
- In Sandy's case he wants to test his hypothesis that teenage girls and boys learn differently thus he has two categories: 'boys' and 'girls'.
- Sandy would use the chi-square test to determine how many participants will fall into each category.
- Note that the chi-square tests an experimental hypothesis (in Sandy's case, that boys and girls learn differently) that predicts how many participants from each group fall into certain categories (e.g. higher or lower scores following the educational intervention).
- This cannot be decided in advance so you will have to test a reasonable number of participants to make sure a sufficient number fall into each category. A rule of thumb is considered to be at least 20 participants.

a desire to know whether there were any differences between male and female participants' responses to the educational intervention, Sandy may organise his data based on sex. He may reasonably hypothesise that teenage boys and girls learn differently, and that a one-size-fits all teaching strategy may not work, and that ultimately, a customised programme for teenage boys, and one for teenage girls, may be more effective. To test this hypothesis as to whether the differences between these two groups (males and females) is greater than the differences within each of these groups, Sandy may still wish to administer pre- and post-tests of knowledge; however, in this case, he will be sorting his data and results based on the sex of the participant.

To deviate from the tests for a moment – increasingly, there has been concern from social science researchers (quite rightly) regarding the use of the sex variable as nominal data, as in the example noted above. While historically researchers have treated sex as a dichotomous, discrete, non-overlapping nominal variable, there is growing recognition that to do so may unfairly force participants into categories that are not reflective of their realities. More about this in the sections related to qualitative research in Chapters 12 and 13. For now, it is reasonable for Sandy to be aware that structuring a research question along dichotomous sex lines may be of general interest and specific importance for him as a researcher, but may actually result in him missing

critical findings relevant to specific individuals because he has forced them into arbitrary categories for his own convenience. This just shows how mindful we must be of social change and the meaningfulness of our research.

Back to Pearson's Chi-square test; this is frequently used when we wish to understand if there are significant differences between pre- and post-test scores for a specific group, or if two groups are actually similar to each other when we ultimately intend to use one group as a control and one group as part of an intervention. It cannot be used when the data themselves are interval or ratio (i.e. parametric).

11.5.2 Tests for Correlation Between Two Sets of Data

Researchers are frequently interested in the influence one variable may have upon another. The magnitude, extent, and direction of these influences can be a powerful tool for predicting future outcomes in similar situations. Inferential statistical tests for correlation are used to examine how important these relationships are by testing two sets of data. These data sets might be from the same individual or from two different groups of individuals who have been categorised based upon a salient demographic characteristic (such as age, occupational status or level of education). Once descriptive statistics have confirmed that one data set moves up or down, the intent is to determine whether the second data set moves in a similarly related – or correlated – manner.

It is important to remember that both sets of data must be continuous because we can't measure sets of data that have been measured differently.

The movement of sets of data is known as the **degree of covariance**. That is the extent to which the two sets of data change together in a particular and predictable pattern in either a positive or negative direction. If both data sets increase together they are said to be positively correlated. If both one set of data increases and the other decreases this is known as negative correlation.

[SANDY EXAMPLE BELOW WITH AN ADDITIONAL DIAGRAM

- For example, in his study of teenage patients with diabetes, Sandy may want to determine if there is any association between body mass index (BMI) and likelihood of receiving a diagnosis of diabetes.
- For each participant, he may then collect both pieces of information and determine the extent, magnitude and direction of the association.
- He may hypothesise that a higher BMI increases the likelihood of diabetes and a diagnosis of diabetes increases the likelihood of a higher BMI: that is, he may hypothesise there is a positive correlation between BMI and diabetes diagnosis because they move in the same direction.

Tests for correlation produce an important kind of inferential statistic called a **correlation coefficient**, usually expressed as 'r' and r values may range from −1 to +1. An r value of −1 indicates a perfect negative correlation (there is no correlation between the two sets of data), while an r value of +1 indicates a perfect positive correlation (the two sets are very highly correlated). As you can see, the closer we are to '1' in either direction the stronger the correlation.

If Sandy's study yields an r value of 0.35 for the association between BMI and diabetes diagnosis, then this would suggest a weak or tenuous correlation between these two variables. We would have to exercise great caution in assuming or predicting that BMI (by itself) was linked with diabetes. The positive direction of the r value suggests there is some (albeit weak) connection here, but it is not strong enough to be predictive in any way.

When running tests for correlation, it is important to remember a key principle of statistics. *Correlation does not mean causation.* It is tempting to oversimplify complex subjects, and some researchers may consciously or unconsciously want to establish the importance of their work by drawing sweeping causal conclusions. Inferential statistics by themselves cannot be used to establish causal links but

they can be used as part of a research programme to establish the associations that warrant further exploration. By using the many methods we have at our disposal we can then achieve greater certainty over time about causes and effects. Let's look at some more statistical tests:

a. Pearson Product Moment Correlation

One of the most common correlation tests is the Pearson Product Moment Correlation, frequently abbreviated to the 'Pearson r'. This test can be used on group or individual data when it is parametric in nature. It is often used to estimate the reliability of a test in a test-retest situation, or between two testers in order to establish inter-rater reliability (go back to Chapter 5 to refresh your memory of reliability). Pearson's r is frequently calculated in academic settings as a way of establishing procedural fairness of testing mechanisms. For example, if as part of his study, Sandy wanted to include material on how to use a glucometer to measure blood glucose levels, then use a performance-based evaluation of his participants to determine whether they had learned anything, Sandy may actually ask the participants to demonstrate how to use the device.

TEACHING AND EVALUATING USE OF A GLUCOMETER

- Sandy would observe them 'in action' and then judge whether they had done it 'correctly' or 'incorrectly'.
- This kind of observational testing of a skill can be prone to bias or error: if Sandy is the tester, he may become momentarily distracted and miss a critical step in the process, or he may see so many people using a glucometer, he starts to get confused and forgets who has done what.
- To enhance the reliability of his evaluation of his participants, he may ask a second rater (or tester) to observe with him, then compare both raters' scores.
- He would then calculate Pearson's r to establish the degree and direction of agreement between the two raters who observed the same thing, as a way of establishing the reliability of the observational method and tools used in the study.

---

b. Spearman Rho

Like Pearson r, Spearman rho is a method of establishing correlation but for non-parametric data when items have been ranked and you wish to compare two sets of rankings to determine if there is any relationship or association. Similar to Pearson r, Spearman rho produces r values that range between −1 and 0–1, depending upon the magnitude, extent and direction of the association.

If Sandy were interested in determining how his participants' subjective satisfaction with the educational programme was correlated with changes in their behaviour, he might proceed as outlined below:

MEASURING RELATIONSHIP BETWEEN SATISFACTION LEVEL AND BEHAVIOUR CHANGE

Sandy could first start by asking them a question such as 'How helpful did you find the information presented in this session?'

- If responses were collected using a 4-point Likert scale (Very Helpful/Somewhat Helpful/Not Very Helpful/Not Helpful), this would represent ordinal data (non-parametric) data.
- Sandy may reasonably hypothesise that the more 'helpful' an individual thought the educational intervention was, the more likely that individual would be to actually apply lessons to his/her daily life (for example, adhering to an insulin dosing schedule).
- One way for Sandy to establish the value of his work may therefore be to compare Likert scale responses to insulin dosing adherence rates (indirectly measured through on-time prescription refill rates).
- Since the data are non-parametric (ordinal), the inferential statistical test that is most appropriate to establish correlation would be Spearman rho.
- If Sandy determines r=0.85, that would indicate a strong positive correlation between participants' subjective satisfaction with the programme and behavioural change, indicating the educational programme had practical impact and value.

For both Spearman rho and Pearson r, the researcher must make important decisions about what value of 'r' is meaningful: at what point or numerical/decimal value does a correlation shift from being 'weak' to 'moderate' to 'strong'? Ultimately, this is a contextual judgment made by the researcher, based upon specific and unique features of the research itself. In general, however:

- 'strong' correlation is arbitrarily defined as $r>0.8$ or $r<-0.8$ (for a strong negative correlation)
- 'moderate' correlation is generally agreed to be $0.5>r<0.8$ or $-0.5<r>-0.8$
- 'weak' correlation is determined to be $r<0.5$ or $r>-0.5$.

These are, however, simply arbitrary numbers and may not be applicable in your specific context. As a researcher it is important to be aware of *generally accepted* bands for weak/moderate/strong correlation but to also understand how – or if – this applies in your specific case.

11.5.3. Regression Analysis

Regression analysis is a technique that is used after a correlation coefficient (e.g. Pearson r or Spearman rho) has been calculated and an association has been established between two variables. There is no point in going any further with statistical tests if two sets of data are not correlated.

The objective of regression analysis is to help us to move beyond correlations towards predictions of future results. **Linear** and **non-linear** regression models exist that allow us to forward extrapolate current data sets using mathematical formulae. In other words they are an attempt to use historical data as a way of predicting a future outcome. As a result, it is one of the most powerful statistical tools available. Regression analyses are neither perfect nor fool-proof as no mathematical model can fully capture all variables that exist in real life. Nonetheless, well-constructed, regression analysis models can provide valuable insights for decision makers, and consequently are widely used in different domains. Caution must always be exercised in placing too much faith in the outcome of a regression analysis. As investors in the stock market are constantly being told, 'past performance is no guarantee of future gain'. Simply because a stock has performed well in the past 6 months in no way guarantees it will perform well in the next 6 months.

There are simply too many confounding environmental variables that *cannot* be predicted and can never be accounted for in a regression analysis model to say with certainty '*this is what the future will be*'. Regression models can provide insights and projections, but these do not substitute for judgment and decision-making.

Few pharmacy practice researchers without advanced statistical training obtained through graduate education have the skills to complete linear or non-linear regression without expert support. While the mathematics and formulae themselves are not overly complicated, their application to an existing data set requires expertise, and consequently details of performing regression analysis are beyond the scope of this chapter. For further information about regression analysis, consult the Further Reading section.

11.5.4. Comparison of More Than Two Variables

Health services research is a necessarily complex activity, as it focusses on real-world experiences of human beings. In many cases, it is simply not possible or realistic to isolate one variable of interest (such as age or sex) as though other variables do not actually influence the outcome. When researchers explore the influence of two or more variables on a study outcome, different kinds of inferential statistical tests are required:

a. Analysis of Variance (ANOVA)

ANOVA is a statistical technique used to compare mean scores of three or more groups within one study. This is useful because we may want to find out the differences in the effects of more than two treatments. This in turn can help us to decide on the most effective treatment to implement in the future, in comparison to other treatments. The ANOVA yields an F ratio, which is then compared to a standardised table to determine whether there is a significant difference between the largest and smallest of the means within the study group. In addition to helping the researcher determine whether there are differences between the means of the study groups, ANOVA can also provide information about differences between individuals within each study group.

SANDY'S OPTIONS

With a new diagram to show potential relationships to be tested, Sandy and a group of researchers working with him may be interested in determining what is the most effective behavioural change to improve blood glucose control in teenagers:

- Improved diet
- Increased exercise
- A new video-game-based glucometer device that is less awkward and more fun to use than the traditional device.

They may construct a study in which there are three groups: 13–15 year olds, 16–18 year olds, and 19–21 year olds, recognising that these interventions may be of differing interest to participants based on age. Within each of these three groups, there could be a further segmentation into male and female. Each group could then be studied on each of the three interventions (diet/ exercise/new glucometer).

As you can see, this is a complicated study, generally beyond the scope of a single pharmacist-researcher. Nonetheless it is a relevant and important study because it recognises that, in the real world, individual patients have different options from which to select, and individual patient demographic characteristics (such as age or sex) may have an influence on preferences, uptake and adherence to a behavioural change. The complexity of this kind of research question will require Sandy to find additional support from a research team. The value of this kind of research question is that it may be more realistic than previous questions that artificially try to isolate one intervention for the convenience of the researcher.

A study such as this would yield an abundance of data that are best analysed using the **one-way ANOVA**. This type

of ANOVA can be used to determine the effect of age and sex on the three different options. It would also allow the research team to determine what interactions exist between age, sex and interventions which could be useful to prompt further investigation.

TYPES OF ANOVA AND THEIR USES

There are a number of types of ANOVA:
- One-way ANOVA (unrelated): used when one variable is tested under three or more conditions and different participants would be used for each of the conditions.
- One-way ANOVA (related): used when one variable is tested under three or more conditions and the same participants would be used for each of the conditions.
- Two-way ANOVA (unrelated): used when two or more variables are tested with two or more conditions for each variable and different participants are used for each of the conditions.
- Two-way ANOVA (related): used when two or more variables are tested with two or more conditions for each variable and the same participants are used for each of the conditions.
- Two-way ANOVA (mixed): this gets a bit complicated! This ANOVA is used when two variables are tests with two or more conditions but for one of the variables. Different participants are used for each condition and for the other variable the same participants are used for each condition.

For most pharmacist-researchers, it is more important to recognise circumstances when ANOVA is appropriate than to know the mathematical formulae themselves. In general, these circumstances will represent a research question and method of sufficient complexity that further support from a research team including a biostatistician may be warranted.

b. Analysis of Covariance (ANCOVA)

Similar to ANOVA, ANCOVA is a valuable tool for studying covariance whilst **controlling for** initial differences between the groups being studied. For example, if there are data to suggest onset of diabetes is linked with puberty and its associated hormonal changes. In this case an extraneous variable (such as age) may influence outcomes of interest related to diabetes diagnosis and management. ANCOVA is a useful tool for taking into account extraneous variables such as this and treating them as covariates, thereby extracting their effects from the data being gathered. In essence, ANCOVA allows the researcher to make the groups being studied more equitable from the outset, thereby allowing for a comparison of final results in a fairer manner. When we use an ANCOVA in this way it accepts that the other variables are important and have an influence on the main variables and mathematically manages their influence to allow the researcher to determine what other correlations may exist.

c. Kruskal Wallis Test

The Kruskal Wallis test is analogous to the one-way ANOVA but is used for non-parametric data. Similar to other non-parametric tests discussed here, this test is based on rankings of non-parametric (nominal or ordinal) data. For example, if Sandy were interested in learning more about the perceptions of diverse stakeholders regarding the pharmacist's role in management and treatment of diabetes amongst young people, he may administer a survey to groups of patients, family physicians, and nurses in which he asked them to respond to a question such as:

'Pharmacists are competent to independently manage insulin dose adjustments for adolescent patients' using a 4-point Likert scale:

Strongly Agree…Agree…Disagree…Strongly Disagree

As far as the example of Sandy's work is concerned comparing this ordinal data collected from three different stakeholder groups would point to use of the Kruskal Wallis test.

d. Multiple Regression

Similar to linear and non-linear regression discussed previously, multiple regression is a complex statistical method generally beyond the scope of most pharmacist-researchers working on their own. As with other forms of regression analysis, multiple regression has as its objective the ability to make predictions or forward projections about a study variable by understanding the effects of two or more independent variables on that study variable of interest. More sophisticated biostatisticians can take this technique even further and actually untangle the relative contributions of each of the independent variables. This type of statistic would allow us to take a set of variables such as age, sex, level of education and family history and discover which one was the best predictor of a diagnosis of diabetes.

The inferential statistical tests presented above are only a sample of the more commonly used techniques within health services research. Few if any researchers perform manual calculations any longer, relying instead upon widely available software programs such as SPSS instead.

11.6. DISTINGUISHING BETWEEN CLINICAL AND STATISTICAL SIGNIFICANCE

In this last but one section we return to the issues of clinical and statistical significance. Findings that just barely meet a

threshold for statistical significance (e.g. $p < 0.05$) may be less likely to have clinical significance in the real world. Similarly, the object of your measurement will also help you to determine clinical significance. If you are measuring 'change in knowledge' that is generally considered a 'softer' or less significant kind of clinical outcome than 'change in behaviour' which in turn is softer than 'change in outcome'. While a change in baseline knowledge may be interesting and important, its importance is premised on the notion that it in turn will lead to behavioural, then outcome, changes which are more important. Clinical significance frequently requires a concrete, observable endpoint (such as a change in a laboratory parameter like HgA1C for a diabetes study), though this will depend upon specific study context.

CASE STUDY EXAMPLE

- To end this chapter on inferential statistics we are going to have a look at how Sandy might make his decisions about which inferential statistics he might use to obtain the evidence he needs to proceed with his research.
- At the end of Chapter 10 we suggested that Sandy might be able to compare BMI with target blood glucose to see if being overweight is related to high blood sugar, so we will look at how he might do this.

The first aim of his research was to find out whether there really was a difference in the blood glucose control of the young people in his care. To do this he has collected data from 250 patients registered to the GP practice where he works. In Chapter 10 we looked at how Sandy might use some descriptive statistics to begin to make some tentative assumptions about his data.

As a reminder here are Sandy's means, SDs and ranges from Chapter 10 and to this table (Table 11.2) we have added the numbers for BMI.

TABLE 11.2 Means, SDs and Ranges for Blood Glucose and BMI

	BLOOD GLUCOSE DAY 1 BEFORE AND AFTER BREAKFAST		BODY MASS INDEX (BMI)
	Reading A	Reading B	
Mean	6.1	8.6	25.6
Standard Deviation	1.69	1.59	6.34
Range	3.6–9.3	5.4–11.4	15–35

11.6.1.   Is There a Correlation Between Blood Glucose and BMI?

Sandy uses a Pearson's Product Moment test of correlation (see Section 11.5.2) which yields an r value of 0.65 for the association between BMI and diabetes diagnosis. This suggests a moderate correlation between the two variables and so Sandy decides to proceed with his inferential tests to see if there is a significant difference between the two. Sandy needs to exercise great caution in assuming that the relationship he is observing is strong enough to be predictive because the correlation is not as strong as he might have hoped.

11.6.2   Test for Significant Difference (See Section 11.5.1) Between Blood Glucose and BMI

Here, we will use artistic license and make a few assumptions ourselves to show how Sandy makes his decisions. We are going to assume that Sandy wants to find out if there is a relationship between BMI and the percentage of time participants are in the target range for diabetes control in his sample. Fig. 11.1 shows a decision tree of how Sandy decides which statistical tests he should be doing.

The decision tree has helped Sandy to come to a conclusion about how to proceed and he has decided that his first step is to find out if there is a relationship between BMI and levels of blood sugar.

Here is a summary of the things that Sandy needed to know:

- Type of data: this is **Interval data** because the data are ordered in a logical sequence and the intervals between numbers are considered equal and represent real and quantifiable amounts (see Section 11.4).
- The data are parametric
- Sandy could use a t-test, an ANOVA or an ANCOVA. Sandy decides to use a t-test (see page 120).

Sandy has hypothesised that patients with a high BMI (over 25) will show poor blood glucose control over the period of 6 months of his study. Therefore he uses a **one-tailed t test** to determine the significance of his results.

Sadly, the results show that the difference between the two variables is not significant ($p > 0.05$) and so Sandy must go back to the drawing board and re-examine his data and indeed his research question. It may be that he can find out more by using qualitative methods, something we will explore in Part III of this textbook.

11.7.   WORKING WITH OTHER RESEARCHERS

We have said this before but working with other researchers on your research project can not only improve the outcomes of your research, it can be an enjoyable and enriching process.

One of the way researchers work together is by choosing the skills they need to be able to conduct their project effectively and identifying colleagues who might be able to help. Many projects require an assessment of the research by a statistician to ensure that the results have been correctly analysed and accurately reported. This doesn't mean to say researchers do not have the skills to do statistics themselves, but it provides an independent assessment that verifies the results.

As you go through your studies your understanding of statistics will increase – often we only really understand something once we have used it, so don't worry if you are early in your studies or training and things seems a little confusing. There are plenty of people in your department or area of work who will be able to help. On large projects it might be worth including a statistician on your team, especially one who has experience in health care and pharmacy practice research.

As this chapter has illustrated, there are many options and decisions that must be considered when using inferential statistics and these can be a little confusing at first. Particularly when making the shift from descriptive to inferential statistics, having a mentor or expert to support your work is of great benefit. Many universities and large employers (including hospitals, pharmaceutical companies and consultancies) have in-house staff statisticians who may be accessible.

However, there are plenty of textbook websites that can help you to develop your knowledge and skills of statistics and some of these are given at the end of this chapter.

Learning to work with other professionals takes time, as does any situation where we work with people from other disciplines. We don't always understand each other and so it is important to work out what other people might mean by certain terms and contexts. Getting to know each other and acknowledging limitations and the strengths you each bring to the research project is as important as is keeping a strong focus on the research questions and objectives themselves. Working together with other professionals is rewarding and, as we have said, can result in better research outcomes.

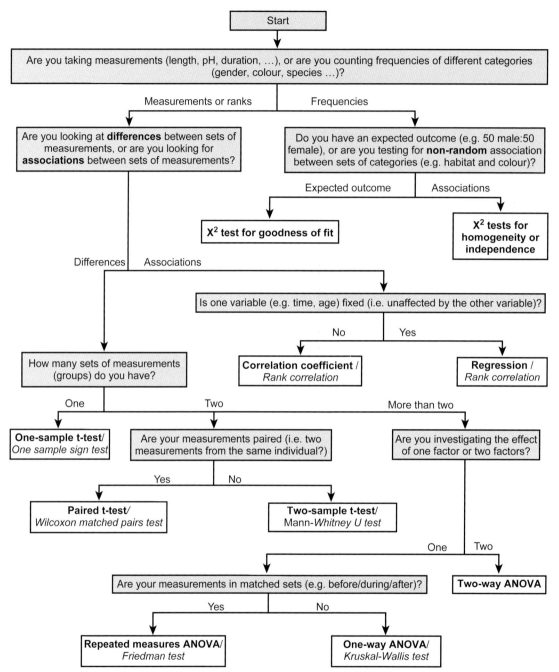

FIGURE 11.1 A simple decision chart for statistical tests in Biol321. Non-parametric options are in *italics.* (Adapted from Ennos R: Statistical and Data Handling Skills in Biology. Harlow, UK: Pearson Education Limited, 2007.)

CHAPTER SUMMARY

- This chapter provided an overview of inferential statistics.
- It recaps types of measurement and how these affect the statistical tests we use.
- It covers some of the most commonly used statistical tests and explains when they might be used.
- It uses our case study pharmacist, Sandy, to illustrate how he might use the tests and why.

FURTHER READING

Statistics

Greene, J., & D'Oliveira, M. (2006). *Learning to Use Statistical Tests in Psychology* (3rd ed.). Oxford: Oxford University Press.

Scott, I., & Mazhindu, D. (2014). *Statistics for Healthcare Professionals: An introduction.* London: Sage Publications.

Veney, J., Kros, J., & Rosenthal, D. (2009). *Statistics for Health Care Professionals: Working with Excel.* London: John Wiley & Sons Ltd.

Introduction to Qualitative Research

LEARNING OBJECTIVES

After reading this chapter you should be able to:
- understand the principles of qualitative research
- describe the differences between quantitative and qualitative research
- understand the ethical issues to be considered when doing qualitative research
- define the concepts of reliability and trustworthiness

12.1 INTRODUCTION

In Chapter 1 of this textbook we introduced you to the whole concept of 'research' and the steps that we felt were important in the research process (see Chapter 1, Section 1.3). We outlined the two main research methodologies – quantitative research and qualitative research and some of the differences between them. Then in Chapter 2 we devoted ourselves to quantitative methodology and methods (see Chapters 4–11), and these were illustrated by our case study pharmacy students – Serena and Rosi – and pharmacists – Sandy and Dorothy. Each of them had a different research question they wanted to answer either as part of a student project or in practice. We saw how they could begin to answer their questions using quantitative methods and suggested that at some point in their research they might find that they couldn't get all of the answers they needed by using quantitative methods alone. They would need to find other research methods to do this. In Table 12.1 below you will find a recap of the research being done by each of our students and pharmacists and the information that they have collected using quantitative methods. In Table 12.4 you will see how they might extend their research using qualitative methods.

Table 12.1, shows that while quantitative research may be the best way to answer questions related to 'what', 'when', 'where' or 'who', what all of our case study researchers have found is that numbers are not enough to do justice to their participants' whole experiences. Numbers alone can't help us to understand 'how' people feel about certain issues, such as giving up smoking or trying to lose weight, and 'why'. The

reasons why people do things that are not good for them are different from person to person, and in order to help them we need to understand those reasons. In this section we will add some new tools to your research toolkit that will help you obtain the richness of data that quantitative methods cannot give. These methods come under the umbrella of 'qualitative research'. We will be bringing back our case study student pharmacists Serena and Rosi and showing how they might use qualitative methods to enrich their research.

New and experienced health care researchers, including pharmacists, will all at some point ask themselves whether they are really answering their research question in a way that matches their observations and experiences of dealing with patients in the real world. Understanding human behaviour which on the surface may appear counterproductive, illogical, and actually risk inflicting self-harm, is a challenge for any clinician. The evidence we use to guide treatment decisions is most frequently derived from quantitative research such as clinical trials (see Chapter 8). When this evidence is used to design health care interventions which are applied at the individual patient level, to deal with a specific issue, it may not necessarily produce the results we expect. Within a world of ambiguity, questions and uncertainty that comes with being human, qualitative research may be of particular value.

Part III of this textbook is about doing qualitative research. This first chapter provides an overview of what qualitative research is, how it is different from quantitative research, and how and when it can be used. We also look at the role of the researcher and the importance of being true to our participants. Chapter 13 'Interviewing Participants' is about

TABLE 12.1 Quantitative Data for Case Studies	
Case Study Researcher	**Quantitative Data Collected**
Sandy	• Age
	• Sex
	• Work status (school or university or employed)
	• Family history
	• Weight
	• Height
	• Data of diagnosis
	• Blood glucose
Dorothy	• Prescribing patterns of doctors, nurses, pharmacists and others
	• Attitudes towards prescribing antimicrobials
	• Barriers and facilitators associated with an antimicrobial stewardship programme
Rosi	• Information about who is on campus, e.g. job, department, age, sex, whether they have any health conditions requiring medication
	• What prescription medication they take
	• What over-the-counter products they use
	• How often they visit a pharmacy off-campus
	• What they visit their pharmacy for
	• Whether they think it would be a good idea to have a pharmacy on campus
Serena	• How long people have been smoking
	• How many cigarettes they smoke per day
	• Have they ever tried to quit smoking?
	• Have they used a smoking cessation aid?
	• If so which one?

learning the key skills that enable us to collect qualitative data, especially the skill of keeping quiet and listening. In Chapter 14 we introduce you to focus groups and how they might be conducted and in Chapter 15 we explore observational research – What can we learn from watching people in certain situations and contexts? In Chapter 16 we give

you an overview of how you might deal with the large amounts of data that can be generated when we use qualitative methods, and we follow this up in Chapter 17 with data synthesis and how we might present qualitative findings. Chapter 18 is devoted to other ways of collecting data with a brief overview of some of the many ways of 'doing' qualitative research. Although the topics we cover in Chapter 18 are important, in our experience they are less likely to be used by pharmacy students.

12.2 WHAT IS QUALITATIVE RESEARCH?

As the name suggests, qualitative research involves methods, techniques and analyses that focus on what observing people and listening to what they say can teach us about a given situation. Qualitative research is most frequently used in an attempt to better understand or explain the underlying causes or reasons for an action, behaviour or observation. Historically, scientifically oriented professions, such as pharmacy, have not embraced qualitative research as fully as other disciplines, such as psychology, political science or sociology. Increasingly, pharmacists and other health care professionals are recognising how complex human behaviours actually are, and how this complexity imposes certain limitations on the extent to which we can rely exclusively upon quantitative research. Within the health professions, there is a growing interest in the role of qualitative research in helping us to better understand complex health and interpersonal situations.

As we have seen in previous chapters, quantitative research produces numerical data which can then be analysed using descriptive or inferential statistics (see Chapters 10 and 11). Well-designed quantitative research, interpreted through the lens of appropriately applied inferential statistics, can allow us to predict with some confidence, future outcomes based on past observations. This type of research provides us with an evidence base to facilitate understanding of the superiority or inferiority of one treatment intervention over another. It is the basis upon which individual therapy decisions, policies and systems are frequently constructed.

With experience in the field, pharmacists and other clinicians begin to recognise that quantitative research (while important and necessary) may be insufficient to explain how things actually work in the real world. In part, this may be due to the lack of continuity between highly structured and controlled study conditions and highly unstructured real-world conditions.

Neither qualitative nor quantitative research alone can presume to actually fully and correctly approximate the truth. As we have said a number of times in earlier chapters, there is a notion that the certainty associated with numbers, statistical tests and mathematical formulae is somehow 'truer'

TABLE 12.2   Comparing Quantitative and Qualitative Research

	Quantitative Research	Qualitative Research
Researcher stance	Objective, unbiased, neutral	Subjectivity is reality and needs to be acknowledged
Reasoning processes	Deductive: moving from the general to the specific – if something is true for a category of things in general, it is true for all members of that category too	Inductive: moving from the specific to the general – we make observations, look for patterns, then infer an explanation, theory or hypothesis
Research focus	Concise, narrow, specified	Complex, broad, open
Role of theory	Tests theories to confirm or refute them	Generates theories for further exploration/study
Unit of analysis	Numbers, statistical methods	Words, narratives
View of reality	A single truth that can be measured and generalised	Multiple truths that are continually evolving with individual interpretations

than other forms of research. Qualitative research provides us with an opportunity to more fully account for the realities of the human beings that are integral to any system, in a way that both honours their experiences and does not presume to pre-judge them.

12.2.1.   Differences Between Qualitative and Quantitative Research

It is tempting to assume that qualitative and quantitative research methods are completely complementary, if not opposing, forms of research. Given the polarity associated with numbers vs words, this may be understandable but the reality is much more nuanced. At the core, qualitative research involves listening to, observing, reflecting upon, and then articulating what participants (e.g. patients) do, say, and think. Qualitative researchers are in some ways investigative reporters, carefully documenting what they see and hear and presenting their findings and analysis in a manner that reflects the narratives of the participants themselves. Much of what qualitative researchers do involves asking questions, then listening to and observing responses. In some cases, qualitative researchers may simply observe participants going about their daily lives and work without direct involvement or questioning (see Chapter 15). In other cases, qualitative research may involve review of artefacts such as written documents (such as policy and procedure manuals, clinical documentation notes, or organisational vision/mission statements) in an attempt to understand the thinking, beliefs and values that informed their development (Table 12.2).

12.2.2.   Background to Qualitative and Quantitative Research

In Chapter 1 we explained that traditionally, quantitative research has been understood to be rooted in the positivist

tradition, while qualitative research is thought to be generally rooted in the constructivist tradition. Positivism is a philosophical stance that highlights the centrality of our sensory experience (what we see, hear, taste, touch) interpreted through human logic and reason, as a means for understanding the world. Positivists place a strong premium on empiricism, the notion that sensory data can be examined, tested and verified leading to the production of truth. To positivists, there actually are real, attainable truths awaiting discovery. Examples of such truths may include 'the sun rises in the east', or '2+2= 4' or 'a measurement of 140/90 indicates high blood pressure requiring treatment'.

In contrast, constructivists believe that knowledge and meaning are not absolute universal truths, but only attain that status because human beings over time have jointly agreed to certain truisms. Why does the sun rise in the east? Because we have agreed that the bright hot yellow object routinely seen in many parts of the world (other than the United Kingdom) is something we will call 'the sun', and that human beings have artificially and arbitrarily forced the label of 'east' onto the direction in which it is first seen. The labels are human creations we all accept, and these in turn have shaped our understanding of the reality we observe, leading us to believe it is 'truth'. To constructivists, truths are neither absolute nor eternal – they simply reflect a temporary agreement about terms that a group or society works with in order to enhance efficiency. From this perspective, truth changes all the time. Thus, a constructivist may see a measurement of 140/90 and recognise that perhaps it indicates high blood pressure requiring treatment, perhaps it indicates high blood pressure not requiring treatment, or perhaps it actually doesn't indicate high blood pressure at all because *we simply don't know enough about the person in whom the measurement has been taken to make such a sweeping judgement.*

It is perhaps easy to understand why positivism has historically dominated health professions like pharmacy. If one believes there is an absolute truth, then decision-making is facilitated. Truths, empirically established and verified, lend themselves to actions, algorithms, treatments and interventions. Pity the poor 'constructivist' pharmacist working in an intensive care unit or emergency room setting; without a firm belief or faith in the existence of truth, how can a decision ever be made? Similarly, pity the poor positivist pharmacist working in an intensive care unit or emergency room setting; with unquestioning belief with the existence of truth comes a tendency to make bold decisions confidently, only to see them not actually work in the real world with remarkable and alarming frequency. Why do patients not lose weight when we advise them to do so, for their own good? Why do people keep smoking even after a first, second or third heart attack? Why would a patient with an infection not take their antibiotic four times a day for 10 days as instructed? As any clinician knows the reality of health care delivery means we cannot simply and simplistically rely upon 'truth', positivism, or quantitative research alone.

12.2.3 Deciding When to Use Qualitative Research

Qualitative research may be uniquely well suited to help clinicians better understand the complex behaviours we actually observe in the real world. It may be tempting to write-off patients who do not comply with our instructions or adhere to our prescriptions, labelling them as uneducated, unmotivated or not worth spending our time with. The reality, however, is that losing weight is difficult, quitting smoking is almost impossible if one's close friends and family still smoke, and that scheduling and remembering to take antibiotics four times a day if one is working and raising a family and having any semblance of a normal life is actually very difficult. For these reasons (and there are many more) it is important to try to find ways of working with patients in what we call a **concordant** relationship. This means we need to listen to their point of view and the difficulties they have fitting health issues into a busy life, and work together with them to find the best way for them as individuals.

Qualitative research helps us to answer questions about *why* things are the way they are, and *how* patients think about and respond to their circumstances. Such information is crucial for clinically oriented professionals like pharmacists who must work in real world situations, not idealised and highly controlled clinical trial conditions.

Ultimately, neither qualitative nor quantitative research alone can fully account for the realities and contingencies of clinical practice. When taken together in a complementary manner, they can help us to better approximate the realities of patients and their circumstances. The greatest strengths of positivism – its emphasis on empiricism, rigour and reproducibility – coupled with the power of quantitative methods and inferential statistics can provide us with confidence in decision-making in difficult or nebulous situations. There are circumstances when both approaches may be appropriate in order to answer our research question, and in Part IV of this textbook we will look at how we can use the two methodologies together in what is called 'Mixed Methods Research'.

In Table 12.3 you will find some ideas about when qualitative and quantitative methods might be used, our reasons why they would be used and some examples. This will help you to make the transition from the material in Section 2 that focussed on quantitative methods to the idea of qualitative methodology. It is not always easy to make that transition when we are doing research. This is because we are moving from methods that provide us with relatively clear cut answers that we can generalise across our study population, to methods that do not enable us to generalise at all.

Qualitative research may have unique contributions to make in helping us to better understand complex human dynamics, but (similar to quantitative research) on its own it may provide an incomplete picture. As will be seen in Chapter 19, mixed-methods research, incorporating elements of both qualitative and quantitative research methods may be the most appropriate approach in many clinical contexts.

For pharmacists involved in patient-facing settings, or for anyone dealing with the messiness of interpersonal situations, qualitative methods are an important part of the research toolkit; consequently an understanding of their foundations, use, applications and implications is essential.

12.3 EXPLORING THE PERSONAL WORLDS OF OTHERS

We have spent quite a lot of time talking about the background to qualitative research, but now it is time to talk about the focus of our attention – our participants.

One of the things that qualitative research study seeks to tell us is why people have thoughts and feelings that might affect the way they behave. For the purposes of this textbook, the focus is on pharmacy practice and the way people behave with regards to their health and to the taking of medicines (e.g. to understand patients' reasons for non-adherence to medications, or to explore the different roles that pharmacists have). The most important point about qualitative research is that it does not seek to generalise its findings to a wider population. We are talking here about individual experiences rather than the effects of health care interventions on populations. Qualitative research is used to gain insights into people's feelings and thoughts which

TABLE 12.3 **When Might One Research Method Be Preferred Over Another?**		
Context	**Qualitative or Quantitative – and Why?**	**Example**
Very little is known about a subject/topic/observation	Qualitative: may facilitate generation of hypotheses or theories which can subsequently be tested or studied	'How do patients interpret and apply pharmacist-initiated medication counselling related to antibiotics?'
When observed behaviour may be driven by individual's feelings, values, emotional needs, or perceptions rather than logic or reason	Qualitative: may support better understanding of complex psychosocial issues and behaviours	'What does "adherence" mean to patients, in the context of antibiotic use?'
Generation of new ideas/ solutions from the grass-roots up	Qualitative: allows participants to share their personal perspectives without steering them in a predetermined direction	'What are patients' perspectives on enhancing pharmacist-initiated medication counselling to optimise adherence to new antibiotics?'
Exploring or testing cause–effect relationship	Quantitative: allows for hypothesis testing and refinement and inferences based on statistical analyses	'Does a written patient information leaflet about antibiotic use improve antibiotic adherence?'
Determining superiority of an intervention based upon objective laboratory parameters	Quantitative: facilitates comparisons between interventions using external benchmarking	'Do patients who take antibiotics as prescribed have reduction in fever more quickly than those who are non-adherent?'

may provide the basis for a stand-alone qualitative study or help researchers to map out survey instruments for use in a quantitative study. (More information about using different types of research in the same study may be found in Part IV of this textbook.) The role of the researcher in qualitative research is to attempt to access the thoughts and feelings of their participants. This is not an easy thing to do as it involves asking people to talk about things that may be very personal to them. Sometimes the experiences being explored are easy for participants to remember and recount, on other occasions reliving past experiences may be difficult or even cause pain or distress. However data are being collected, the primary role of the researcher is to safeguard participants and their stories. Mechanisms for such safeguarding must be clearly articulated to participants and approved by a relevant research ethics review board prior to embarking upon research. For this reason, researchers and practitioners new to qualitative research should seek advice from an experienced qualitative researcher before they start. In the next section we outline some of the ethical issues that must be considered when doing qualitative research.

12.3.1   The Ethics of Qualitative Research

Qualitative research provides unique and highly personal insights into individual's experiences in the real world. This intimate, subjective insight may be as psychologically invasive

and dangerous to participants as taking blood or tissue samples may be physically risky. As a result, there are unique ethical burdens and responsibilities researchers must be mindful of when engaging in qualitative research. A good place to start is to put yourself in your participant's shoes and ask how you would want to be treated. Major ethical issues to consider in qualitative research include:

a. Anonymity: The objective of ensuring anonymity is to protect the identity of the individual participant wherever possible. Techniques to ensure anonymity include, for example, allocating pseudonyms or participant numbers to each participant rather than using their real name, or not presenting any unique identifying demographic characteristic that would allow a reasonably informed person to deduce a participant's identity. In some cases, it may not be possible to fully ensure participants' anonymity (for example if interviewing high-profile individuals with unique roles or experiences). In such cases, it is essential that participants be informed that attempts will be made to ensure anonymity but these cannot be assured or guaranteed. They then have enough information to decide whether they want to take part or not.

b. Confidentiality: Of necessity, qualitative researchers will have access to identifying information about their participants including items such as telephone numbers, email addresses as well as personal health, medical or psychological data. Such information must be protected carefully by the researcher to ensure that only those with an absolute need to access such information can do so. Casual research staff, administrative personnel, or others who do not have an absolute need for such information must not be allowed access to it.

c. Ask or observe only that which is absolutely necessary: Interviews, focus groups and observations are not social excursions designed for the gratification of the researcher – they are targeted information collecting sessions which should have clarity of focus and remit. While it may be tempting to argue 'we must cast the net wide since we don't know exactly what we are looking for', it is more important to respect the time and vulnerability of participants. Research that is simply a fishing-trip without specific purpose not only wastes participants' time, it also exposes them to disclosing information that may be irrelevant to the ultimate research question or objective.

d. Respect and honour the participants' involvement: Participants are essential for your research and consequently need to be respected. Scheduling around their timetables and needs (not yours), providing a comfortable environment for meetings or interviews, providing refreshments and support for travel costs/parking, etc., is expected. Increasingly, there is an expectation that participants receive some kind of financial compensation for the time involved in the research; most frequently this may be a small gift card or other honorarium that is indicative (not necessarily representative) of the time and effort involved for participation.

e. Option to withdraw: At any time during the research process, participants must be fully aware that they can 'drop out' of your study; while this may be problematic and irritating to you as a researcher it is an essential safeguard designed to protect participants' rights. Participants need to be fully informed that they can leave the study completely, request that a particular response or data set be removed from the analysis, or simply choose not to answer or participate in some or many portions of the research itself.

f. Opportunity to review: Particularly for interviews and focus groups, participants should be given the opportunity to review your raw data (e.g. interview transcripts, focus group field notes). During this review process, they should also be provided with the opportunity to ask for portions of the data set to be removed without cause of explanation provided. Participants should also be given the opportunity to review and comment upon any other published or presented materials that flow from their participation in your research.

g. Secure storage of raw data: All data collected in the study must be securely stored and eventually destroyed pursuant to research ethics board requirements. The exact nature of this process will vary depending upon context, institution and research ethics boards practices; familiarising yourself with these requirements in your local context prior to embarking upon research is essential.

h. Informed consent: Participants must be fully aware of and capable of providing consent to their participation in your study. They must understand its rationale, objectives, methods, confidentiality/anonymity provisions, storage/disposal of data practices, and their rights in terms of withdrawal and review of data. Signed consent is generally a requirement for most studies.

i. Safety netting: It should be made clear to participants exactly who they should go to if they have any concerns about any part of the research in which they have participated. This is not just in the immediate aftermath but in the future too. Participants may remember something they have said during an interview and focus group and want to talk it over. It is essential to draw up a list beforehand so that participants can be signposted on to further expert help if necessary.

Unfortunately, there are no commonly agreed-upon checklists or protocols to guide qualitative researchers in the design and implementation of their projects. The general principle of all research, 'first, do no harm', fully applies here. In general, research ethics committees (RECs) are an important safeguard in the process, ensuring potential risks to participants are managed and minimised. It may be tempting to think 'all I'm doing is talking to people, what's the risk here?' Of course, the risk involved in qualitative research may involve the vulnerability and disclosure that emerges through observation and interview. The feeling of being watched and judged by another person (even if the researcher him/herself is not being judgmental) can have devastating psychological consequences. Further, depending upon the research question itself, certain sensitive or private issues may emerge. For example, a pharmacist may believe she/he is conducting 'safe' qualitative research about antibiotic use, but for a participant the REASON for the antibiotic use may be quite personal (e.g. involving sexual health). In some cases, seemingly innocuous questions may trigger participant's memories about previous unpleasant or dangerous situations, which in turn could provoke considerable psychological distress. While it is impossible to completely prevent such occurrences, it is necessary to understand they may arise and to identify strategies to manage and mitigate harm that may result. More information about the ethics of doing qualitative research may be found in the 'Further Reading' section at the end of this chapter.

12.4 GETTING STARTED WITH QUALITATIVE RESEARCH

We deliberately spent some time on the differences between quantitative and qualitative research (Section 12.2) because the ways of doing them are so different. If you can set out on your discovery of qualitative research accepting that you are not trying to achieve the same outcomes as you would with quantitative research, then taking the time to read about the differences will be time well spent.

For scientifically trained clinicians such as pharmacists, qualitative research may initially require some cognitive flexibility. Truisms related to 'generalisability', 'reliability' and 'objectivity' which we have been trained to accept as part of good research may appear differently in the qualitative realm. In the chapters that follow we will describe in some detail three different ways of approaching qualitative research. For each we will tell you how to go about doing the research itself using, for example, interviews or focus groups, how to record your data and how to manage the output and analysis. However, there is one thing that we feel is essential to getting started in qualitative research and that is the development of an awareness of our own and others' points of view. You may not have expected to begin with yourself, but as a researcher who is trying to understand and interpret other peoples' viewpoints it is an essential place to begin. At the end of Part III we want you to be thinking like a qualitative researcher!

12.4.1 Understanding Different Perspectives

For the novice qualitative researcher, an important starting point in the process is to accept that we all have an opinion about things. In technical terms we can call this our 'position' or 'standpoint'. The idea of having a position about things (sometimes called 'positionality' is rooted in the constructivist foundations of qualitative research, and requires the researcher to mindfully and honestly self-appraise and articulate his/her interests, biases, and assumptions. The reason that this is important is that qualitative research involves interpreting what participants who might be patients or pharmacists or other health care professionals, really mean by what they say or do. That is a big responsibility and as researchers we have a duty to be true to our participants standpoint – not our own. Without an understanding of this it is easy to slip into interpreting other people's narratives from our own viewpoint – rather than theirs.

So, we have to learn to acknowledge our own standpoint and put it aside whilst we pay attention to our participants'. However, our own viewpoint will be of great value when we come to interpreting what participants mean because we have the knowledge and experience of our own profession to help inform that interpretation. In Chapters 16 and 18 we will look at qualitative methodologies that have 'meaning' or 'phenomenology' as their foundation.

An example of this might be a pharmacist, seeking to better understand problems with adherence, who may not fully recognise or acknowledge that she/he actually thinks adherence is a good thing, and that it is better than non-adherence. During your training to become a pharmacist you are likely to have developed opinions about medicines and their use and believe them to be true. These values and norms regarding behaviours associated with medication seem to take root and we rarely think about where they came from or what effect our opinions might have on the decisions we make about patient care.

In many respects the practice of pharmacy is very black and white. It is essential that some medicines are taken in a certain way and there is no alternative. In learning this you will have also learned that there are good reasons why you follow the rules and that **compliance (or adherence)** is better than non-compliance. When we observe non-adherence in the real world with patients, our previous experiences, education and trajectory through life all conspire to lead us to a value-laden judgement about the non-adherent patient. Even if it is for the most noble (albeit paternalistic) of reasons, most pharmacists are simply wired to assume adherence is better than non-adherence.

12.4.2 Problematising

Social scientists refer to this as 'problematising' an observed behaviour, and it can be a useful tool for helping us to understand why people do the things they do. Problematising means that we assume that the behaviour we are witnessing is – in fact – a problem. Indeed it may be a problem…but to whom? Let's look at some viewpoints:

- For pharmacists, non-adherence may be seen as and feel like:
1. professional failure:
   'I didn't do my job properly, so the patient isn't doing what he is supposed to do.'
2. character deficiency:
   'Well if the patient was intelligent, of course he would listen to me and do as he was told…so if he isn't adherence, perhaps he's not that smart…'

Problematising an observation is intimately connected to the worldview or general set of beliefs/values/norms of the person doing the observing:

- An alternative medicine health practitioner who does not believe in antibiotic interventions – may observe the same non-adherent patient and think:
  'What a sensible person, not allowing himself to be poisoned by artificial substances.'
- Yet another observer – let's say an environmentalist – may observe this non-adherent patient and think:

'How great – knowing that antibiotics excreted in the urine are fouling our precious water reservoirs, he is willing to endure an infection longer than necessary to save the planet.'

In the meantime, from the patient's perspective perhaps adherence is really just not an option. If we think back to the earlier example of the patients trying to struggle with working full time, raising a family, managing a household then remembering to take a capsule every 6 hours on an empty stomach! The patient may have every good intention to comply – but life just gets in the way. There are no sweeping principles around environmentalism, evidence-based medicine or drug-as-poison involved, simply the day-to-day struggle of a busy parent just trying to stay ahead of things.

We hope you are beginning to see that there is more than one perspective at play in qualitative research: the focus of the research from the participants' perspectives and the standpoint of the researcher. As can be seen, the perspective of the researcher in framing the problem and starting the entire research process is critical. If, as researchers, we have not taken the time and energy required to actually and honestly self-reflect and appraise our underlying positions on the observations we define as problems, we cannot undertake qualitative research in any meaningful way.

12.4.3 Reflection

To truly understand the complexity of different peoples' viewpoints on health issues we need to first admit to ourselves our own positionality as researchers. A pharmacist-researcher may therefore need to articulate his/her values around adherence, compliance to authority, evidence-based medicine, and other relevant factors.

Reflecting then articulating one's positionality is a complex and time-consuming process, and is absolutely essential for qualitative research. Many would argue it is equally essential (though rarely undertaken) for quantitative research, as similar biases and stances may interfere with problematising and data collection, analysis and interpretation. Reflecting and eventually writing down where we stand on the topic of our research can help to clarify our thoughts and the writing of this is sometimes called a 'Positionality Statement'. In thinking and writing about this there are several questions which should be addressed:

a. Why am I interested in this topic? What is driving your enthusiasm, energy or interest in researching this subject – this is often a clue as to your underlying values and beliefs.

b. What do I actually think the answer is going to be? The veneer of objectivity and dispassionate disinterest that is seen as the pinnacle of scientific behaviour can be stripped away by honestly acknowledging that, in starting a research project, most of us have preconceptions as to what we will find. Articulating these preconceptions can provide a safeguard during the research process and when presented to readers of your work, help them to understand where you are coming from in the first place.

c. What am I expecting to get out of this? In some settings, the researcher may not have any particular interest in their work – instead it is an employment or academic requirement and just a job. Alternatively, the researcher may have an axe-to-grind, a desire for vindication or self-congratulation. In both these extreme circumstances the psychological needs of the researcher cannot help but influence the direction of the research, the depth to which the researcher is willing to go to find information, and the way the research itself will be conducted.

d. What do others in my professional community think? We all live and work in a highly social world; one in which peers and colleagues may affect our behaviours in subconscious ways. Taking unpopular stances even when such stances truly reflect our beliefs can be difficult if we wish to maintain collegial relationships. Acknowledging the influence and importance of peers in shaping our values, beliefs and norms and how this may inhibit or affect us is essential.

e. How will I handle dissonant information and results? How open are you – truly – to not simply finding but honestly reporting results that do not conform to preconceptions. Will you be able to 'see' and 'hear' data that do not actually conform to your expectations, or will you subconsciously ignore it? How will you even know if you are subconsciously ignoring such data?

It is neither possible nor desirable to write a comprehensive checklist for developing a positionality statement; your positionality will be constantly evolving and becoming clearer to you during the course of the research itself. These preliminary questions are merely a good place to start the process. Equally essential is the imperative of documenting this process: simply reflecting without writing does not provide sufficient accountability to you as a researcher or transparency to those who will read your work.

12.4.4 Reliability and Trustworthiness

One of the questions that arise regarding qualitative research is about the reliability of the interpretation and representation of the participants' narratives. There are no statistical tests that can be used to check reliability and validity as there are in quantitative research. However, there are other ways to establish whether we can be confident about the way we have written up the things participants have said or done. In the context of qualitative research this is called 'trustworthiness' and more about this topic can be found in the 'Further Reading' section of this chapter.

Trustworthiness is assessed at different points during the research process. For example,

- Clarifying what a participant has said by asking them what they meant or by recounting to them what you heard them say, in an interview or focus group.
- Ensuring that we take an accurate account of what is said during the collection of data through interviews and focus groups by audio or video recording the session. This provides us with a record of what was said and can be listened to or viewed afterwards.
- Coding transcriptions of our audio or video recordings by more than one researcher and discussing any similarities and differences in our own and another's coding. This simple act can result in revisions to the codes and help to clarify and confirm the research findings.
- Inviting participants to read and comment on what we have written once we have written up our data.

The concept of reliability and trustworthiness will be discussed in more detail in Chapters 13–18 where they will be related to the individual research methods.

12.4.5 Using the Experiences of Individuals to Inform Practice

In many cases, qualitative researchers will use multiple research methods aligned with their methodological orientation. Further, and particularly within health services research, the use of mixed qualitative-quantitative methods research is growing. In both cases, this illustrates the recognition that no single method and neither qualitative nor quantitative research on its own can reasonably be expected to fully address the complexities associated with clinically relevant research in the health professions.

As consumers of research – whether qualitative or quantitative – it is essential for you to understand the consequences of choices made by researchers and how this influences the weight you place on their findings in your day-to-day clinical work and decision-making. One particularly important issue for clinicians involves the concept of generalisability.

Recall from earlier chapters the premise of most quantitative research is to facilitate generalising from the specific to the general (i.e. extrapolating from the experience of a representative sample or subset to the broader, general population of interest). Qualitative research aimed at, for example, understanding 'barriers and facilitators' is often purported to produce a similar kind of generalisability. This becomes a daunting task if, for example, only a dozen, or twenty, or thirty patients have actually been interviewed.

A key concept in most qualitative research is the notion of indicativeness, rather than representativeness. Recall from earlier chapters the importance of sampling from a population as a way to support generalisability in quantitative research.

By assembling a representative sample, the researcher is able to concentrate efforts on a smaller group but still benefit from the opportunity to extrapolate findings to the general population of interest. Representativeness is crucial for this process: the sample must be demographically similar to the general population and contain, in representative proportions, the characteristics of interest and relevance to the study.

For practical reasons, it is almost impossible to construct qualitative 'samples' that are representative: the sample size required for statistical representativeness would mean hundreds if not thousands of interviews or observations might be required, an impossibility for almost any qualitative researcher. Since generalisability is not the usual intent of qualitative research, another barometer has been used to establish the quality and rigour of the research itself: indicativeness. Indicativeness does not require the study participants to be demographically representative of the study group, nor does it require a sample frame of a certain number of participants. Instead, indicativeness is an indicator of quality in qualitative research. Within health professions, we rely heavily upon indicativeness as a diagnostic tool: for example, in diagnosing a heart attack, we rely on signs and symptoms that are characteristic (or indicative) of a heart attack to guide treatment decisions. So long as our study participants are indicative – or characteristic – of the population of interest they need not be strictly and statistically representative of it in order to still generate valuable findings and hypotheses.

The methodology you chose as the foundation of your research is closely connected to your positionality as a researcher. Consequently, the identification and selection of most appropriate methodologies to guide your research should generally occur during or after the process of self-reflection and articulation of your biases and stances.

12.5. SOME COMMONLY APPLIED METHODOLOGIES

There are numerous qualitative research methods from which to select, once a methodology has been identified. Note that most of these methods can be applied within any of the methodologies; it is the *way* in which the method is used that is defined by the methodologies, not the actual selection of a particular method itself. We can conduct interviews with participants (Chapter 13) and focus groups (Chapter 14) and around those we can observe and document particular processes. Whatever method we choose it must enable participants to express themselves openly and without constraint.

To end this chapter we shall return to our case study students and pharmacists (see Table 12.1) and see how they might proceed with their research by using qualitative methods (Table 12.4).

TABLE 12.4   Qualitative Data Options for Case Studies

Case Study Researcher	Quantitative Data Collected	Qualitative Data That Might Be Collected
Sandy	• Age • Sex • Work status (school or university or employed) • Family history • Weight • Height • Data of diagnosis • Blood glucose	• How participants feel about having type II diabetes • What difference it makes to their lives • Would they like to change their diet and lifestyle
Dorothy	• Prescribing patterns of doctors, nurses, pharmacists and others • Attitudes towards prescribing antimicrobials • Barriers and facilitators associated with an antimicrobial stewardship programme	• Influences on prescribing • How do prescribers make their choices • The effect of barriers and facilitators on their practice • How they would feel about implementing an antimicrobial stewardship programme
Rosi	• Information about who is on campus, e.g. job, department, age, sex, whether they have any health conditions requiring medication • What prescription medication they take • What over-the-counter products they use • How often they visit a pharmacy off-campus • What they visit their pharmacy for • Whether they think it would be a good idea to have a pharmacy on campus	• Convenience issues of having a pharmacy on campus • Confidentiality • Why they think it would be a good idea or not to have a pharmacy on campus
Serena	• How long people have been smoking • How many cigarettes they smoke per day • Have they ever tried to quit smoking? • Have they used a smoking cessation aid? • If so which one?	• How people feel about smoking • How they feel about giving up • How they feel if they have failed to give up in the past

CHAPTER SUMMARY

- This chapter has described the differences between quantitative and qualitative research.
- It has outlined the principles of qualitative research and how and when it might be used.
- It has set out the ethics issues involved in asking people to talk about themselves.
- It has highlighted the importance of reflective practice in qualitative research.

FURTHER READING

A number of our recommendations about doing qualitative research come from the discipline of psychology. This is because most of the methodologies and methods have their roots there.

Doing Qualitative Research

Quinn Patton, M. (2015). *Qualitative research and evaluation methods: Integrating theory and practice* (4th ed.). Thousand Oaks: Sage. **Includes a section on ethics.**

Willig, C. (2013). *Introducing qualitative research in psychology* (3rd ed.). Maidenhead: Oxford University Press.

Qualitative Health Research

Murray, M., & Chamberlain, K. (Eds.), (1999). *Qualitative health psychology: Theories and methods.* London: Sage.

Qualitative Interviewing

13.1. INTRODUCTION

As we said in Chapter 12, numbers alone can't help us to understand 'how' people feel about the health issues that affect their lives and 'why', and 'how' and 'why' the ways people cope with illness and health differ from person to person. Also, individuals can sometimes find it harder or easier to cope with health changes depending on how they are feeling at the time and what else is going on in their lives. In order to help them as much as we can we need to understand the reasons why people can cope with some things and not others, how they feel and why.

Although there are a number of ways of collecting qualitative data, e.g. asking people to write free text answers to open questions in a questionnaire, talking to participants is a good way of collecting information about their experiences. For this reason we will be concentrating on interviews as a method of data collection throughout Chapters 13 to 17. In Chapter 19 we will outline some other ways of collecting and analysing qualitative data and we will point you towards some further reading on this subject.

Interviews are amongst the most common qualitative research methods used. As a method for gathering information from individuals, interviews have significant advantages because they are like having a conversation with your participants. Sometimes it is hard for participants to say all they want to say in answer to a questionnaire but in a well thought through interview, rich details can be elicited through carefully honed interviewing skills.

Since most human beings have significant experience with conversations, it is sometimes tempting to believe we are already experts at qualitative research involving interviewing.

As will be outlined in this chapter, interviewing is both an art and a science, and must be selected and implemented with care and forethought. Interviews may or may not be easy, practical and the most appropriate choice of method – all of this needs to be determined as part of the research planning process. In this chapter we will give you some ideas on how to get started with your interviews, how to build your interviews into your research design, how to design an interview schedule and some tips on how to conduct the interviews themselves.

In this chapter we will rejoin Sandy Sullivan, one of our case study pharmacists. Here is a reminder of what he was trying to do.

But let's leave Sandy for a little while and look at some more theory about interviewing.

CASE STUDY

Sandy Sullivan is our pharmacist working in a primary care collaborative practice. Sandy has an office within the practice, and spends most of his time meeting with patients to educate them on the most appropriate use of their medications; he also is available to consult with the GPs and other team members on issues related to pharmacotherapy, prescribing and medication use.

For the past year, he has been noticing more and more patients being diagnosed and treated for type II diabetes within the practice. This is particularly concerning since so many of these patients are young, typically less than 25 years of age. Even more concerning is his sense that, despite all the best efforts of the entire practice team, a large number of these young, newly diagnosed type II diabetes patients do not appear to be stabilising appropriately. Sandy believes he and his colleagues are following guidelines and providing the care required … yet his observations about the patients in the practice are troubling to him.

At the end of Chapter 11 we left Sandy with the results of the quantitative part of his study. Sandy had hypothesised that patients with a high BMI (over 25) would show poor blood glucose control over the period of 6 months of his study. There was no conclusive evidence of this so Sandy decided to go back to the drawing board and re-examine his data and indeed his research question. It may be that he could find out more by using qualitative methods. Sandy has been discussing his research question with colleagues and has decided that he really needs to find out what his patients think and feel about their blood sugar control before going any further. Perhaps he could use qualitative interviews to elicit more information. In the table at the end of Chapter 12 we showed you how Sandy and his colleagues might use qualitative methods to help achieve their research aims and we will show how Sandy might do this as we go through this chapter.

13.2. GETTING STARTED WITH INTERVIEWS

As outlined in Chapter 4, the choice of research method needs to be thought through at every stage of your research planning. Before starting to design your interview schedule there are a number of things you need to consider and we will look at those in detail throughout this chapter. We have already discussed (in Chapter 12) the importance of establishing right from the beginning of your research how you as a person actually feel about the topics you will be discussing. We called this your 'positionality' and recommended that you write a statement of your interests, biases, assumptions and stances based on your personal history, education and experience. Committing your positionality in writing, then frequently referring to it and amending as necessary during the research process is an important mechanism for enhancing the quality of your research, and for increasing the transparency of your work to your readers. Understanding yourself as the researcher is critical to the success of your work. Your positionality statement may then be useful in informing your methodological choices. As outlined in Chapter 12, methodology provides us with the overarching framework within which the research will be undertaken.

Clarity and specificity around methodology will help you to then select the most appropriate research method to achieve your research objectives. Accepting your own feelings about your topic and your participants will also go a long way to reducing **bias** in your research. Remember, it is your responsibility to let your participants tell their stories in their own ways and to recount these in the most honest and accurate way you can.

13.2.1. From Methodology to Interview

As you saw in the section on quantitative research (Chapter 2) it is essential for you to have a **research protocol** that specifies your research question, research aims and objectives and the design of your study. The framework within which your research is situated will guide not only the decision to select interviews as a method in the first place, but the way in which you will carry out the interview. In some cases, e.g. grounded theory (see Chapter 18) interviews provide the researcher with an opportunity to gather data unencumbered by any pre-existing guiding theories or hypotheses. Gathering data for the purpose of generating theory requires a certain openness of mind, the ability to honestly approach a situation without preconception or bias and allow the words of the participants to actually shape and direct both the interview itself and the subsequent analysis of the data. This may not be possible in some cases, depending upon your positionality. For example, if you were interested in determining the success of your efforts in patient counselling, and chose to interview patients whom you had counselled, it would not be realistic to assume a grounded theory methodological stance. This is because as the person who did the patient counselling in the first place, you have too much at stake and are too invested in the process to truly allow you to hear what your participants are saying. No matter how open and willing you may think you are to receive honest feedback about your work, it is unlikely that your participants are going to feel comfortable telling their counsellor the truth. Further, when the interviewer is also one of the subjects of the interview, grounded theory cannot apply – having been part of the patient counselling process itself, you will already have developed a series of ideas and assumptions about the process and the patient which will taint your interpretation of the data.

In other cases, the methodological choice will guide the emphasis you place on the interview process. For example, if you are situating your research within the **symbolic interactionist** tradition, you may have particular interests in the contextual clues provided by your participants. The words they speak will of course be relevant, but in this methodological framework, other cues (including non-verbal gestures, references to social contexts, etc.) may be of particular emphasis to you.

An interview – like most research methods – is simply a technique for gathering information and data from participants. The methodological framework which informs your interviews will help you to prioritise and emphasise what parts of the interview are of more or less relevance to you. This is an important thing to consider and plan in advance of your first interview: without a guiding methodology, data collection and analysis may become haphazard and improvised. Without a methodology, you may prioritise non-verbal cues for your first participant, verbal responses for your second participant, and incorrectly assume a grounded theory stance for your third interview. Interviews as a data-collection method work best when there is consistency of approach throughout the project: without methodology, you run the risk of having a sequence of self-contained interviews that were all executed in a different way, thereby limiting your ability to see patterns across the entire pool of interviews.

13.2.2. Why Choose to Do Interviews?

Interviews are frequently selected as a method of choice because of their conversational quality; through the process of interviewer and participant engaging in a social context it is more likely that thoughts and ideas can be explored. The to-and-fro of conversation in a comfortable environment intellectually stimulates both interviewer and participant to recall details, make connections and synthesise ideas in a way that simple self-reflection cannot accomplish. As a result, interviews are particularly well suited to exploratory research around concepts or ideas that are not well understood, described or articulated.

The opportunity to actually hear from participants – in their own words – is one of the greatest strengths of interviews. Within health care, there are circumstances where well-intentioned paternalism can create havoc. With their education and general desire to help, health care professionals can sometimes jump to conclusions about what is best for patients without truly taking the time to understand their perspectives, needs and wants. Qualitative interviewing provides an opportunity for participants to use their own words to describe these perspectives, needs and wants, rather than having them inferred rightly or wrongly by the health care professional. In circumstances where we recognise the importance of the patient's voice but do not have ready access to it, interviews can be a most useful method to achieve this objective.

Interviews are well suited to facilitate richness and depth: their conversational quality allows participants time and space to elaborate on their perspectives which in turn may seed further thoughts and conversations. Interviews are rarely brief affairs – in most cases, they will last at least 30–45 minutes, which provides significant opportunities to explore many different facets of a conversation in depth. The key to this process is effective use of elicitation techniques such as open-ended questions. Interviews may not be the most appropriate choice of method for a series of closed-ended questions which are perhaps better answered through survey methods. Closed-ended questions (i.e. questions that are generally answered with 'Yes' or 'No') may be used as part of an interview process, so long as time and space are provided to allow the participant to elaborate on his/her answer, and answer the question of why 'Yes' or 'No' was selected. In Section 12.3 we describe different types of interview and when they might be used.

Research interviews are complex time- and resource-intensive activities, and should not be embarked upon lightly. They are not simply about having a chat with your participants. Interviews are well-designed, information-gathering activities requiring a great deal of knowledge and skill for successful implementation. With this in mind the next section is devoted to thinking about the practicality of finding the right interview environment. It is important to think about this right at the beginning because it may take some time to find the right location.

13.2.3. Recruiting Participants for Your Interviews

Unlike quantitative research methods, there is no burden of 'representativeness' in selecting participants for your interviews. Indeed, it is likely mathematically impossible to assemble a sample frame for interviews that is statistically representative of your population of interest. As discussed in Chapter 12, the objective instead is to demonstrate indicativeness of your sample frame, finding participants who share important demographic characteristics of your population of interest but who also are ready, willing and able to share their stories, articulate their ideas, and be honest in their commentary. Purposive snowball sampling methods, in which participants refer other participants to you to contact for future interviews, is most frequently used in this context. Since there is no expectation of generalisability of findings beyond the sample group, the approach to recruitment of participants can focus on important issues such as convenience, logistics of travel, willingness to speak, etc.

In Chapter 12 we outlined the ethics issues associated with doing qualitative research and we urge you to look at these and to seek advice from your supervisor before beginning your research. Interviewing involves asking people to talk about themselves and needs to be done with care, placing your participants at the centre of all you do.

13.2.4. The Interview Environment

Interviews are a popular and common research method within most qualitative research methodologies. At the core of the interview process is the concept of 'elicitation'. Our aim is to make sense of or interpret life events in terms of the meanings people bring to them. Sometimes the people we interview don't really understand how they feel, and so gentle and respectful elicitation can create an atmosphere that enables the participant to explore his/her thoughts and feelings with the help of the researcher. It is essential that we create a comfortable environment so that participants feel free to actually share their thoughts with us without fear of judgment or retribution.

Creating this 'comfort zone' is one of the most important jobs for the interviewer: as part of your positionality statement it is critical to consider your capacity and ability to actually do this well – both in personal and practical terms. While most of us like to think we make other people comfortable, the reality may be different. For example, you will need to find the right location that suits the needs of participants and your needs as a researcher. Let's bring our practice pharmacist, Sandy, back and look at how he might think about the interview environment.

SANDY'S INTERVIEW ENVIRONMENT

- Sandy has his own office in the GP practice in which he is based
- Sandy's patients are used to coming to see him in the practice
- Is his office too formal?
- Would coming to his office for an interview make his patients feel they were coming for a routine consultation?
- There is a meeting room in the practice with comfortable chairs and tea and coffee-making facilities.

Sandy realises that he wants the patients he interviews to see him as a person who is interested in them rather than just the pharmacist who checks their blood sugar and weight. Of course, he is always going to be that pharmacist but perhaps by changing locations to the more informal meeting room he might be able to make the environment more relaxed.

Here are some key points about setting the scene of your interviews:
- Give participants information in advance about what to expect during the interview – the more information they have the more comfortable they will feel.
- Set the interview space somewhere that is easy for participants to get to.
- Make the interview space look and feel comfortable.
- Help your participants feel at ease with you. Interviews work best when interviewer and participant can feel relaxed in each other's company.

13.3. FORMS OF INTERVIEW DESIGN

Interviews are not simply on-the-fly casual conversations you make up as you go along. Instead, they are well-considered structured opportunities to gather thick and rich data from participants, using conversation as an opportunity for elicitation and 'riffing' (the process of building new thoughts by bouncing ideas off one another).

Interviews are usually guided by an **interview schedule** (see Section 13.4) and can range from fully structured interviews to fully unstructured with what are known as semi-structured interviews somewhere in the middle. Structured is generally set by the extent to which the questions are fixed or the fixed nature of the answers possible. Fully structured interviews constrain both questions and answers. Each of these formats has specific advantages and disadvantages in terms of information/data collection as well as knowledge and skills required.

13.3.1. Fully Structured Interviews

As the term implies, these interviews are very structured and detailed in terms of wording and sequence of questions. For this reason they are also called 'standardised interviews'. All participants in the interview process are asked the same questions, in the same order, regardless of their unique circumstances or interests. Each question in the **interview schedule** (see Section 13.4) which is used to guide the interviewer through the interview is carefully worded and, commonly, participants may be asked to choose a response from a set of options given to them by the researcher. Response options may be given in a number of formats including 'Yes'/'No', rating scales or multiple choice. The benefit of this type of interview is that the information it yields can be readily quantified, e.g. how many participants said what. This means that responses can be compared and contrasted across your study population. This method can be used when the researchers have a clearly defined study population and have the time and resources to spend interviewing each one individually. It also has the advantage that it can be done either face-to-face or on the telephone (think of market research companies who telephone you and ask you to take part in a survey) (Table 13.1, Box 13.1).

13.3.2. Unstructured Interviews

The interview schedule for a semi-structured interview is generally a list of talking-points or topics rather than specific questions so is sometimes referred to as a 'topic guide'. There are no precise questions and the order in which they are asked is not fixed. Where specific questions are noted in the topic guide they tend to be prompts for the researchers on ways to phrase a question, not a specific direction of how to conduct the interview with each participant. Some

TABLE 13.1	**Advantages and Disadvantages of Face-to-face and Telephone Interviewing**	
	Face-to-Face	**Telephone**
Time	Very time consuming	Less time consuming
Cost	Can be costly in both researcher time and participant access and travel expenses	Cheaper to administer and the researcher can stay in one place and telephone a list of participants
Accessible groups	Participants can be contacted in advance and a date for the interview set	Participants are only those who answer the telephone on the day so some groups of people may be missed
Quality of response	Can act on non-verbal cues, e.g. when someone is silent because they are thinking about their answer	No non-verbal cues
Quantity of response	Longer	Shorter

BOX 13.1 Example of Fully Structured Questions

How old are you?

What is your school or employment status? __School __full-time employment __part-time employment

Your age when you were diagnosed with diabetes? ____

Do any of your family members have diabetes? ___Yes ___No ___ Don't know___

Do you think your blood sugar is under control?___Yes ___No ___ Don't know___

Do you think your weight affects your blood sugar control? ___Yes ___No ___ Don't know___

BOX 13.2 Example of Unstructured Interview Content

I would like to chat to you today about your diabetes.

Tell me how old you are? It must have been quite hard to be diagnosed with diabetes, how did it make you feel?

Do any of your family have diabetes? If the answer is 'yes' then we could explore who they are and if they helped the interviewee with their diagnosis.

How do you feel about your blood sugar control?

---

questions or topics may not be covered or may be covered in a different way for each participant. The idea behind unstructured interviews is for the interviewer to respond to the verbal and non-verbal cues provided by the participant, using these cues to create questions and opportunities for dialogue in a way that enhances the comfort of the participant. At the far end of the 'unstructured' scale is a completely spontaneous interaction between participant and researcher which relies heavily upon the natural curiosity of both interviewer and interviewee. This is the most complex form of interviewing and relies heavily on the experience and the expertise of the researcher. With this approach, there are no specific questions and no interview schedule or topic guide. Instead, the interviewer must take note of verbal and non-verbal cues of the participant and shape the interview in real time. The lack of structure helps facilitate a natural, comfortable environment and supports elicitation. Such interviews are characterised by extraordinarily rich 'in the moment' experiences that can be invaluable in understanding a situation or a problem.

Analysis of unstructured interviews is time-consuming and can be difficult. Researchers using this method of qualitative research tend not to use quantitative means of any kind (although it is possible to count the number of times words or phrases are used in a form of '**content analysis**'). Analysis tends to involve audio-recording and transcription of interview data followed by an in-depth exploration of themes that emerge. The aim of such research is to tell the participants' stories using their own words in the form of direct quotations from interviews. These themes may or may not be interpreted by the researcher but such interpretation must be done with care to preserve the integrity of participants' narratives. In Chapters 16 and 17 we will describe the process of analysis of the output from qualitative interviews (Box 13.2).

13.3.4. Semi-Structured Interviews

This format is more structured than an informal conversation but less formal than a fully structured interview. For this reason it tends to be the method of choice for many health care researchers. There are many variations of semi-structured interviews that can be used according to the nature of the topic being discussed, the experience of the researcher-interviewers and the ultimate aim of the research. This type of interview will almost always be guided by an interview schedule or topic guide and this will be determined by the researcher at the start of the interview design process. The analysis of this type of interview can be either quantitative or thematic or a mixture of the two.

13.3.5. Making a Choice

The art in any face-to-face interviewing is to read the participant correctly, respond appropriately and use language and non-verbal cues to create the comfort zone we talked about in Section 13.2.4. This will help the participant feels at ease and encourage conversation. By not dictating specific questions that must be asked, there is greater flexibility for the interviewer to probe certain issues of relevance in greater depth. For inexperienced interviewers, this can be daunting, as it means each interview takes on a life of its own. It is a good idea to practice interviewing and being interviewed by fellow students or colleagues, and many of you will have done this already as part of your MPharm degree programme. With unstructured interviewing there is generally no need to worry about covering the same topics with every participant. For example, if you wanted to explore individuals' perceptions of a diagnosis of diabetes (as we think Sandy might want to do) then each participant's experience will be unique. However, we may think that participants might share some common feelings and thoughts about their diagnosis and in this case semi-structured interviews would be the method of choice.

Research interviewing is about finding the balance between responsiveness and flexibility to each participant's unique characteristics, but we may want to ensure that the same general areas of interest are explored with each and every interview participant and that a core set of data is collected from each interview, while also permitting a reasonable degree of flexibility and adaptability to respond to each participant's unique reality. In standardised open interviews, the interviewer is clearly in charge and directing the interview; in semi-structured interviews, the interviewer may still be 'driving the bus', but is more responsive to suggestions from the participant for what direction to follow.

Let's pause for a moment and look at how Sandy might make decisions about the best way to interview his participants.

13.4. DEVELOPING AN INTERVIEW SCHEDULE

One of the most important preparatory steps for interviewers is to develop a standardised open or semi-structured interview schedule or topic guide. This schedule will guide the interview process and provide you with a memory-jogger in case you lose your way in the interview or if the conversation slows down. In developing an interview schedule, there are several key considerations:

a. Use open-ended questions as much as possible, to facilitate and build the conversation, e.g. *How do you feel about that*? Closed questions shut down conversation and send a message to the participant that their words and voice don't really matter all that much, e.g. *Do you feel unhappy about that*?

b. Be careful about using terminology that is too complex – or too simple – for your participants, particularly when dealing with anatomical terms or bodily functions. Be respectful of how others may talk about sensitive issues. The term 'mirroring' is used to describe the technique of using the words the participant himself/herself uses to move the conversation along. If your participant uses the term 'pee' to describe urination, use that term. If she/he uses the term 'make water', use that term. Do not allow your own squeamishness to interfere with mirroring, but also be respectful of your own boundaries in terms of words you simply don't feel comfortable using.

c. Avoid use of judgemental or value-laden words and concepts. It can sometimes be easy in an interview to lapse into an overly familiar conversational style and say something like 'You don't really believe that, do you?' or 'Seriously, you did that?' These should be avoided as they are cueing to participants and judgmental. Similarly be careful about assuming you and your participant share similar values about what is 'good' or 'better': for example, you may assume that adherence to prescription directions is a 'good' thing but your participant may have different ideas. The objective of interviewing is to explore such diverging thoughts and ideas in depth, so do not shut them down by making assumptions.

d. Ask only one question at a time. Be careful about overwhelming your participant with too many questions – you are not running an inquisition! Give sufficient time for the participant to reflect before speaking and don't force them to answer something for which they do not have an opinion. This will undermine the quality of the data you collect.

e. Be careful about overusing the question 'Why?' In an attempt to better understand what a participant is saying, you may wish to probe more deeply. 'Why' questions are well suited for such probing but (as any parent knows) they become extremely tiresome after a while. A few 'why' probing follow-up questions during an interview are to be expected, but don't overdo it!

f. Writing good interview questions is as much art as science; finding the right balance between specificity and flexibility

SANDY – CHOICE OF DESIGN AND WHY

At the beginning of this chapter we gave you a summary of Sandy's research and said that he had been unable to find evidence for why people with a higher body mass index (BMI) had poorer control over their blood glucose levels, using quantitative methods. This could be for a number of reasons including how he designed his study in the first place or that he needs a larger number of patients in his study. It could also mean, of course, that high BMI is not a reason for poor blood glucose control amongst his study population. Sandy thinks that his early thoughts that blood glucose and weight (as measured by BMI) may not be right so he thinks through what he should do next:

- Look back at his results and in particular what his participant demographics are. Here is the table from Chapter 10 that shows some of these:

ID	Age	Sex	Work Status	FH	Weight	Body Mass Index (BMI)	Date of Diagnosis	DAY1 BG1 A	DAY1 BG1 B	DAY1 BG2 A	DAY1 BG2 B
1	17	m	school	Yes		25		4.2	7.4		
2	16	f	school	No		28		5.6	8.4		
3	22	f	uni	No		19		7.9	9.2		
4	19	m	work	No		29		6.2	9.3		
5	25	m	work	No		15		3.6	5.4		
6	19	m	unemp	No		33		6.0	8.7		
7	18	m	school	Yes		31		5.4	8.0		
8	24	f	school	Yes		22		4.1	7.1		
9	21	f	work	Yes		35		9.3	11.4		
10	20	f	uni	Yes		19		7.6	9.3		
11	18	m	work	No		26		7.2	9.9		

- Looking at the table above Sandy can see that a similar number of males and females had high BMIs at the start of his study.
- Those with higher BMIs are also in a variety of situations, e.g. school, university and work.
- Some of those with higher BMIs have a family history of diabetes.

Sandy can see that there are some unanswered questions here such as what do these patients eat and when. It may be that it is the type of diet rather than the amount they are eating that is responsible for the poor blood glucose control. It may also be that being brought up in a family with a history of diabetes may make a difference to diet, weight and blood glucose control.

These are things that Sandy could not have put in his questionnaire – it would have taken far too long for his participants to reply. He knows now that if he had done some qualitative background work before his survey then he might have had a better picture of the reasons for the lack of blood glucose control.

Sandy is determined to find out the answers to his research question and decides to design a small qualitative study. He bases his study on the following things:

- He could talk to his patients individually using one-to-one interviews to find out about them and their lives. This would mean that what they say won't be shared with anyone else.
- Or he could talk to his patients as a group, using a focus group technique, which means that what his patients say will be shared with others.

There are advantages and disadvantages to both methods so we will show you how Sandy might proceed with one-to-one interviews and then in Chapter 15 we will show you how he might use focus groups to explore the perceptions of his patients further.

Sandy decides to use semi-structured interviews (Section 13.3.4) to keep his options open about what he asks and how. More importantly, he wants to give his patients the chance to talk freely without constraining them to answer particular questions in a particular order.

We will return to some theory now and at the end of the next section we will give you an example of a guide that Sandy could use for his interviews.

is crucial but difficult to do. Within a health services context, and particularly for pharmacists, it is sometimes challenging to write questions that do not lead participants to your own foregone conclusions. Leading questions are those where a desired answer is implicit in the phrasing of the question. For example, asking 'How did antibiotic side effects like diarrhoea influence your decision as to whether to take the medication as prescribed?' may lead participants towards a specific negative response. The inclusion of such a significant and negative side effect like 'diarrhoea' in the question sets a tone at the outset of something distasteful to be avoided, which puts participants in a negative frame of mind at the beginning of the question. Instead, it may be useful to break this question up into smaller components, for example 'What was your experience with side effects with the antibiotic?' then, 'How did these experiences influence your thinking about whether to take the medication as it was prescribed?'

g. Think about your follow-up and redirecting prompts in advance: even the most carefully constructed and pilot-tested interview schedule may not perform as expected in the real world. Interviewers need to be constantly on their toes to be able to gently nudge participants back on to task if they start to veer off in directions that may be unhelpful to the research objective. Polite and affirming redirecting statements such as, 'That's such an interesting observation! I wish we had time to explore all of these important points but with your permission I'd like to return to the focus for our interview today', must be prepared and rehearsed in advance to be sincere and effective. Similarly, follow-up prompts (other than the ever-present 'Why?' question) must also be considered. Examples of follow-up prompts may include, 'And how did that make you feel?' or 'And what did others think about your decision?' Follow-up prompts help you to probe deeper into the significance of a participant's response or focus on a meaningful aspect of that response in greater detail.

Getting back to Sandy and the development of his topic guide, there are a number of ways Sandy might design the guide for his interviews. We will call this a 'topic guide' because the interview is semi-structured and Sandy wants to leave it as open as possible. We are sure you can think of other things you would like to ask and in different ways, but below is one example of a topic guide Sandy could use. You can find out more about designing interview schedules in the Further Reading section at the end of this chapter.

If you go online to the material that supports this textbook you will have the opportunity to design your own interview schedule/topic guide.

13.5. CONDUCTING INTERVIEWS

In general, novice interviewers will find standardised open interviews to be most effective at managing nervousness and inexperience with the process. Only the most seasoned interviewers will feel comfortable and confident using informal conversational interviewing; in many cases, the most practical middle-ground will be use of semi-structured interviews. Once the interview format has been established, there are important next-steps to consider to optimise the likelihood of success with the research, including (a) preparing for the interview; (b) constructing questions/items for a semi-structured or standardised interview schedule; and (c) actually conducting the interview.

13.5.1. Before the Interview

Preparing for the interview is arguably the most important step of the process, proving again the research adage that 'well begun is half done'. Key aspects to consider in organising yourself in advance of the interview include:

a. Select an appropriate setting for your interview: Finding a place that is comfortable, private, and with minimal distraction is important. Do not simply arrange to meet participants at a local coffee shop or restaurant – it is not private enough and there are too many environmental distractions that will compromise elicitation. In general, a participant's home ground (e.g. their office or classroom) is preferred – it minimises inconvenience for the participant and can make them feel more comfortable. However, there are times when participants may find it easier to be in a completely anonymous location – in which case you should accommodate that as best you can. In most circumstances, though, you should avoid a completely private location, like the participant's home. It is important to be mindful of your own safety and security since, in many cases, you may be meeting a participant for the very first time and know very little about them. Ensure you let other people know about your whereabouts, keep a mobile phone with you at all times and be aware of potential risks to safety. You could arrange to meet in a very public location – such as a coffee shop – for initial introductions, and then move to a more private but not isolated location for the actual interview itself. When in doubt, never compromise your safety and security, or the perception of safety of the participant, even if it means the interview ends up being conducted in a less than ideal public location.

b. Ensure the participant understands the objective of the interview: In some cases, participants may agree to be interviewed without fully understanding your objectives and their responsibilities. Prior to even starting the interview, confirm this understanding with the participant and allow them opportunities to ask questions about the purpose of the interview, and how the data will be used and managed. If there is an honorarium provided or expenses paid to the participant, ensure relevant paperwork and documentation for financial auditing purposes are completed at this point.

c. Explain how confidentiality will be protected and anonymity will be maintained: Research ethics boards will require you to outline a coherent system for protecting the identity of all participants in your research to the best of your abilities. Commonly used techniques will include use of pseudonyms or number codes rather than actual real names, and secure storage of raw data including consent forms that may identify who participated in the research. All these procedures need to be explained to participants. If the nature of your research is such that the kind of participant being interviewed is so unique it is not possible to anonymise them, this should be fully disclosed in advance.

d. Outline the process of the interview: Let the participant know how much time is going to be taken, whether you are audio-taping and/or maintaining field notes, and how the interview process will play out. If, as part of the interview, you are going to present hypothetical cases or other activities to spur discussion, let the participant know about this in advance.

e. Clearly explain the rights of participants: All participants have the right to withdraw some or all of their comments and data at any time from your research. They may inadvertently say something they didn't mean to say, and then ask you to delete that from the record; conversely, they may ask you to turn off the tape recorder at a certain point so as not to be recorded saying something. Several days after the interview, the participant may have a change of heart and ask you to strike a comment from the record. All of these are rights of participants – you must inform them of these up-front so they are aware of their options. You should also consider mechanisms for follow-up, allowing your participants to review their own comments at a later date and to review summary manuscripts or reports that flow from the research.

f. Provide clear follow-up contact information: Ensure participants know how to contact you by email and/or phone if they have questions or concerns following the interview. If you are a student researcher, ensure your supervisor's contact information is also included, as well as contact details for the research ethics board that approved the project.

g. Provide sufficient opportunities for questions from participants to address topics you have not discussed.

h. Only when you are happy that your participant is happy should you invite them to sign a consent form to take part in the interview. This should be signed by both participant and interviewer and each should have a copy.

As can be seen, this process can be time consuming and is not the sort of thing that can be left to the last minute. In some cases, it may be preferable to schedule two meetings with your participants so these preliminaries can be dealt with first, allowing sufficient time for the actual interview itself.

Another key aspect of interviewing preparation involves rehearsal with your interviewing format. Most researchers will pilot-test interview schedules as a way of enhancing their confidence in using them, as well as to ensure the schedule performs as expected. There are no rules governing the number of pilot interviews that should be done – in large part, this will depend on your own comfort with interviewing. In general, novice interviewers should expect to pilot-test interviews with 3–5 people prior to launching the interviews for real; more experienced interviewers may only need to pilot test on 2–3 individuals. Learning to interview effectively is more than just reading off a schedule or topic guide; it also means learning how to ask questions, listen to responses, observe non-verbal cues and respond in real-time, all while looking natural and composed.

13.5.2. During the Interview

Careful preparation in advance of the interview can save significant time and stress during the interview itself. During the interview, however, there are certain techniques that are important to use to keep you and your participant on task, on track, and on time:

a. Ensure your recording equipment is working during the interview itself. It is important to verify, in real time, that you are actually recording the interview (if that is part of your protocol) and that your equipment is functioning properly. Do not assume that a pre-interview check is all that is needed. You do not want to end the interview only to learn there was a problem half-way through the interview and in fact no data were actually recorded! You must also ask your participants to give their consent to the interview being recorded. An example of a Consent Form is given at the end of this section (Box 13.3).

b. Stay as neutral as you can during the interview, and be mindful of your 'tells'. Tells are social cues (usually non-verbal) that communicate to a participant what you are actually thinking and feeling even if you use no words. For example, an arched eyebrow, a surprised look, or an uncomfortable cough all convey a message of discomfort that will be picked up by the participant. Such cues do not help you to set a comfortable environment and in

---

BOX 13.3   Participant Consent Form

Project Researchers   **University of Maghull**
Sandy Sullivan and Professor Sutton-Austin

Study Into Young People and Diabetes
Interview Consent Form
Please tick all boxes that apply to you

1.   I confirm that I have read and understand the information sheet dated 1st February   _____(Initial)
        2017 for the above study.
2.   I understand that my participation is voluntary and that I am free to withdraw at   _____(Initial)
        any time up until the analysis of the information from the interview.
3.   I agree to be audio recorded during the interview.   _____(Initial)
4.   I understand that all data collected during the study will be anonymous and my   _____(Initial)
        participation kept anonymised.
5.   I agree to the anonymised transcript from my interview being made available for   _____(Initial)
        use in future research, by the same research team.
6.   I agree to be quoted in academic journals or magazines and understand any   _____(Initial)
        quotes will be anonymised so that I cannot be identified from them.
7.   I agree to take part in the study.   _____(Initial)

_____   _____   _____
Name of participant   Date   Signature
_____   _____   _____
Name of researcher   Date   Signature

---

fact will shut down elicitation as they may be interpreted as judgmental.

c. Use encouraging non-verbal cues to keep the dialogue going. Nodding your head, or the occasional 'uh-huh' are non-verbal signals of interest and engagement and used in natural conversations as techniques to continue a dialogue. Such non-verbal signals are the opposite of the judgmental ones discussed in (b) above.

d. If you are taking your own handwritten field notes during the interview (to complement or replace an audio recording) tell your participants what you are doing and then make sure you do so in a natural and unobtrusive way. Keep your eyes on the participant and not on your notebook. Failure to maintain appropriate eye contact is a strong social cue that you are uninterested or distressed by something you have heard and will shut down conversation.

e. Mirror the non-verbal and verbal communication of your participant, particularly when it comes to things like smiling, laughing, and facial cues. Such mirroring helps to establish a comfortable environment and reduces risk that you will be perceived as judgmental or authoritarian, which in turn will enhance elicitation and improve the quality of data you gather.

13.5.3.   After the Interview

After concluding the interview and thanking your participant, the real research work can begin! If you have used an audio recorder to capture data, you will need to produce transcripts of the interview. Verbatim transcripts are word-for-word scripts of what exactly was said during the interview. Be sure to anonymise your transcripts to protect the confidentiality of your participant: using a pseudonym or numerical code can be helpful here. Summary transcripts are excerpts that are produced from the audio tape, frequently containing a combination of both exact verbatim quotations in key instances and a summary of a discussion in less critical parts of the discussion. Verbatim and summary transcripts, taken together with your field notes maintained during the interview itself, become a significant data repository for your future analysis.

In most cases, particularly for novice researchers, it is recommended that you do your own transcriptions rather than getting a professional transcriber to help you with this work. In producing your own transcripts, you will re-live or re-experience the interview and this will provide you with important and unique insights that will be valuable during analysis. Additionally, the person completing the interview is best able to address recording flaws (e.g. mumbling) and fill in gaps that an outsider would not be able to do. Software such as Dragon Dictation may sometimes be used to expedite the transcription process; however, even the best transcription software will still make errors and will not be able to provide the context that you as the interviewer can provide during transcription. Remember that your transcripts are your most valuable data source – poor transcripts will frustrate your attempts at data analysis and synthesis, so taking the time and care needed to produce the best-quality transcripts possible will enhance the outcome of your work.

In many cases, interviewers use the process of generating transcripts in an iterative way; they learn how to be better interviewers the next time by transcribing an earlier interview. This type of development is particularly valuable for making sure that you follow-up interesting topics in subsequent interviews, and another reason why producing your own transcripts is generally desirable.

A critical question for many interviewers relates to the number of interviews you are required to do in order to demonstrate rigour in your processes. Unlike in quantitative research, where a sample size calculation can be undertaken to determine how many participants are required, there is no mathematical formula indicating how many interviews are required to provide confidence of indicativeness. Instead, qualitative researchers rely on the notion of saturation.

Saturation is generally defined as the process of ensuring adequate, necessary and sufficient data have been collected through the interview process to facilitate attainment of research objectives. Words such as 'adequate, necessary and sufficient' may be interpreted differently by different people; in general, we use the term *saturation* to mean nothing new is learned or added through additional interviews. It can be challenging to know at what point this occurs; for all researchers there is always a belief in the possibility that one more interview may yield something new, different or important. Of course, this can result in endless 'one more interviews' being undertaken for no additional gain. The researcher must rely upon a thorough process of analysis and coding, complemented by his/her intuition, to make the declaration of saturation. Traditionally, qualitative researchers have suggested that 8–15 interview participants is needed before the declaration of saturation can be made (see the Miles and Huberman book in Further Reading). As we have said before, there is a lot of work involved in qualitative research. For example, you can expect 1 hour of recording to take about 8 hours to transcribe. The transcription can run to 20–30 sides of A4 paper, depending on how much each participant has to say. For this reason if you try to do too many interviews, your data will become very difficult to manage. We will talk more about this and other issues about managing your data in Chapters 16 and 17. In the following chapter we will concentrate on collecting research data using focus groups.

CHAPTER SUMMARY

- This chapter has outlined some of the key principles of research interviewing.
- It has described recruitment procedures.
- It has outlined the importance of the interview environment.

- Finally, it has provided guidance on what to do before, during and after the interview.

FURTHER READING

Doing Qualitative Research

Quinn Patton, M. (2015). *Qualitative research and evaluation methods: integrating theory and practice* (4th ed.). Thousand Oaks: Sage. *Includes a section on research interviewing.*

Willig, C. (2013). *Introducing qualitative research in psychology* (3rd ed.). Maidenhead: Oxford University Press.

Research Interviewing

Mishler, E. G. (1991). *Research Interviewing: context and narrative.* USA: Harvard University Press.

Qualitative Health Research

Murray, M., & Chamberlain, K. (Eds.), (1999). *Qualitative health psychology: theories and methods.* London: Sage.

Focus Groups

LEARNING OBJECTIVES

After reading this chapter you should be able to:
- understand what a focus group is
- describe some of the challenges faced by researchers when running focus groups
- understand the effect of social interaction on the focus group
- describe how and when to use a focus group

14.1 INTRODUCTION

Focus groups are an increasingly popular form of qualitative research with roots in the marketing and business world. Focus groups involve a small number of individuals sharing their perceptions, opinions, beliefs and attitudes with one another, generally within a facilitated discussion environment. One of the great advantages of a focus group process is the opportunity for individuals to 'riff' off one another. Riffing is the process by which ideas are generated and built through highly engaged and interactive conversation. One person's thought triggers another person's idea which in turn produces other perspectives that further amplify and refine a discussion. Unlike interviews which are limited to **dyads** (a dyad is something that consists of two parts), where one person is clearly the 'researcher' and the other is clearly the 'participant', focus groups facilitate more dynamic interactions which can result in great synergies – or produce significant chaos! Similar to interviewing, the process of facilitating a focus group discussion is complex and requires knowledge and skill. In this chapter we will continue to follow our case study pharmacist Sandy, and see how he might use a focus group in his research.

14.1.1. What Is a Focus Group?

The use of a focus group is a method of bringing together individuals for a facilitated group discussion. Although it's use has a long history in marketing, business and social sciences, the term 'focus group' itself is relatively new. One of the most extensive examples of the use of focus groups was in the United States of America during World War II, when groups of civilians were asked to comment on the success and value of different forms of wartime propaganda designed to inspire patriotism and motivate young men to join the war effort. From its outset, the focus group has had a behavioural change orientation, one that is in part related to persuasion and understanding what motivates individuals to behave in certain ways.

Focus groups represent a type of interview that is based on discussions amongst individuals, but this is not just another variation of an interview. It is not a more time-efficient way of running interviews by saying *'let's interview 8 people at the same time and call it a focus group!'* The focus group is its own, unique qualitative research method that will generate distinct and different data than interviews would. Interviews and focus groups are not interchangeable methods but frequently are complementary and can help the researcher better understand a situation or problem.

14.1.2. Social Interaction

The increase in understanding of complex issues that focus groups can bring comes from the interaction between the members of the group. Methodologically, focus groups are more firmly grounded within the **symbolic interactionist** paradigm, since the explicitly social milieu of the focus group requires individual participants to effectively navigate peer relationships as part of the process. Focus groups are generally less suited to the grounded theory methodology (see Chapter 18). This is because in order to actually be functional and useful, the facilitator needs to assume some leadership to ensure control and order during the proceedings. This control and leadership presumes a level of knowledge and awareness of the situation itself. A facilitator who knows nothing about the content of the focus group (as would be expected for grounded theory work) would not be able to manage proceedings effectively, and the focus group itself would likely devolve into a situation where the loudest voices prevail.

Focus groups may be used for many different purposes, both constructivist and positivist in their orientations (see Chapter 1, Section 3.4). On the one hand, focus groups can be used for consensus building purposes, to take a group of individuals with their own unique viewpoints then, through the process of discussion, build some kind of agreement, in a positivist-oriented manner. Conversely, focus groups can also be used to elicit a number of different ideas and perceptions from the group members with no attempt to reconcile or unify them into agreement. Such a constructivist-orientation can allow the focus group to be a spring board for discussions and a free-flow of idea generation.

Given the multiple ways in which focus groups can be used, and the multiple options available for facilitators, it is essential that researchers using focus groups have a clear understanding of their remit, a strong set of interpersonal and communication skills to allow them to act effectively as a facilitator, and alignment between research objectives, methodologies, and this method.

14.2 HOW DO FOCUS GROUPS WORK?

The essential core of the focus group is the idea that group discussion produces insights that could not be triggered through one-on-one dialogue or self-reflection alone. The process uses **riffing** or **cascading**. This is where group members listen to each other and the ways thoughts and feelings are expressed and are stimulated to add to the discussion. This passing on and stimulation of ideas relies on the intensely social nature of human cognition and emotion. Symbolic interactionism is a particularly well suited methodology for focus group methods given its emphasis on the social construction of realities. However, there are alternative methods, for example, participant observation, which uses ethnographic and action research principles. These are discussed in Chapter 15 (Observational Research) and Chapter 18.

The psychology that underpins the success of focus groups is both complex and fascinating, and it is critical for the researcher to understand this psychology prior to using this method. While interviews rely heavily on the notion of a comfort zone to foster elicitation (see Chapter 13), focus groups work through a more combative or confrontational process, where discomfort and disagreement are the catalyst for conversation, discussion and idea generation. Focus groups where all participants are constantly agreeing with one another may actually raise doubts as to their value and the quality of data generated. Not all potential research

participants will be comfortable in the hurly-burly environment of a focus group; for some individuals, the simple thought of speaking out in front of a group of strangers is daunting. For others, the need to be liked is so strong that they may simply agree to whatever anyone else says simply to avoid confrontation, and as a result, will not actually disclose their true thoughts and feelings. For yet others, there may be great susceptibility to simply go along with what the crowd says and does. The unique nature of focus group interactions requires participants have a particular kind of psychological make-up to make them successful. The ability to speak up, the ability to listen, the ability to think on one's feet and respond in real time, and the ability to psychologically manage a socially complex and inherently combative environment are all necessary attributes for focus group participants.

14.2.1. Group Dynamics

The term 'group dynamics' refers to the behaviours and psychological processes that happen within (**intra**group dynamics) or between (**inter**group dynamics) social groups. It is something that has been studied since the end of the nineteenth century and has an impact on our understanding of social prejudice and discrimination, e.g. racism or sexism. In focus groups we are interested in intragroup dynamics, and they can help us to understand the group process in two different ways:

- At the intrapersonal level we can learn about the thoughts, feelings and attitudes of the individuals who make up the group.
- At the intragroup level we can learn about how members of the group interact and communicate with each other.

In everyday society groups tend to form naturally say as a result of an interest, e.g. playing football and supporting a particular team, or an occupation, e.g. working as a pharmacist in a particular pharmacy sector. In these cases people can be part of different groups at different levels. In the first example this might be 'all football supporters' and 'all supporters of XXX football team' and the individuals concerned are likely to behave differently when interacting in each group. So, all football supporters might show solidarity when a TV channel suggests dropping coverage of important matches, but that solidarity disappears when they are supporting individual teams. In fact, as we have often seen, solidarity can readily turn to conflict and aggression before, during and after football matches – sometimes with disastrous consequences.

When we set up focus groups we are, in a sense, forcing people to become members of groups that are new to them. This is in spite of the fact that they may have been drawn from the same participant pool, e.g. pharmacists, and will have volunteered to take part. Understanding the way people can behave when in groups is important if you are going to be an effective facilitator. You must be able to recognise the different dynamics going on between group members and both use them to your advantage or use your understanding to divert group members who might be heading for disagreement. Sometimes focus group members just all seem to get on very well together and you will witness a sense of group cohesion, especially if as a facilitator you show and lack of understanding of the topics being discussed. This can result in the whole group disagreeing with what you have said and being quite vocal about it. On the other hand there may be one person in the group who consistently differs from the others in their attitudes or values. This is sometimes called the 'black sheep effect' and can be difficult to deal with as it can create conflict within the group. It is the role of the facilitator (as you will see in Section 14.6) to use the differences between group members to explore ideas and issues about the topics under discussion, but not to allow these to escalate into argument and unpleasantness. Finally, in most groups there will be those who talk a lot and those who do not talk very much. There will also often be one person who emerges as a leader or 'star'. This person may have very little to say but when they do speak, they say things that seem to resonate with the rest of the group – almost as if they represent the group's views. There is a huge amount of literature on group dynamics, and you can find some references to this in the Further Reading section at the end of this chapter.

14.2.2. How and When to Use a Focus Group

There is a long tradition of use of focus groups in politics, business and marketing, particularly when researchers are interested in complex issues related to motivations and intentions to behave. More than interviews, focus groups used in such contexts are explicitly purported to be generalisable to the population of interest, even though methodologically this is quite unlikely. Advertisers run focus groups prior to launching national campaigns with the desire to 'test' how their product placement will be perceived by the general public. Similarly, politicians use focus groups as a way of evaluating whether a specific stance on a particular issue can be expected to gain or lose votes come election time. Using focus groups in isolation as a tool for predicting population-based outcomes and behaviours is quite risky. This is because it is mathematically very difficult to actually build focus groups that are representative samples of their populations, given the unique characteristics required for successful and effective functioning within a focus group setting itself.

Focus groups are perhaps most effectively utilised at critical points within a research project where decisions must be made but clear direction is unavailable. For example,

focus groups can be effective tools for helping researchers interpret the words and thoughts of participants, as a prelude to development of a survey for more general distribution. Alternatively, focus groups can be effective as a way of helping researchers interpret the results of a survey and can bring quantitative data to life using participants' own words. When researchers simply feel 'stuck' and unable to generate ideas or determine a direction for research, a focus group can provide a valuable springboard (and sounding board) for where a project needs to go. This is a good point to take a break from the theory and see how Sandy might use focus groups as part of his research.

CASE STUDY: SANDY

In Chapter 13 we learned how Sandy could use semi-structured interviews to help him to find out more about his young patients who have type II diabetes. As we saw, face-to-face, semi-structured interviews would give his patients the opportunity to talk privately about their condition. Sometimes, though, it can be helpful to have a group discussion so that people can bounce ideas off each other, to hear about other people's experiences and even to help people feel they are not alone in those. Sandy thinks that it might be useful to get some of his patients together in small groups to talk about some of the issues he has heard about during the course of his consultations with them. Using a focus group technique means that what his patients say will be shared with others, and he could use his understanding of diabetes management to develop his focus group topic guide. Sandy will need to follow the advice contained in the next sections, and we will embed some specific ideas for Sandy as we go along.

14.3. FOCUS GROUP DESIGN AND PLANNING

Contrary to what some may think, focus groups are both time consuming and resource intensive, and they can require significant planning, effort and resources in order to be successful. It is essential, therefore, that they be used appropriately and in the most effective way possible.

For focus groups to function effectively there are certain key elements that are required, and we will explore these in the following sections.

14.3.1. Facilitation

A facilitator is someone who can moderate the discussion and keep the group on time, on task and on track. This is not an easy job and in many cases researchers themselves may lack the skills and confidence to fill this role. In such cases, it is often possible to recruit an external individual to actually moderate the focus group session itself, though this will require significant training to ensure alignment with your research objectives. If you lack confidence in acting as the facilitator for your own focus group, and if there is no budget to bring in external expertise, the focus group method may not be an appropriate choice for your needs. We will talk in more detail about facilitator roles and responsibilities in Section 14.6.

> Sandy will be the facilitator for his focus group and fortunately he has done this before. He helped a colleague run a focus group for people with high blood pressure and has a reasonably good idea of what he should do.

14.3.2. Participants

Focus groups should be constructed to minimise previous professional or social interactions amongst participants. At their best, focus groups generally consist of groups of strangers with no awareness of each other and consequently minimal personal 'baggage' which may interfere with or affect proceedings. At times, it simply may not be possible to build focus groups where each participant is unknown to all others; in such cases, it is advisable to ensure strong facilitators are available to manage potential previous relationships and to use a more structured focus group protocol to guide discussions. Where this is not possible, it may be prudent to consider an alternative data-collection method such as interviews to prevent contamination of results through previous social relationships.

> All of the people who will be part of the focus groups will know Sandy and some will know each other from coming to the clinic. This may or may not help; Sandy knows that a couple of them don't get on very well so it might be good to make sure they are not in the same group!

14.3.3. Ground Rules

The facilitator needs to clearly establish – and enforce – certain ground rules around the operations of the focus group. Issues related to turn-taking, managing disagreement/ dissent, speaker order and air-time to prevent one person from monopolizing discussion are all complex aspects of focus-group management. At the outset, it is important the facilitator indicates how these sorts of issues will be managed

during the focus-group proceedings – and to follow through and manage them as outlined. Failure to do so will undermine the credibility of the facilitator and the process and will likely lead the focus group to devolve into chaos. Once again, without a strong facilitator empowered to establish and enforce ground rules, an alternative data collection may be required.

Be clear on what the remit of the focus group will be: is it attempting to find commonality and consensus/agreement, or is it about using riffing and cascading techniques to generate and build ideas out of disagreement? Clarifying this in advance, and ensuring both facilitator and participants are clear will help the focus group to succeed.

14.3.4. Focus Group Effectiveness

Focus groups are generally most effective and appropriate in the following circumstances:

a. Participants are authentically engaged and interested in the topic of the research – selecting the right participants to contribute to a focus group is essential. Unlike other forms of quantitative research, a representative sample of the population is not necessarily a requirement for a focus group. While a focus group that is indicative of the population of interest is desirable, the ability to actually keep up with and contribute to the proceedings of the focus group is as important an attribute of success as any other demographic characteristic.

b. When something – but not a lot – is known about the subject. Focus groups are generally less appropriate within a grounded theory methodological framework. To simply manage the logistics of a focus group means the facilitator must have some pre-existing knowledge or experience with the content area, which in turn will mean the facilitator will enter the focus group with some preconceptions. In order to organise and operationalise a focus group, it is usually helpful to know something and have some pre-existing ideas, theories or hypotheses about the research subject of interest. Conversely, if a lot is already known about the subject of interest, focus groups may not be the most efficient way of gathering information; consider a survey or other method instead that can reach more individuals.

c. Some theory generating and some theory testing are both required. Focus groups may be most effective when researchers are midway through a project and require support for both theory generation and theory testing simultaneously. The unique structure of focus groups means it is possible to use them as both a sounding board for testing of 'trial balloons' as well as to help researchers sort through complex data sets and ideas to start to generate and refine hypotheses for subsequent testing.

d. When there is a power or hierarchy difference: The group aspect of focus groups can provide some powerful insulation for those seeking to speak truth to power. While a single individual within a one-on-one interview setting may be hesitant to truly speak his/her mind where large power differentials exist, a consensus-building focus group distributes responsibility (and blame) across a larger number of individuals – which in turn may make it more likely in some cases that honest responses will be provided. Similarly, when confronting power differentials based on professional status, focus groups can be a powerful tool for addressing differences in the ways in which patients and practitioners think, act, and behave.

e. When there is a need to be respectful of the audience: Focus groups can be the safest type of qualitative research method for some individuals because of the notion of 'safety in numbers'. When participants outnumber researchers – as they do in focus group – a measure of power and control rests with the group, and this can be a valuable tool to generate honest discussion and dissent.

14.4.   FOCUS GROUP IMPLEMENTATION

A well-run focus group is both an invaluable tool for researchers and a pleasure for participants. At their best, focus groups provide participants with a stimulating opportunity for discussion and self-reflection in an environment where their opinions and thoughts matter.

14.4.1.   Sample Size

Here we are talking about the number of people in total who are going to be included in your focus groups.

Importantly, it is extremely rare that only one focus group on a topic is sufficient to address a research question. As with interviews, the end point of focus group work is the concept of saturation, the point at which no or little new information/thoughts/ideas are forthcoming from the participants. There is no magic number or formula of how many focus groups or how many participants are needed to achieve saturation; careful and defensible data analysis is required in order to make the call that saturation has actually occurred. In general, few researchers expect saturation to occur with anything less than three or four focus groups of 6–10 individuals.

Remember, focus groups are neither debates nor a form of group therapy. They are intended to be an opportunity to collect data in order to answer a research question. In most focus groups, conflict and disagreement are valuable tools for advancing a discussion and forcing individuals to dig more deeply to consider and defend their position; at times focus groups may become uncomfortable, and it is the facilitator's responsibility to find the right balance between creative disagreement and unhelpful argument.

> The likely number of people in Sandy's target group will be 20 (based on the number of his patients with diabetes who are between the ages of 16–25), so he will need to identify those and decide how many he wants to include in his focus groups. The likely number of people in Sandy's target group will be XX (based on XX) and so he decides to ask them all if they would like to take part and see what sort of response he gets. The final number of people who take part will be his sample size.

14.4.2.   Group Size

Focus groups typically consist of 6–10 individuals. The group needs to be large enough to generate rich discussion and to encourage the riffing and cascading that are hallmarks of the process, but not so large that some participants feel left out and others feel they need to shout in order to be heard. As discussed previously, selecting individuals for a focus group is less about representativeness and more about indicativeness. More than interviews, focus groups require participants who possess a series of attributes which in fact may NOT be representative of the general population of interest. Some of these attributes include self-confidence in stating one's opinions, English-language skills to articulate complex ideas, the ability to manage other people's criticisms of one's ideas and the ability to critically reflect on others' opinions, the ability to 'read' an audience and fit into a discussion, the ability to listen and respond effectively in real time, and an open attitude towards changing one's mind. Of course, we cannot know which of these attributes our group members have until the day of the focus group!

14.4.3.   Length of Session

Typically, focus groups last about 45–90 minutes. Anything longer than 90 minutes and participants may become restless or bored and the productivity of the group will diminish significantly. Anything less than 45 minutes will not leave sufficient time for the group to learn to work together effectively and establish its own way of interacting. The focus group should in general be guided by a carefully constructed series of predetermined questions – usually no more than 10 questions within a 90-minute session. Similar to interview questions, the focus group prompts should be carefully framed to be open-ended, value-neutral, and not leading in any manner. Questions should facilitate the free flow of discussion and riffing that will result in a successful session. Remember that focus groups are not debates; the objective is not for participants to tenaciously argue one predetermined point of view throughout, but instead to examine the way in which a social milieu shapes thinking and attitudes and how the discussion itself fosters evolution of thinking. Ideally, a homogenous group of strangers should be selected for a focus group. A heterogeneous group, with individuals of different levels of self-confidence, verbal skills or education can cause some participants to feel uncomfortable. Inevitably, participants in a focus group will compare themselves to other focus group participants; where social distance is great between participants, some individuals may actually feel intimidated and inhibited and consequently will not share as freely as they could. It is generally advisable where possible to have groups of strangers – inhibitions to free exchange of thoughts and ideas will be reduced when people do not know each other and likely will never see each other again.

Sandy cannot ensure that all of his focus group participants are strangers because some of them may have met at clinics, or know each other because they live locally. So, Sandy will make sure that if there are any who he knows do not get on together (and we have mentioned before that he knows of at least two), they are placed in different focus groups.

14.5. DEVELOPING THE FOCUS GROUP TOPIC GUIDE

Similar to the interview protocol, focus group protocols are an important tool to help guide the focus group, support the facilitator, and ensure alignment between research question, methodology, and method. Focus group protocols generally consist of three types of questions:

1. Engagement questions: These are questions designed to introduce participants to one another and to the research topic of interest, as well as to help them see where others are coming from. Engagement questions provide an opportunity for leveling or creating a common understanding of terminology and concepts that will be important during the focus group itself. Engagement questions are generally uncontroversial and ask people to simply report personal experiences rather than to draw inferences or solve problems. Within a typical focus group 20% of questions and time should be allocated to engagement questions.

2. Exploration questions: These questions are in essence the heart of the discussion itself. They are structured to be somewhat more controversial as a prompt for reflection and interaction. Exploration questions should be focussed and singular in their remit: they must be clear and

comprehensible with a minimal amount of subjective interpretation required. Given their central role in the focus group process, exploration questions should typically account for 70% of questions and times within the protocol.

3. Exit questions: These are questions that allow participants an opportunity to fill in blanks or to build on previous discussion for the purpose of pointing to future focus groups. Exit questions should also provide sufficient opportunity to ensure any strong emotion generated as part of the focus group is dissipated. Typically, exit questions account for no more than 10% of the questions and times in the protocol.

Topic guides are rarely if ever verbatim scripts for facilitators to follow. Instead they are generally phrased topic ideas, and it is usually left to the facilitator to find the correct wording and timing to introduce them within the time allocated for the session. It is usually very difficult to pilot-test focus group protocols, since a single individual's interpretation of the protocol will not be the same as a group of 6–10 individuals; consequently, the first iteration of the focus group is often the pilot-test for the protocol.

Within the focus group protocol it is usually important to consider important issue with respect to logistics of the focus group itself. Key issues to consider include the following:

a. Physical placement of participants: Traditionally, as a way of deemphasizing hierarchy, a round table is used to seat participants with the facilitator outside the circle to minimise proximity hierarchy. Other configurations may be required depending upon the space and furniture available. Generally it is advisable to not use rectangular tables that have a head seat occupied by the facilitator as this will subconsciously reinforce notions of authority and hierarchy. Unless there is a compelling reason, participants should be free to select their own seats around the table or in the room; overly-engineered seating arrangements may prompt concerns from participants about the intent of the facilitator and thus may inhibit conversation.

b. Transcripts: Verbatim transcripts are sometimes kept of focus group proceedings, but much less frequently than with interviews. Verbatim transcripts from audiotaped recordings are difficult to produce since most focus groups will involve multiple speakers talking simultaneously, and it is difficult for a transcriber to attribute specific quotations to specific individuals as many voices sound similar. Rather than transcripts, it is customary to ensure a second observer-researcher is in the room carefully documenting interactions, discussions and specific verbatim quotations where appropriate. The observer-researcher remains uninvolved in the proceedings themselves, and is only there to capture and record what transpires during the focus group. In general, facilitators themselves should not be expected to act as recorders; the job of facilitation is challenging enough without also recording who said what.

c. Video-taping: More common than audio-taping, video-taping of focus groups can provide a rich source of subtextual data around non-verbal responses and communication. In a large and boisterous focus group with 6–10 strong-willed and articulate individuals, even the most experienced observer-researcher will miss important social cues and context; video-taping of the proceedings can provide researchers with opportunities to review specific moments within the focus group at a later time. Placement of video cameras is crucial for this purpose, to ensure as many participants' faces as possible are captured by the camera.

d. Time and task-keeping: Many facilitators use a large countdown clock or stop watch to keep themselves – and the group – on time and on task. Since the time in a focus group can move quickly, it is often helpful to post at the beginning flipchart pages outlining ground rules for behaviour, research objectives, etc., to save time during the focus group itself. In general, facilitators should neither require nor expect that focus group participants will actually complete pre-readings or homework prior to attending the focus group; instead, all that needs to be accomplished should be achievable within the 45–90 minute time frame allocated.

Sandy's topic guide is shown below (Box 14.1). He has used his experience of running the clinics to inform the questions he would like to ask. He has come up with three main areas for the conversation and thinks that these will be enough to keep the group talking. He wants to avoid getting too personal about weight so intends to keep the conversation to diet and if the participants talk about their weight then that will be fine.

14.6. FACILITATOR ROLES AND RESPONSIBILITIES

The facilitator has unique responsibilities in managing the conversation of the focus group. Several techniques can be useful to ensure conversation flows and time and task are respected. Attributes of an ideal focus group facilitator will include the following:

a. The ability to actively listen to and respond sympathetically and in real time to changes in participants' mood and affect

---

BOX 14.1 Example of Informed Consent Information Sheet

University of Maghull
Patients' Views on Having Type 2 Diabetes
We are interested in finding out your views and beliefs on having diabetes. We are also interested in finding out how you feel about your blood sugar control and the things that make a difference to this.

All information from this focus group will be treated in the strictest confidence – so we will not use your name or refer to any people you might mention directly by their name. Any identifiable place names will also be removed. We would like to audio-record this session. The recordings will be assigned a number and you will be assigned a letter, e.g. Person A, Person B, and that is how we will refer to you when we present this information in any way.

1. Background
   Brief discussion as an ice-breaker – weather, travel to get to focus group. Set some ground rules
2. Diagnosis of diabetes
Can you remember how you felt about being diagnosed with diabetes?
3. Blood sugar control
   Do you think your blood sugar is under control? (PROMPT: what are the numbers like? Are they generally the same from day to day?). This may include some of the following:
   • How often do you measure your blood sugar?
   • How easy/difficult/convenient is this?
   • How does having to test your blood sugar make you feel? (PROMPT: embarrassed/angry/upset/no problem)
   • Would you like to change the way you manage your blood sugar?
   • If so, what would help you do this?
4. Do you think your diet affects your blood sugar?
   • What sort of food do you eat? (PROMPT: how many meals a day? When do you eat? What do you eat?)
5. Finally: Any other issues?
   Is there anything else you would like to talk about today? THANK YOU

---

b. The ability to listen, think and speak – all at the same time. Facilitators must be able to multitask and manage complex communication dynamics while still appearing cool, calm, and confident.

c. Genuine belief that each group participant has something valuable to offer to the discussion, and keep his/her own personal opinions out of the discussion.

d. The facilitator should have some general knowledge but no actual expertise in the research topic of interest. Without general knowledge of the topic, it is challenging for the facilitator to distinguish between relevant and extraneous conversations and responses, and impossible for the facilitator to redirect discussion and probe for further information when warranted. A facilitator with too much expertise, however, may have an overly developed sense of what is right or wrong within the discussion context and may betray their own biases and assumptions.

e. Facilitators must be individuals all participants can relate to in a convivial manner, but also project some sense of gravitas or importance. This can be particularly challenging and important in some situations: for example, no matter his personal qualifications and skills, it may be inappropriate to use a male facilitator to lead a discussion around sexual harassment with a group of women.

It is important to ensure basic logistics are covered by either the facilitator or the observer-recorder. Name tags for each participant (first names only), tent cards for seating and refreshments should be made available.

One of the important first jobs for the facilitator is to have participants complete an informed consent form. Consent within the context of a focus group is somewhat different than in an interview setting. Firstly, the very nature of a focus group means that anonymity and confidentiality cannot be fully protected as there will always be other participants in the focus group who will see and hear what is done and said. Anonymity can be attempted for any reports or manuscripts that flow from the focus group, but participants need to be aware that it cannot be guaranteed given the nature of this research method. As with interviews, focus group protocols need to be reviewed and approved by a relevant research ethics board/committee, and this information must be included in the informed consent form. Where demographic information is required, it should not be collected publicly; instead, each participant should complete a separate form with this information. Caution should be exercised in collecting demographic information; collect only that information which is essential for the study objectives. General questions related to age, marital status, country of education, etc., may be interesting but unless these items are directly germane to the research objectives, they should not be asked.

Most focus group facilitators develop a formal script to guide their introductions for the group. Key items to include in the introduction are the following:

a. General welcome and thank you to participants for their time and commitment

b. Logistics information – length of the focus group, location of toilets, etc.

c. Introduction and background of facilitator, observer-researcher and any other research staff

d. Succinct statement regarding purpose of focus group and research objectives

e. Summary of ground rules, including: (i) emphasis that participants should be doing most of the talking, not the facilitator; (ii) respectful disagreement and polite turn-taking are expected; (iii) there are no right or wrong answers and there is no test at the end of the session; (iv) speak up, whether you agree, disagree, or have no opinion at all – silence is very difficult to interpret at a focus group; (v) what is said in the room should stay in the room; and (vi) indicate the manner in which data will be collected (e.g. audio recording, video recording, observer-researcher field notes, etc.) … while attempts will be made to protect confidentiality and support anonymity, participants also need to be aware that focus groups are by their nature public and social, and consequently the research team is limited in terms of what they can actually do to protect participants.

f. Successful moderators often develop a mildly amusing icebreaking activity or joke to lighten the mood and enhance participant's comfort. Don't overdo this – trying too hard to make people comfortable can sometimes make them even more uncomfortable.

Facilitators also need to demonstrate sophisticated interpersonal communication skills, particularly when managing challenging participants. Common challenges for facilitators will include the following:

a. Participants who genuinely believe they are an expert in the issue and that all others should naturally defer to their opinions. Simply saying, 'Thank you for your perspective – what do other people think about this opinion?' sends a strong but subtle message that all voices at the table should be considered equal.

b. Speakers who will dominate a conversation and not let others get in a word; this can be managed by a facilitator interrupting if necessary to say 'Great thoughts – let's hear now from someone else in the group'.

c. Some individuals may have a tendency to drone on, taking 20 words to say something that should be said in five words. Non-verbal techniques for addressing this behaviour may include stopping direct eye contact with the individual, looking at the watch in the room, or simply waiting for the speaker to pause to inhale before jumping in and asking for another person to speak.

d. Participants who feel intimidated or shy may respond well to direct eye contact from the facilitator, encouraging smiles, and a clear invitation to share their thoughts.

Facilitators must actively use their excellent communication skills to keep conversations going. Three skills in particular are relevant:

1. Summarising – to provide confirmation of facts or opinions in a concise manner, to ensure all participants are 'on the same page'.
2. Paraphrasing – to capture the essence but not the details of what has been communicated, as a way of moving a discussion along, preventing long-winded participants from dominating conversation, and cutting to the core of an issue in the interests of time management. When paraphrasing it is important to not interject one's own opinions or thoughts but to, as accurately as possible, reflect the essence of the participant's ideas.
3. Probing – as a tool for eliciting further discussion and deeper thinking about an idea or statement. Examples of probing comments include 'Can you give me an example?', 'Help us all to better understand the point you're trying to make', or 'Can you tell me a little bit more?'

Facilitation is a complex and exhausting job – in general, facilitators can only perform well running two 90-minute sessions in a single day; any more than this will likely lead to deterioration in their performance and substandard data collection.

Wherever possible, the facilitator should NOT ask the observer-researcher to participate in any conversation; do not ask this person to repeat what was said, summarise a comment or in any other way contribute to the discussion. Observer-researchers should not be put on the spot and instead should focus their attention on accurately recording proceedings. It is usually advisable for the facilitator and the observer-researcher to allocate 30–45 minutes at the end of the session (once all participants have left) to debrief with one another (while the video/audio recorder is still running) to collect preliminary insights and thoughts about the session. When multiple focus groups are run, it is easy for both facilitator and observer-researcher to forget who said what when.

As can be seen, focus groups are complex social processes to organise and to run, but when well organised they can yield abundant rich information in a unique manner. We will discuss data management, analysis, coding and synthesis in Chapters 16 and 17.

CHAPTER SUMMARY

- This chapter has described the focus group as a qualitative method of data gathering.
- It has described how group dynamics can affect your focus group.
- It has outlined facilitator roles and responsibilities.
- It uses the example of our case study pharmacist Sandy and how he might use a focus group technique.
- It gives an example of Sandy's topic guide.

FURTHER READING

Millward, L. J. (2006). Focus groups. In G. M. Breakwell, S. Hammond, C. Fife-Schaw, & J. A. Smith (Eds.), *Research methods in psychology* (3rd ed.). London: Sage.

15

Observational Methods

15.1. INTRODUCTION

In Chapter 1 of this textbook we described the purpose of doing research as being to find the answers to things that are at least of interest to us and at best can result in innovations that can change people's lives. This statement holds true for research in any field but this textbook is all about doing research in pharmacy practice and so we are most interested in research that can improve people's health through interventions based on research. In other words – we want to 'do' evidence-based practice.

As we have seen so far evidence can be difficult to find even when we have chosen to use what we think are the most useful tools in the research toolkit. The problem is that human beings do not always behave in the ways we expect them to: they don't take their medicines in the way they have been advised, they do things that can be both good (healthy eating) and bad (overeating) for their health. To complicate matters even more, what is healthy for one person may not be healthy for another.

As you learned in Part I of this textbook, the research process begins with a question that arises either as a result of other research or as a result of events and behaviours we observe in practice. In essence all research involves some level of observation. We read existing research and observe the effects of it translated into practice; we conduct our own surveys and audits and observe the results to see if they compare with what we have seen in practice. But as human beings ourselves and as health care professionals we observe human beings experiencing all the emotions that go hand in hand with receiving good and bad news about their health, which is personal and specific to them.

We watch for particular signs of behaviour all the time because that is how we get through life. We must observe the behaviour of others in order to understand them and be able to respond accordingly. In this chapter we are going to explore how observing people can help us to understand them better and how such observation is used in research methods. For this chapter we will have the help of our pharmacist – Dorothy, whose research is about antimicrobial stewardship. In Chapters 6 and 7 we saw how she might use different research methods to answer her research question and suggested that she might think about doing some qualitative work to enrich her research outcomes. We will refresh your memories about Dorothy's research as we go along. However, before we continue with observational research here is a reminder of the ethics of doing research.

15.1.1. Standards of Conduct, Ethics and Performance for Pharmacy Professionals

As we pointed out in Chapter 1, the General Pharmaceutical Council (GPhC) is the statutory regulator for pharmacists and pharmacy technicians and is the accrediting body for pharmacy education in Great Britain. The GPhC is responsible for setting standards and approving education and training courses which form part of the pathway towards registration for pharmacists. The GPhC is also responsible for setting the standards of conduct, ethics and performance for qualified pharmacy professionals (pharmacists and pharmacy technicians). Although the expectations of the way pharmacist-researchers conduct themselves is the same for all research, we felt this was a good point to again mention the ethics of conducting research. This is because clinician-researchers who are involved in observational research have unique issues to consider given their dual roles.

While many forms of observational research emphasise a somewhat detached stance between researcher and participants, there may be situations faced by clinician-researchers that require them to explicitly acknowledge their professional practice responsibilities. Consider for example a situation where a pharmacist-researcher is undertaking research involving patients' understanding of their medications, and in the course of this research, notices a significant drug–drug interaction that has been undetected by other clinicians involved in this patient's care. A non-clinician researcher would not necessarily know about such interactions and consequently would likely not even be aware of a problem. A pharmacist-researcher, however, would have the burden of such knowledge and a unique responsibility to act within his/her code of ethics to ensure no harm came to patients. In such a case, the pharmacist-researcher may have to balance his/her interests in rigorous research methods with professional responsibilities associated with knowledge of potential harm that could occur. Clinician researchers of all sorts need to consider such possibilities when developing research protocols and devise methods to allow them to ensure that the role of researcher and ethical responsibilities as a practitioner can both be maintained. Including specific processes for addressing clinical problems that arise as part of research activities can be useful; at the very least, thinking in advance about how such a situation may be handled and documenting this within the research protocol should be considered.

To remind you of the things you must consider, here are the seven principles you must adhere to as a pharmacy professional:
1. Make patients your first concern
2. Use your professional judgement in the interests of patients and the public
3. Show respect for others
4. Encourage patients and the public to participate in decisions about their care
5. Develop your professional knowledge and competence
6. Be honest and trustworthy
7. Take responsibility for your working practices.

15.2. WHAT IS OBSERVATIONAL RESEARCH?

Observational methods are ways of *collecting data*, as are all the methods we have included in this book. In fact if you think back over what you know now about research, many of the methods available to us use observation. For example, in the last two chapters we described how to conduct interviews and focus groups. In both, we are using our skills

as observers to know when to speak and when to keep quiet, we are watching our participants for signs of misunderstanding or distress and in focus groups we are watching for conflict and ways to avert or channel it. But observational research is a research method of its own and is sometimes called '**Field Research**'. This is because researchers doing this kind of research generally engage with the people they are interested in observing, in their own natural setting, e.g. where they live or work. This differs from the experimental research you read about in Chapter 8 where researchers manipulate an environment in order to control certain variables. There are three main types of observational research, 'controlled observation', 'naturalistic' or 'non-participant' observation and 'participant' observation and we describe these in more detail below. The choice of method will depend to some extent on whether we want to be an onlooker, a participant or both in our role of researcher.

Before we begin the next sections we are going to re-introduce you to Dorothy and her research.

Dorothy Tseng is a hospital pharmacist and part-time MSc in Health System Improvement working in a community hospital. As part of her MSc degree programme, she is required to complete a research-based thesis; her workplace interests and needs have highlighted a potential are of focus for her work.

Through her years of experience and observation in the hospital pharmacy environment, Dorothy recognises that appropriate use of antibiotics is a particular challenge, both from a budget and quality perspective. In Chapter 6 we saw Dorothy develop her research question which is:

'What are the barriers and enablers to implementation of an antimicrobial stewardship programme in my hospital?'

She then went on to set out her research objectives:
1. Describe the attitudes of the interprofessional team towards antimicrobial stewardship
2. Compare the views of doctors, nurses, pharmacists, microbiologists and others involved in the antimicrobial prescribing decisions made at XX hospital
3. Identify barriers to implementation of an antimicrobial stewardship programme
4. Identify the enablers to implementation of an antimicrobial stewardship programme
5. Develop a draft programme

When we left Dorothy in Chapter 6 she had decided she needed to gather more information about her target population prior to writing her recruitment strategy. The purpose of this additional work was to identify everyone in the hospital who is involved in antimicrobial prescribing and decision-making. Dorothy made a list of those people who are involved. So far, on the list Dorothy has staff involved with:

- prescribing and administering, e.g. doctors, pharmacists, nurses
- infection prevention, e.g. patient safety and quality assurance team
- higher level decision-making, e.g. department heads
- pharmaco/epidemiology, e.g. staff involved in auditing, analysing and reporting data
- laboratory services, e.g. staff involved in the use of tests and the flow of results
- information technology, e.g. staff involved in integrating protocols at the point of care.

Dorothy's study is very complex because of the number of people and processes that she wants to explore. Although her survey will provide her with a significant amount of information, there are going to be many issues that will not be revealed by quantitative methods alone. Let's look at how Dorothy might help inform her survey and supplement her survey findings using different observational methods. There will be other ways that Dorothy could answer her research question, so please treat what follows as examples.

15.3.   CONTROLLED OBSERVATION

Controlled observations were most often carried out by psychologists in laboratory type conditions. Some of you might be familiar with the work of Albert Bandura known as the Bobo Doll Studies (see Further Reading at the end of this section). This research was carried out in 1961 with the aim of observing the development of aggressive behaviour in children. The children in this study were observed in secret through a one-way mirror so that they were unaware that they being watched. It is unlikely that this research would be acceptable today because it raises a number of

ethical concerns. You can read more about this in the reference we have given you.

If you wanted to do something like this in a pharmacy practice study you would not be able to observe people **covertly** but there are modifications of this method that might be possible in a health care setting that would be carried out with the participants' full knowledge and consent. At the end of this section we will look at how Dorothy might use this method to explore the antimicrobial prescribing process.

Another famous observational study was carried out by Mary Ainsworth in 1971. This was about how children develop relationships and was called the Strange Situation Study. Ainsworth used an interview schedule to record each time the researcher-observer observed a particular behaviour. The schedule from this research is reproduced in Table 15.1. Each time a researcher observed a behaviour event they ticked one of the boxes.

15.3.1.   When Would We Use This?

This type of study has been used in health care research to assess the quality of care given in different situations. For example, researchers might observe video recordings of doctor–patient consultations and record on an observation schedule how often doctors pick up cues from patients. The controlled observation study would be useful in this situation because the volume of video recordings would mean that a number of different researchers could assess the consultations using the previously agreed schedule. This would reduce costs in terms of research time and effort.

15.3.2.   How Could Dorothy Use This?

Dorothy could use controlled observation to assess the decision-making process of the clinicians prescribing antibiotics. The hospital Dorothy works in has a protocol

TABLE 15.1 **Strange Situation Study**				
OBSERVATIONS WERE MADE EVERY 15 SECONDS				
Intensity	**Proximity & Contact Seeking**	**Contact Maintaining**	**Proximity & Interaction Avoiding**	**Proximity & Interaction Resisting** **Seeking**
1				
2				
3				
4				
5				
6				
7				

From Ainsworth M. 1971.

for the management of patients infected with **clostridium difficile**. The protocol specifies how such patients should be treated from the diagnosis to recovery. The diagram below shows the first steps that are specified in the protocol (Fig. 15.1).

Dorothy could convert the steps in the protocol to an observation schedule and ask different groups of clinicians,

e.g. doctors, pharmacists if they would agree to be observed making clinical decisions. She could tick boxes in the schedule each time a decision was made. Once all of the observations were complete Dorothy could enter her results on to a database and compare the decision-making of each group of clinicians. This would tell her (a) if the protocol was being followed and (b) if not why not? It would also

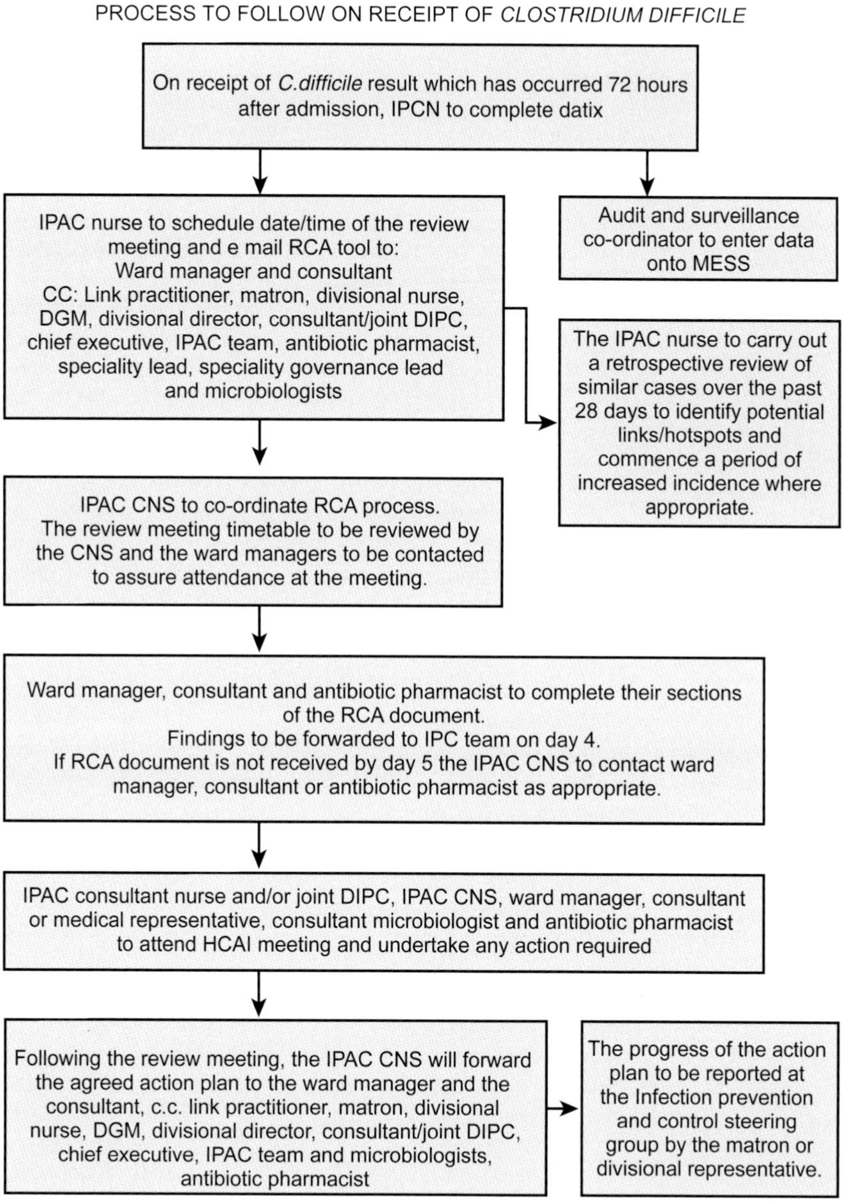

PROCESS TO FOLLOW ON RECEIPT OF *CLOSTRIDIUM DIFFICILE*

FIGURE 15.1 Diagram of protocol. (Adapted from Prevention & Management of Clostridium Difficile Infection Policy, V5. Royal Cornwall Hospitals NHS Trust. http://www.rcht.nhs.uk/.)

contribute to her understanding of the attitudes of the inter-professional team towards antimicrobial stewardship and give her an idea of how different clinicians prescribe for this condition.

15.3.3. Strengths

a. Controlled observations tend to have an observation schedule like the one above. For this reason it is easy to have more than one researcher involved in the study because they can all use the same schedule. They can all be trained to recognise specific behaviour events and so it is possible to establish a degree of inter-rater reliability.

b. The data derived from the observation schedule is in numeric form, e.g. the number of times a behaviour event is noted. This can be placed on a database and analysed quantitatively. This can provide a quick and easy summary of the number of times behaviours were observed.

c. As the collection and analysis of data are relatively quick it is possible and cost-effective to gather large amounts of data. This can establish a degree of generalisability.

15.3.4. Limitations

a. Controlled observation can lack validity because when people know they are being watched their behaviour changes. Remember the **Hawthorne Effect** described in Chapter 5, Section2 where the accuracy of observation of workers in the Hawthorne factory could not be assured because they behaved differently when the researchers were watching them.

15.4. NATURALISTIC OBSERVATION

Naturalistic observation involves the study of people in their own surroundings. There is nothing structured about this observation and the interest of researchers who use this method is in spontaneous behaviour. In contrast with controlled observation – there is no control; the researcher has not initiated any kind of behaviour nor does he/she manipulate the situation. This sort of research is where we think of the researcher as 'the fly on the wall', but it can be challenging to become integrated into the social group being studied. This is a prime example of where the Hawthorne Effect can interfere with the researcher's findings!

One of the most 'naturalistic' pieces of research was conducted by Margaret Mead who spent a lot of time living with people in the South Pacific in order to study their behaviour. You can find more about Mead's work in the Further Reading section at the end of this chapter. Naturalistic observation in its purest form is about as far away as it is possible to get from the positivist tradition of research that we focussed on in Part II. To summarise the differences between positivist research and naturalistic research we have reproduced this Table 15.2 from the work of Lincoln and Guba (1985).

15.4.1. When Would We Use This?

It is possible to use naturalistic observation in a health care setting inasmuch as it would be defined as the observation of behaviour in its natural or 'real-life' setting. However, it would be very difficult for a researcher to become so integrated into the context that is the subject of research, that the people being observed could become completely

TABLE 15.2 **Contrasting Positivist and Naturalistic Axioms**[1]		
Axioms About	**Positivist Paradigm**[2]	**Naturalist Paradigm**
The nature of reality	Reality is single, tangible and fragmentable	Realities are multiple, constructed and holistic
The relationship of knower to the known	Knower and known are independent, a dualism	Knower and known are interactive, inseparable
The possibility of generalisation	Time and context-free generalisations (nomothetic statements) are possible	Only time and context-bound working hypotheses (idiographic statements) are possible
The possibility of causal linkages	There are real causes, temporally precedent to or simultaneous with their effects	All entities are in a state of mutual simultaneous shaping, so that it is impossible to distinguish causes from effects.
The role of values	Inquiry is value-free	Inquiry is value-bound

[1]An axiom is a principle; [2]A paradigm is an example or pattern of something.
From Lincoln, Guba: 1985.

unaware of the researcher's presence. On the other hand, observing the things that happen in say an outpatient's clinic has helped to inform the outpatient experience. It could also be used to observe how people make decisions in policy or patient care meetings.

15.4.2. How Could Dorothy Use This?

Dorothy's hospital is part of an NHS Trust which has a specialist pharmacist who is responsible for advising on antimicrobial use. One of the roles of this specialist is to attend ward rounds on specialties of high antibiotic use. Dorothy is interested in understanding who influences whom with respect to antibiotic decision-making so she wants to actually observe the process at the point of prescribing. To this end, she decides to undertake some field work observing surgical teams doing their bedside rounds. She can then document the process by which decisions around antibiotic use are made within an inter-professional acute care setting.

Dorothy could seek permission to join a series of ward rounds as an observer-participant for the next month and use naturalistic observation to find out more about how the decisions regarding antibiotic prescribing are made. It might give her some insights into the attitudes of clinical staff to antimicrobial stewardship and any barriers or enablers that might be evident at the ward rounds. Dorothy's role as an observer would mean that she was detached from the group and would not contribute to it in any way, but she would be able to ask questions with the permission of the group members.

The goal of Dorothy's observation would be to keep a full and detailed account of what happened at every ward round. She would not be looking out for anything in particular. Rather she would be recording as much of what was said as possible by taking '**field notes**'.

Dorothy's specific goals would be to:

* describe the setting, the events and the people observed
* analyse what happened and interpret that data
* explain what happened using the data
* use specific events that happened during the ward rounds to explain and support any conclusions she draws.

(We will describe how to take notes and record observational data in the last section of this chapter. We will explore how to manage qualitative data in general including analysis and synthesis of findings in Chapters 17 and 18.)

15.4.3. Strengths

a. Being able to observe people in their own environment increases ecological validity. Ecological validity refers to the extent to which the findings of research can be applied to real-life settings. In naturalistic observation because the data have come from the setting that is being studied it is more likely that the findings will have relevance to that setting.

b. Naturalistic observation can help researchers to generate new ideas that can help with their overall study design. By observing the topic of study in a real-life setting researchers can obtain a better understanding of the study topic than they might have had.

15.4.4. Limitations

a. All such observations are based on a very small sample of a much larger system. For this reason it is not possible to generalise findings to a wider population.

b. Researchers have no control over the environment they are studying and have to record what happens when it happens. It is therefore unlikely that another researcher would be able to replicate their work and so reliability of findings is reduced.

c. There are no variables and no control and so establishing cause and effect is impossible.

d. Researchers undertaking naturalistic observation must have a clear idea of what they are recording and why so that they can recognise significant events when they happen.

15.5. PARTICIPANT OBSERVATION (SEE CHAPTER 18 FOR MORE DETAIL ABOUT THIS FORM OF OBSERVATION)

Participant observation is similar to naturalistic observation, but the researcher-observer can be involved in different ways. Most often participant observation refers to the observer becoming part of the group and participating in its activities (see (a)):

a. As a **participant observer** the researcher becomes a part of the group he/she is observing. With this method the researcher is generally known to the group being observed and can act as a member of the group because he/she has the background knowledge and skills to do so.

b. As **observer participant** the researcher joins the group with the specific intention of observing (similar to naturalistic observation). This type of observer is not as active of the participant observer and the method may provide access to information that would otherwise be unavailable to the researcher

c. As a **complete observer** the researcher would be totally detached from object of the observation who may be aware of his/her presence but unable to see the observer. An example of this is in clinical training where medical students might watch an operation through one-way glass but the operating theatre staff would be unable to see the students.

15.5.1. When Would We Use This?

Given the different levels of participation available using this method it lends itself well to health care research that involves the interpretative skills of the researcher. A pharmacist-researcher could use participant observation to study their own multidisciplinary team to find out about roles and responsibilities; he/she could be an observer participant and remain detached from the group in order to make a more objective assessment of the group's activities. Finally a pharmacist-researcher could use complete observation to observe the steps in the dispensing process.

15.5.2. How Could Dorothy Use This?

Dorothy could use participant observation to join other clinicians in her hospital who are involved in the prescribing process, to talk through some of the issues involved in antimicrobial stewardship at their regular multidisciplinary team meetings. Dorothy would be able to use her knowledge and training as a qualified pharmacist to participate in discussions and to ask questions relevant to her research. This would be challenging as Dorothy would be both participant and observer and would need to keep really focussed to be able to fulfil the two roles.

15.5.3. Strengths

a. Participant observation can be of particular use when the researcher has a similar degree of knowledge of the tips as the group being observed. They can use that knowledge to explore real-life issues from the standpoint of one who understands.

15.5.4. Limitations

a. It can be difficult to participate in the group activities and make an accurate record of what is said and done, at the same time. This means the researcher would have to rely on memory to make notes after the event.
b. The group members may not be as open about their views.
c. The researcher may become too involved in what is being said and thus introduce bias to the research, e.g. by having his/her own view about antimicrobial prescribing.

15.6. CASE STUDY RESEARCH

Case studies are used in many research settings but most often in those whose aim is to understand complex social phenomena. A case study is not a method it is a strategy for research that must be built into your research design. Case study research can include single or multiple case studies, is not limited to qualitative methods of data collection and can use mixed methods. Part IV of this textbook is devoted to mixed-methods research but an introduction and example here will help you to see how the qualitative elements of case study research might be carried out. A 'case' can be an individual, a group or an organisation. A case study is an empirical inquiry which means an inquiry based on, concerned with or verifiable by observation or experience. Its focus is on something that is happening in real-life but it may not be clear how the real-life event or process came about. Thus the use of case studies to thoroughly describe what is going on. A case study can be conducted over an extended period of time in order to document processes and events that might change or be treated differently due to the circumstances of the case study setting.

15.6.1. Types of Case Study

Case studies can include many sources of evidence such as documentation, archival records, interviews, direct observation, participant observation and physical artefacts. There are also several different applications of case study methodology, the main ones being exploratory, descriptive and explanatory:

a. Descriptive case study

     The purpose of this type of study is to describe in detail a research phenomenon and the real-life context in which it takes place, e.g. observation of the dispensing process in a community pharmacy.

b. Exploratory case study

     This type of case study is used to explore situations where the researcher has no knowledge of what the outcome might be, e.g. a pharmacist–patient consultation.

c. Explanatory case study

     This is a more complicated case study that would be used to find answers to questions about real-life interventions in which it is thought that there are causal links, but these are too complicated to be investigated by quantitative means (i.e. survey), e.g. pharmacy student online training programme.

     In the next section we are going to use as an example, one aspect of antimicrobial prescribing that should be at the centre of all stewardship and decision-making – the patient. First we will tell you a little more about Dorothy and her experience as a pharmacist.

15.6.2. Treatment Decisions for One Patient: A Descriptive Case Study

Dorothy has a good working understanding of antimicrobial prescribing because she has been working in hospital pharmacy for many years. Through her years of experience and observation in the hospital pharmacy environment, Dorothy recognises that appropriate use of antibiotics is a particular challenge, from both budget and quality perspectives.

Antibiotic prescribing is challenging: while best practice indicates that culture and sensitivity tests should be done prior to prescribing, the practical reality is that it is often difficult to get results back in time to support informed prescribing. As a community hospital, there are many time lags and process delays associated with ordering C & S tests, processing them in the lab, and communicating results back to the prescriber. As a result, many physicians rely on their intuition and experience and prescribe antibiotics 'empirically' without C & S test results. Frequently, this means that 'over-prescribing' is done: a more powerful, expensive, broad spectrum antibiotic may be used just to be safe, when a more conventional, cheaper, and targeted antibiotic may be actually needed. When the results do come back, it can be very difficult to change, discontinue or modify the antibiotic that was initiated: there seem to be few good mechanisms for communication and effective process between the clinical laboratory, the prescriber, and the pharmacy, and everyone in the system seems loath to change something that appears to be working. As a result, Dorothy believes there are opportunities for improving prescribing, saving money and enhancing process without compromising quality of patient care. As this project will serve both as her MSc thesis and as part of her day-to-day work responsibilities, Dorothy wants to ensure she approaches this problem and her ideas in a scientific, rigorous and defensible manner. Dorothy decides that she needs to follow the process for one patient at her hospital and what follows is a protocol for a descriptive case study of a hypothetical journey from diagnosis to patient outcome.

To help Dorothy understand what happens when a patient is suspected of having an infection, Dorothy has received permission from both a patient and their doctor to follow the patient's treatment journey from diagnosis to recovery. The case study will be descriptive because at this stage Dorothy just wants to know what happens in the process (Table 15.3).

In the next section we will outline the key principles that apply to all forms of observation.

15.7.   KEY PRINCIPLES OF OBSERVATION

Whatever type of observation you are doing you must give yourself time to understand what observation is and how to do it effectively and in this section we will summarise the key principles of observation. So far we have described what observation is and broken it down into three main types, along with examples and the strengths and limitations of each. We then went back to Dorothy's research and focussed on how she might combine different methods of observation using a case study approach to answer part of her research question. We now move back out to a broader

level and describe the main principles of observational research whatever method you choose to use. We will refer back to Dorothy's protocol in Table 15.3 to give you some examples.

15.7.1.   Define Research Question

All through this textbook we have talked about the need to define and refine your research question. Apart from your overall research question it is useful to write down which part of your question you intend to answer using observational methods. For example, Dorothy has an overall research question (see Table 15.3) and a case study research question. This helps her to contain her expectations of the extent to which she can answer her overall research question using a case study approach.

15.7.2.   Decide on the Purpose of Your Observation

You have to be clear to yourself about what you are trying to achieve and what you cannot. For example, Dorothy knows that the information she collects will help inform the other phases of her research and give her an idea about the barriers and enablers to implementation of an antimicrobial stewardship programme in her hospital. What the data she collects will not do is allow her to generalise any of her case study findings to a wider population.

15.7.3.   Specify How Your Observation Can Contribute to the Answering of Your Research Question

Associated with (2) in Table 15.3, once you have decided on the purpose of your observation you can set out which specific observations can contribute to answering which parts of your research question. For example, Dorothy can use her controlled observation of how the phlebotomist collects the blood sample from the patient to see whether a procedure is followed. She can then compare the procedure used to policies and procedures in place in her hospital.

15.7.4.   Choose Your Participants

The setting of your case study will determine your participants. This is because the people who work in the setting of interest will be defined by that setting. However, there may be other people who influence the activities that occur in the case study setting and you might want to include some of these in your research. For example, Dorothy may find that there is no clear procedure for collecting blood samples and their transport to the laboratory. She could identify who is responsible for the production and dissemination of these and interview them in another part of her research.

TABLE 15.3   Case Study Protocol

Overall research question	What are the barriers and enablers to implementation of an antimicrobial stewardship programme in my hospital?
Case research question	What are the treatment decisions and actions taken by staff involved in the prescribing and administration of antibiotics?
Purpose of case study part 1	To describe the treatment decisions and actions taken by staff involved in the prescribing and administration of antibiotics
Study design	a. A single case study will be used to describe the treatment decisions and action to provide the researchers with an understanding of the process from diagnosis to outcome b. The focus of the study is one patient recovering from a total hip replacement who is suspected of having a wound infection
Participants	a. Patient b. Prescriber c. Phlebotomist d. Laboratory porter e. Laboratory receptionist f. Laboratory technician g. Microbiologist h. Ward nursing staff
Data collection (method in brackets)	a. Introduction of researcher to patient (**face-to-face conversation**) b. Naturalistic observation of doctor–patient consultation (**field notes**) c. Controlled observation of phlebotomist (**observation checklist**) d. **Field notes**: documentation of process of requesting laboratory porter to arrival of sample in laboratory e. Controlled observation of laboratory reception process (**observation checklist**) f. Naturalistic observation of laboratory technician (**field notes**) g. Naturalistic observation of microbiologist (**field notes**) h. Participant observation of nursing staff (**field notes**) Field notes of patient's progress and repeat of case study part 1 if patient infection does not respond to first-line antimicrobial therapy
Analysis: criteria for interpreting case study findings	This will depend on the data collection method used and will be covered in Chapter 16

15.7.5.   Decide What to Observe

What you observe will also be determined by the setting and what goes on there during the periods of your observation. However, you should begin with a plan of who and what you are going to collect information about. Dorothy has done this in Table 15.3 above so she knows, for example, that she will be doing a naturalistic observation of the patient–doctor consultation where she will be looking at the way the doctor and patient interact and what they ask and tell each other.

15.7.6.   Decide How to Observe

How to observe is connected to what you want to achieve. Again, this is specified in Table 15.3 above where Dorothy has decided, for example, that the best way to learn about the doctor–patient consultation is to sit back and watch and listen.

15.7.7.   Design Coding Scheme

Decide how you are going to define and code a piece of behaviour. For example, Dorothy may think that when a consultant crosses his/her arms over his/her chest they are indicating that they are not interested in what the patient is saying or they disagree.

15.7.8.   Specify How Data Will Be Recorded

After Dorothy has identified the behaviours she is interested in it will be a simple job to enter these into a report chart. She could then tick each time she observes each behaviour and under what circumstances.

TABLE 15.4	**OPTION Rating Scale**
Score	**Description**
0	The behaviour is not observed.
1	A minimal attempt is made to exhibit the behaviour.
2	The behaviour is observed and a minimum skill level achieved.
3	The behaviour is exhibited to a good standard.
4	The behaviour is exhibited to a very high standard.

TABLE 15.5	**OPTION Instrument Item 1**
Score	**The Clinician *Draws Attention to* an Identified Problem as One That Requires a Decision-Making Process**
0	The behaviour is not observed.
1	A minimal attempt is made to exhibit the behaviour.
2	The behaviour is observed and a minimum skill level achieved.
3	The behaviour is exhibited to a good standard.
4	The behaviour is exhibited to a very high standard.

15.8. KEEPING RECORDS

If you have read this chapter up to here you have probably realised that recording the information you collect during the observation process is extremely important. To end this chapter we are going to return to the three types of observation we defined earlier, to show how data might be collected for each type.

15.8.1. Recording Controlled Observation

Recording controlled observations is probably the most straightforward data recording method of all the observation types. This is because, like fully structured interviews (see Chapter 13) the controlled observation conforms to a previously agreed and developed format. In Section 15.3 we referred to the 'Strange Situation Study' and gave you an example of a format for record keeping used by researchers in the study.

Controlled observation has been used in many settings in health care too and the OPTION instrument is one that has been used to observe the behaviour of clinicians in patient consultations.

There are 12 items in the OPTION instrument and all of them are scored using the rating scale in Table 15.4.

Following extensive background work involving many members of a multinational research team the researchers arrived at a set of behaviours and their definitions that they would expect to take place during a patient consultation. Each of the observers was then trained in what to look for. Here is an example of item 1 (Table 15.5).

The behaviour referred to here is very specific. It is expected that the clinician will 'draw attention' to an identified problem that requires a decision-making process. It is worded to be used by any clinician involved in patient consultations. For example, a surgeon may want to discuss treatment options for a patient with a prolapsed intervertebral disc ('**slipped disc**') so might begin by saying: '*So, we have looked at all of the X-rays and scans and you have seen that you have a slipped disc, there are a number of things that we can do about this that we can talk about today*'. This would be a good example of the behaviour and might score 3 or even 4 depending on what has been decided by the researchers.

The behaviour in question includes not only the words but the way the clinician sits in relation to the patient and how comfortable they seem to be making the patient feel. The observer would be watching for signs of all of these things and if they were all present then the score would be higher. If the surgeon did not draw the patient's attention to the fact that some decisions needed to be made and just said '*I've looked at your scans and I intend to operate to remove the disc*', this would probably score '0'.

Another example might be a pharmacist-prescriber who is talking to a patient with newly diagnosed hypertension ('high blood pressure'). The pharmacist might begin by saying: '*Hello Mr Smith, now that you have used the blood pressure monitor and we have found that your blood pressure is higher than we would like, we need to think about what choices of treatment you have*'.

15.8.2. Recording Naturalistic Observation

As you will remember from Section 15.4, naturalistic observation is almost at the opposite end of the spectrum to controlled observation. Rather like an unstructured interview (see Chapter 13) the observer makes no attempt at control. The difference between an interview and an observation is that the person being interviewed knows that a conversation of some sort will take place and that there are some boundaries, e.g. the participant will know what the topic of conversation is. In a situation where people are being observed in their natural setting they will usually be aware that there is someone amongst them who is not normally there and that can create its own set of problems for accurate record-making. For example, the people being observed may feel inhibited by the presence of a stranger who might just be sitting, listening and watching – and taking the occasional notes. This means that their behaviour will change and this is called '**reactivity**' (back to the Hawthorne Effect).

Weber and Cook did some research in 1972 (see Further Reading at the end of this chapter), and they identified four different roles that people being observed might adopt. Please note that psychological research in those days was very science based and so the people who took part in this research were known as the '**subjects**'. This is actively discouraged in most parts of the world today as it is dehumanising and does not acknowledge the role of the participant as one who takes part with their full knowledge and consent. In the list below we have put 'participant' in square brackets after 'subject' and then used participant in the remaining text. Weber and Cook also used the word 'experimenter' to describe the 'researcher' and we have highlighted this too:

1. **The Good Subject [Participant] role**: The participant tries to validate the anticipated result. Give the experimenter [researcher] the result they want.
2. **The Faithful Subject [Participant] role**: The participant attempts to be honest and faithful, even when they can anticipate the expected result.
3. **The Negativistic Subject [Participant] role**: The participant produces responses or behaviour that is in the opposite direction of the anticipated result.
4. **The Apprehensive Subject [Participant] role**: The participant feels uncomfortable about being evaluated. Because of evaluation apprehension, the participant tries to behave in a socially desirable way. They don't want to look bad. They may give the socially desirable response, even if it's not what they really think, or if it's not what the investigator [researcher] expects to see.

So, alongside the problems already inherent in trying to get an accurate idea of how people behave in their natural setting, we have the problem of how to make a record of what was said and done whilst affecting the behaviour of participants as little as possible.

There are only really two ways of avoiding reactivity and they are either not to tell people they are being observed or not to tell the people being observed the real reason for the observation. Either way this is deception and would be against the ethical guidelines for research in most countries.

So, what we have left is two options for making records of naturalistic observations that minimise the impact of the observer on the participants:

1. Taking written notes of the narrative involved in the observation and making prompts for ourselves about any significant events that we can write up later. Taking written notes can be an arduous process, and it is very difficult to make a record of everything that is said and done in a specified period of time. For example, if we go back to Dorothy in Section 15.4.2 we find that she was using naturalistic observation to note what happened when members of the multidisciplinary team went on ward rounds to review patient's medication. Dorothy will need to think through the practicalities of note taking whilst she is walking around the ward. She could have a small notebook and record what happens for one patient in the first instance. That would give her an idea about whether her system was working and help plan for future ward rounds. The key thing to remember about making records of observations is to be selective about what to record in whatever form. For example, on a ward round, Dorothy could decide to make a record of the actual point at which a decision is made about the prescribing of an antibiotic and what led to that decision. This would enable her to make some comparisons with other ward rounds.

Table 15.6 shows some examples of the notes Dorothy might take.

2. Make video or audio recordings of the events. Seeking the permission of participants to record either in video or audio is another option. However, it would be very difficult to get ethics approval to video record what went on in a ward in real-time. There are so many other people who would enter and leave the ward, not to mention the ethics of recording unwell people and their relatives. Using video or audio-recording might be possible if, for example, Dorothy decided to take part in a multidisciplinary team meeting, and we will explore this in Section 15.8.4.

It is hard to say which of these options is the least intrusive because every situation is different. Back in the days when Margaret Mead (see Section 15.4) was conducting research into the people of the South Pacific, she went to live amongst them, eventually becoming an accepted member of the community. The people knew she was there but seemed to forget the purpose the more integrated she became. However, in a workplace setting such as Dorothy's, where she might be known to some of the participants it might be as close to a true naturalistic setting as she can get. It might also mean that her colleagues may accept her presence more readily and reactivity might be reduced because of their familiarity with her.

15.8.3. Recording Participant Observation

The practicalities of making a record of a piece of participant observation are similar to those above. However, in participant observation the researcher is not trying to become a 'fly on the wall'. Rather he or she is trying to capture information about a system or process that is not affected by participant reactivity to the same extent as naturalistic

TABLE 15.6	Note Taking			
Prescriber	**Ward**	**Patient ID and Indication**	**Discussion About Treatment**	**Decision Point**
Jackson Finch	General Medicine	ID: 215755 Cellulitis left leg	Initial Rx for Ceftriaxone without culture/sensitivity – no anaerobic coverage?	Empirical tx started Follow-up once C & S done
Mayellen Wu	General Surgery	ID: 225463 Hip replacement MRSA	Concern re: vancomycin as patient has experienced 'red-man' previously	Discussion with RN regarding appropriate IV administration protocols
Feng-Xi Philpott	Intensive Care Unit	ID: 678282 Septicemia	Patient ordered tobramycin tid; no levels ordered	Appropriate to change to once-daily dosing? – follow-up on renal function tests needed
Pestonji Dhunshakwalla	A & E	ID: 347272 Fever not yet diagnosed	Requires ID service approval for ordering restricted antibiotics (imipenem)	ID service to follow-up one assessment completed

To help Dorothy record key events she might design a form that she could use to enter information. This would provide her with a record of the actual point at which a decision is made about the prescribing of an antibiotic and what led up to that decision. This would enable her to make some comparisons with other ward rounds.

observation. As we mentioned above, if Dorothy were known to her participants they might accept her more readily and relax in her presence. Dorothy could make herself a checklist of the behaviours or events she wants to make a record of and this might be easier to use in the context of a team meeting where everyone remains in one place (rather than moving from patient to patient in a ward round). Regardless of this Dorothy must ensure that she recognises that she may have had an impact on the behaviour of the participants and make some reflective notes about this when she writes up her research findings. We will be talking about analysis and writing up of qualitative data, including observations, in Chapters 16 and 17.

15.8.4. Documents and Other Written Evidence

In this section rather than continue to give you descriptions of the types of record you could make we will give you some examples of the additional documentation that you might collect as part of your observation.

In health care research it is possible to gain access to a large number of documents that can be anonymised and used to add richness to the report of your observation. Here are some of the documents you could collect and some examples:
- Diagnostic criteria used for decision-making:
  - Results of culture-and-sensitivity assays to determine antimicrobial use
  - X-rays, ECGs or other diagnostic tests
  - Complete blood count, neurovitals and other routine laboratory and physical assessment findings.

- Hospital policies about prescribing:
  - Hospital formulary
  - Hospital or health-region specific prescribing guidelines
  - Consensus guidelines for prescribing generated by expert advisory panels
  - National formularies and prescribing guidelines (e.g. National Institute for Clinical Excellence (NICE) guidelines).
- Patient notes, e.g. records of what was prescribed for what patients, when and by whom. Here's an example:

EXAMPLE

Surname: JONNESON
Given Name(s): HELGA OLGA
DOB: 1955 04 20
Gender: Female
Phone: 01234 567890
Email: prefers phone contact only
Physician: Dr Mackay Gregory
Home Address: 15B Station Approach Road, Merseyside, Liverpool
Health Insurance: 57663T367R
Allergies: Penicillin (rash – reported by patient when she was a child)
Past Medical History:
Hypertension x 5 years Notes: uses home blood pressure monitoring, target is 130/85
Hypercholesterolemia x 3 months

TABLE 15.7 Medications

Prescription	Prescriber	Dispensed Date	Dispensed Amount	Notes
Ramipril 5 mg po daily	Dr Mackay Gregory	June 14 2016	90	
Hydrochlorothiazide 25 mg po daily	Dr Mackay Gregory	June 14 2016	90	
EC-ASA 81 mg daily	Dr Mackay Gregory	August 15 2016	90	
Atorvastatin 40 mg daily	Dr Mackay Gregory	August 15 2016	90	
Ramipril 10 mg po daily	Dr Wanda Severide	September 6 2016	30	BP 140/90 – no adverse effects reported
Hydrochlorothiazide 37.5 mg po daily	Dr Wanda Severide	September 6 2016	30	Ensure 25 mg HCTZ tablets split for patient

- Laboratory report:

Laboratory reports can be somewhat difficult to interpret, and you will need to know what the normal values are for each test. If you follow this link you will find these at the end: http://www.stedmansonline.com/webFiles/Dict-Stedmans28/APP17.pdf

Here is an example of a report:

EXAMPLE

Surname: JONNESON   Given Name(s): HELGA OLGA
DOB: 1955 04 20
Gender: Female
Phone: 01234 567890
Email: prefers phone contact only
Physician: Dr Mackay Gregory
Home Address: 15B Station Approach Road, Merseyside, Liverpool
Health Insurance: 57663T367R
Allergies: Penicillin (rash – reported by patient when she was a child)
Physical Examination:
Ht: 145 cm
Wt: 68 kg
Temp: 37.0   Temp Site: Oral

Pulse: 72   Rhythm: Regular
BP: 140/90 (measured twice)
General Appearance: well developed, well nourished, no acute distress
Eyes: conjunctiva and lids normal, PERRLA, EOMI, fundi WNL
Ears, Nose, Mouth, Throat: TM clear, nares clear, oral exam WNL
Respiratory: clear to auscultation and percussion, respiratory effort normal
Cardiovascular: regular rate and rhythm, S1-S2, no murmur, rub or gallop, no bruits, peripheral pulses normal and symmetric, no cyanosis, clubbing, edema or varicosities
Skin: clear, good turgor, colour WNL, no rashes, lesions, or ulcerations

Albumin, serum	40 g/L	N=32–46 g/L
Bicarbonate, serum (venous)	24 mmol/L	N=22–29 mmol/L
Creatinine (plasma)	69 mcmol/L	N=53–97 mcmol/L
Fasting blood glucose	5.0 mmol/L	N=3.5–5.3 mmol/L
Glycated hemoglobin A1c	0.05	N= 0.042–0.059
Iron, serum	12.4 mcmol/L	N=9.0–30.4 mcmol/L
LDL-cholesterol, plasma	4.12 mmol/L	3.37–4.12 mmol/L = borderline
Potassium, plasma	4.1 mmol/L	N=3.4–4.4 mmol/L
Sodium, plasma	140 mmol/L	N=136–145 mmol/L
Trigylcerides	5.65 mmol/L	>5.65 mmol/L = hypertriglyceridemia

(N= is the normal reference range)

CHAPTER SUMMARY

- This chapter has outlined some of the ways of collecting data through the use of observational research.
- It has emphasised the standards of conduct, ethics and performance for pharmacy professionals.
- It has looked back at some observational research from the past.
- It has used the example of our case study pharmacist, Dorothy, to show how some of the key observational methods might be used.

REFERENCES

Ainsworth, M., Bell, S., & Stayton, D. (1971). Individual difference in strange-situation behaviour of one-year-olds. In H. R. Schaffer (Ed.), *The origins of human social relations* (pp. 17–58). London: Academic Press.
Lincoln, Y., & Guba, E. (1985). *Naturalistic inquiry*. Newbury Park, CA: Sage Publications.

FURTHER READING

Bobo Doll Experiment
Bandura, A., Ross, D., & Ross, S. A. (1961). Transmission of aggression through imitation of aggressive models. *Journal of Abnormal and Social Psychology*, 63, 575–582.

Naturalistic Inquiry
Lincoln, Y. S., & Guba, E. G. (1985). *Naturalistic Inquiry*. California: Sage.

Margaret Mead
http://psychology.jrank.org/pages/401/Margaret-Mead.html.

Roles of Research Participants
Weber, S. J., & Cook, T. D. (1972). Subject effects in laboratory research – examination of subject roles, demand characteristics, and valid inference. *Psychological Bulletin*, 77(4), 273–295.

16

Data Analysis and Coding

LEARNING OBJECTIVES

After reading this chapter you should be able to:
- understand some of the key principles underpinning qualitative research
- describe different methods of data analysis
- understand what coding is and some ways of doing this
- define 'trustworthiness'

16.1. INTRODUCTION

In this chapter, we will review some principles of qualitative data collection, analysis and management to help pharmacists interested in doing research in their practice to continue their learning in this area. Qualitative research can help researchers to access the thoughts and feelings of research participants, which can enable the development of an understanding of the meaning people ascribe to their experiences. Whereas quantitative research methods can determine how many people undertake particular behaviours, qualitative methods can help researchers to understand how and why such behaviours take place. Within the context of pharmacy practice research, qualitative approaches have been utilised to examine a diverse array of topics, including perceptions of key stakeholders regarding pharmacists prescribing and post-graduation employment experiences of young pharmacists (see Further Reading).

In this chapter we will refer to three commonly used methodologies: ethnography, grounded theory and phenomenology. Briefly, **ethnography** involves researchers using direct observation to study participants in their 'real life' environment, sometimes over extended periods of time. **Grounded theory** (see Chapter 18) and later modified versions (e.g. Strauss and Corbin 1990 – see Further Reading), use face-to-face interviews and interactions such as focus groups to explore a particular research phenomenon and may help to clarify a lesser understood problem, situation or context.

Phenomenology shares some features with grounded theory (such as an exploration of participants' behaviours) and uses similar techniques to collect data but focusses on understanding *how* human beings experience their world. It provides researchers with an opportunity to put themselves in another person's shoes and understand the subjective experiences of participants. Some researchers use qualitative methodologies but adopt a different standpoint (see Chapter 12, Section 12.3.1) and an example of this is in the work of Thurston et al (see Further Readings) discussed later in this chapter. As we suggested in Chapter 12, qualitative work requires the researcher to both reflect upon and articulate their worldview, perspectives and biases before and during the research process as a way of providing context and understanding for readers. When being reflexive, researchers don't try to simply ignore or avoid their own biases (as this would likely be impossible): instead, reflexivity requires the researcher to reflect upon and clearly articulate his/her position and subjectivities so that the readers of the research can better understand the filters through which questions were asked, data were gathered and analysed, and findings were reported. From this perspective bias and subjectivity are not inherently negative but they are unavoidable: as a result, it is best to articulate these upfront in a manner that is clear and coherent for readers.

16.1.1. The Participant's Viewpoint

Let's just recap what we are trying to achieve by doing qualitative research. What qualitative study seeks to tell us is **why** people have thoughts and feelings that might affect the way they behave. This may be in a number of contexts but for the purposes of this textbook, the focus is on pharmacy practice and the way people behave with regards to medicine's use (e.g. to understand patients' reasons for non-adherence to medications, or to explore resistance from physicians to pharmacists' clinical suggestions). As suggested in Chapter 12, an important point about qualitative research is that it does not seek to generalise its findings to a wider population. Qualitative research is used to gain insights into people's feelings and thoughts, which may provide the basis for a future stand-alone qualitative study or help researchers to map out survey instruments for use in a quantitative study. Using different types of research in the same study is known as 'mixed-methods' research, and Chapter 19 is devoted to using different research methods in one study.

At the risk of becoming repetitive it is important to understand that the role of the researcher in qualitative research is to attempt to access the thoughts and feelings of their participants. This is not an easy task as it involves asking people to talk about things that may be very personal to them. Sometimes the experiences being explored are fresh in the participant's mind, on other occasions reliving past experiences may be difficult. Regardless of how data are being collected, the primary role of the researcher is to safeguard participants and their data (which of course represents their thoughts, feelings and beliefs). Mechanisms for such safeguarding must be clearly articulated to participants and approved by a relevant research ethics review board prior to embarking upon research. Researchers and practitioners new to qualitative research should seek advice from an experienced qualitative researcher before embarking on their project (see Chapter 12 for more on the ethics of doing qualitative research).

16.2. DATA COLLECTION

In Chapter 12 we pointed out that, although there are different ways of collecting qualitative data, e.g. by asking participants to give free text answers to a questionnaire or by observing how people behave in certain situations, one of the most commonly used methods is interview or focus group.

Whatever philosophical standpoint the researcher is taking and whatever the data-collection method (e.g. focus group; one-to-one interview) the process will involve the generation of large amounts of data. If the researcher is audio-recording data collection then the recordings must be transcribed verbatim prior to the commencement of data analysis. As a rough guide one 45-minute audio-recorded interview can take 8 hours for an experienced researcher/transcriber to transcribe, resulting in 20–30 pages of dialogue. Many researchers will also maintain a folder of field notes to complement audio-taped interviews. Field notes allow the researcher to maintain and comment upon impressions, environmental contexts, behaviours, or non-verbal cues that may not be adequately captured through audio taping, and

are typically hand-written in a small notebook at the same time an interview takes place. Field notes can provide important context within which to interpret audio-taped data and can help remind the researcher of situational factors that may be important during data analysis. Such notes need not be formal, but they should be maintained and secured in a similar manner to audio tapes and transcripts, as they are sensitive information and relevant to the research. For more information about qualitative data collection please see and the Further Reading section at the end of this chapter.

16.3. DATA ANALYSIS AND MANAGEMENT

If, as suggested earlier, doing qualitative research is about putting oneself in another person's shoes and seeing the world from their perspective, the most important part of data analysis and management is to be true to one's participants. It is their voices that we are trying to hear so that these can be interpreted by the researcher and reported on for others to read and learn from. To illustrate this point, consider the anonymised transcript extract presented below, which has been taken from a research interview conducted by one of the authors (JS). This is referred to throughout the remainder of this chapter to illustrate how data may be managed, analysed and presented. In Sections 16.5 and 16.6 we will rejoin Serena and Rosi, our pharmacy students, to see how they might make some sense of the data they have collected.

As you read the transcript (Box 16.1) try to imagine what the person being interviewed might have felt at the time of the events they are describing and during the interview. This is what it means to begin to put yourself in someone else's shoes.

16.3.1. Interpretation of Data

Interpretation of the data will depend on the theoretical standpoint taken by researchers. For example, some research conducted by Thurston et al. is entitled '*Discordant indigenous and provider frames explain challenges in improving access to arthritis care: a qualitative study using constructivist grounded theory.*' As the title suggests this research was conducted taking into consideration at least two theoretical standpoints. The first is the culture of the indigenous population of Canada and their place in society, and the second is the social constructivist theory used in constructivist grounded theory method. In the first case, to have decided to conduct the research, the researchers must have felt that there was anecdotal evidence that there were differences in the access to arthritis care for patients from indigenous and non-indigenous backgrounds. In the second case, social constructivist theory was used because it assumes that behaviour is socially constructed, e.g. we do things because they are expected of us by those in our personal world or

---

BOX 16.1 **Sample Interview Transcript**

This participant was in their late 50s and had suffered from a chronic mental health illness for 30 years. They had become a 'revolving door patient' which refers to someone who is frequently in and out of hospital. They talked about their past experiences and the researcher asked:

1   What was treatment like 30 years ago?
2   *Umm – well it was pretty much they could do what they wanted with you because I was put into the err, the err*
3   *kind of system err, I was just on endless section threes.*
4   Really
5   *But what I didn't realise until later was that if you haven't actually posed a threat to someone or yourself they*
6   *can't really do that but I didn't know that. So wh-when I first went into hospital they put me on the forensic ward*
7   *'cause they said 'We don't think you'll stay here we think you'll just run-run away'. So they put me then onto the*
8   *acute admissions ward and – er – I can remember one of the first things I recall when I got onto that ward was*
9   *sitting down with a er a Dr XXX. He had a book this thick [gestures] and on each page it was like three questions*
10   *and he went through all these questions and I answered all these questions. So we're there for I don't [know]*
11   *maybe two hours doing all that and he asked me he said "well when did somebody tell you then that you have*
12   *schizophrenia" I said "well nobody's told me that" so he seemed very surprised but nobody had actually [pause]*
13   *whe-when I first went up there under police escort erm the senior kind of consultants people I'd been to where*
14   *I was staying and ermm so err [pause] I.... the, I can remember the very first night that I was there and given*
15   *this injection in this muscle here [gestures] and just having dreadful side-effects the next day I woke up [pause]*
16   Oh
17   *.....and I suffered that akathesia I was swear to you, every minute of every day for about 20 years.*
18   Oh how awful.
19   *And that side of it just makes life impossible so the care on the wards [pause] umm I don't know it's kind of, it's*
20   *kind of hard to put into words [pause]. Because I'm not saying they were sort of like not friendly or interested*
21   *but then nobody ever seemed to want to talk about your life [pause] nobody asked me any questions about my*
22   *life. The only questions that came into was they asked me if I'd be a volunteer for these student exams and*
23   *things and I said 'yeah' so all the questions were like 'oh what jobs have you done', err about your relationships*
24   *and things and err but nobody actually sat down and had a talk and showed some interest in you as a person you*
25   *were just there basically [pause] um labelled and you know there was there was [pause] but umm [pause] yeah......*

---

in the wider society in which we live. (Please see Further Reading at the end of this chapter for more about social constructivist theory.)

Thus, these two standpoints (and there may have been others relevant to Thurston et al.'s research) will have affected the way in which the researchers interpreted the experiences of the indigenous population participants and those providing their care. Being aware of the standpoints being taken in one's research is one of the foundations of qualitative work. Without such an awareness it is easy to slip into interpreting other people's narratives from our own viewpoint – rather than that of the participants. To analyse the example extract we will adopt a phenomenological approach because we want to understand how the participant experienced their illness and try to see that experience from their perspective.

16.3.2.   Transcribing and Checking

For the purposes of this chapter it is assumed that interviews or focus groups have been audio-recorded because this is

the most practical way of collecting an accurate account of what was said. Transcribing is an arduous process, even for the most experienced transcribers, but it has to be done in order to translate the spoken word into the written word to facilitate analysis. It is essential that anyone new to conducting qualitative research transcribes at least one interview and one focus group in their life as a researcher. It is only by doing this that researchers realise how difficult the task is, and this affects our expectations when asking others to transcribe. If your research project has sufficient funding then a professional transcriber can be employed to do the work. If this is the case then it is a good idea to sit down with them if possible, and talk them through the research and what the participants were talking about. This is important in research where people are using jargon or medical terms (as in pharmacy practice). Involving your transcriber in this makes it both easier and more rewarding for them as they will feel part of the team. Transcription editing software (e.g. ELAN) is also available but is expensive (see Further Reading at the end of this chapter).

In the first instance, all audio recordings should be transcribed verbatim regardless of how intelligible this may be when reading them back. Lines of text should be numbered. The researcher should then read the transcription and listen to the recording simultaneously and do the following:

- Correct any spelling or other errors
- Anonymise the transcription so that the participant cannot be identified from anything they say (e.g. names, places, significant events)
- Add in pauses, laughter, looks of discomfort
- Add in any punctuation such as commas and full stops (see the transcription above for examples of these)
- Include any other contextual information that might have affected the participant, e.g. temperature or comfort of the room (this is where your field notes will help you).

Dealing with the transcription of focus groups is slightly more problematic as multiple voices are involved. One way of transcribing such data is to 'tag' each voice, e.g. 'Voice A', 'Voice B', etc. Researchers will usually have two focus group facilitators to help with the process of making sense of the data. Whilst one facilitator guides participants through the topic the other can make notes about context and group dynamics. More about group dynamics and focus groups can be found in Chapter 14 and in Further Reading at the end of this chapter.

16.3.3. Reading Between the Lines

During the above process the researcher can begin to get a feel for the participant's experience of the phenomenon in question and start to think about things that could be followed-up in subsequent interviews or focus groups (if appropriate). In this way one participant's narrative informs the next and the researcher can continue to interview until nothing new is being heard or, as it says in the textbooks, 'saturation is reached'. Whilst continuing with the processes of coding and theming it is important to consider not just what the person is saying but what they are not saying. For example, is a lengthy pause an indication that the participant is finding the subject difficult or are they just deciding what to say?

The aim of the whole process from data collection to presentation is to be able to tell the participants' stories using examples or '**exemplars**' from their own narratives,

thus grounding the research findings in the participants' lived experiences.

Smith J (1996) suggests a qualitative research method known as **Interpretative Phenomenological Analysis** (IPA) which has two basic tenets. First, it is rooted in phenomenology in that it attempts to understand the meaning individuals ascribe to their lived experiences and second, the researcher must attempt to interpret these meanings in the context of the research. That the researcher has some knowledge and expertise in the subject of their research means that they can have considerable scope in interpreting the participant's experiences. IPA (or any qualitative research for that matter) is not just about providing a description of what participants say. Rather, it is about getting *underneath* what a person is saying to try to truly understand the world from their perspective. This process is extremely important if you are to be true to your participants and tell their story – not yours.

16.3.4. Coding

Once all of the research interviews have been transcribed and checked it is time to begin coding. Field notes compiled during an interview can again be a useful complementary source of information to facilitate this process, as the gap in time between an interview, transcribing and coding can result in memory bias regarding non-verbal or environmental context issues that may affect interpretation of data. Coding refers to the identification of topics, issues, similarities and differences which are revealed through the participants' narratives and interpreted by the researcher. This process enables the researcher to begin to understand the world from the participants' perspectives. Coding can be done by hand on a hard copy of the transcript, e.g. by making notes in the margin or highlighting and naming sections of text. More commonly, researchers are using qualitative research software (e.g NVivo™ qualitative data analysis software; QSR International Pty Ltd.) to help manage their transcriptions. It is advised that researchers undertake a formal course in the use of such software or at the very least seek supervision from a researcher experienced in these tools.

Returning to our transcription and reading from lines 23–27, a code from this section might be 'diagnosis of mental health condition' but this would just be a description of what the participant is talking about at that point. If we read a little more deeply we can ask ourselves how the participant might have felt about the doctor assuming they were aware of their diagnosis or indeed that they had only just been told the diagnosis. There are a number of pauses in the narrative that might suggest that the participant is finding it difficult to recall that experience. Later in the text, the participant says '*nobody asked me any questions about my life*' (lines 43–44). We could just code this as 'health care

---

> **ACTIVITY** Look at the transcription and see what you think the pauses between lines 18 and 22 might mean. The participant is reliving the time that they were first diagnosed with schizophrenia – how might they be feeling?

professionals' consultation skills' but that would not reflect how the participant must have felt never to be asked anything about their personal life, about them as a human being. At the end of this extract the participant just tails off as they recall that no one showed any interest, which makes for very moving reading. As practitioners in pharmacy it might also be pertinent to explore the participant's experience of akathesia and why this was left untreated for 20 years.

16.3.5. Trustworthiness

One of the questions that arises regarding qualitative research is about the reliability of the interpretation and representation of the participants' narratives. There are no statistical tests that can be used to check reliability and validity as there are in quantitative research. However, work by Lincoln and Guba (1985) suggest that there are other ways to 'establish confidence in the "truth" of the findings' (p. 218). They call this criteria 'trustworthiness' and more about this topic can be found in the work of Lincoln and Guba references to which are given in the Further Reading section at the end of this chapter. One way of establishing 'trustworthiness' of our coding is to ask another researcher to code the same transcript and then to discuss any similarities and differences in our own and another's coding. This simple act can result in revisions to the codes and help to clarify and confirm the research findings (see Chapter 12 for more on the topic of trustworthiness).

16.3.6. Theming

Theming refers to the drawing together of codes from one or more transcripts in order to present the findings of qualitative research in a coherent and meaningful way. For example, there may be examples across participants' narratives of the way they were treated in hospital such as 'not being listened to', 'lack of interest in personal experiences' (as we have in the extract). These may be drawn together as a theme that runs through the narratives that could be named 'The patient's experience of hospital care'. The importance of going through this process is that at its conclusion, it will be possible to present the data from the interviews using quotations from the individual transcripts to illustrate where the researchers' interpretations come from. Thus, when organising the findings for presentation, each theme can become the title of a section in one's report or presentation. Underneath each theme will be the codes, examples from the texts and the researcher's own interpretation of what themes mean. Implications for real life, e.g. the treatment of people with chronic mental health problems, should also be given.

In the final section of this paper we will describe some ways of drawing together or 'synthesising' research findings to represent, as faithfully as possible, the meaning that participants ascribe to their life experiences. The work by Latif et al. referenced in the Further Reading at the end of this chapter, gives an example of how qualitative research findings might be presented.

16.4. DATA SYNTHESIS

Synthesis refers to drawing together into a whole, and this is the aim in the final stage of qualitative research. There are a number of ways that researchers can synthesise and present their findings, but any assumptions made must be supported by relevant quotations from the participants. In this way it is made clear to the reader that the themes under discussion have emerged from the participants' interviews and not the mind of the researcher. In Part IV we will look at mixed-methods research and some of the issues involved in combining data from different sources.

16.4.1. Report Planning and Writing

As we suggested above, if researchers code and theme they will naturally find the headings for sections of their report. Qualitative researchers tend to report 'findings' rather than 'results' as the latter imply that data have come from a quantitative source. The final presentation of the research will normally be in the form of a report or a paper and so should follow the accepted academic guidelines for this. In other words, there should be an introduction including a literature review and rationale for the research. There should be a section on the chosen methodology and a brief discussion about why qualitative methodology was the most appropriate and why, for example, IPA was chosen over grounded theory to guide the research. The method should then be described including ethics approval, choice of participants, recruitment and method of data collection, e.g. semi-structured interviews or focus groups. This is followed by the findings of the research which will form the main body of your report or paper. The findings should be written as if a story is being told and as such it is not necessary to have a lengthy discussion section at the end. This is because much of the discussion will take place around the participants' quotes so that all that is needed to close the report or paper is a summary, limitations of the research and the implications the research has for practice. As we have said many times, it is not the intention of qualitative research to be able to generalise the findings, therefore this is not, in itself, a limitation.

16.4.2. Presentation of Findings

Planning out the way findings are going to be presented is helpful. It is useful to put in the headings of each section (the themes that emerged from the data) and then make a note of the codes that exemplify the thoughts and feelings of your participants. It is generally advisable to put in the quotations that you want to use for each theme using each quotation only once. After all this is done the telling of the story can begin as you give your voice to the experiences of the participants, as you write around their quotations. Do not be afraid to draw assumptions from the participants' narratives as this is necessary to give an in-depth account of the phenomena in question. Discuss these assumptions, drawing on your participants to support you as you move from one code to another and from one theme to the next. Finally, as appropriate it is possible to include examples from literature or policy documents that add support for your findings. As an exercise, you may wish to code and theme the extract in Section 16.3 and tell the participant's story in your own way. Further Reading about 'doing' qualitative research can be found at the end of this chapter. In Chapter 17 we will look at how data might be drawn together and presented.

Qualitative research can help researchers to access the thoughts and feelings of research participants, which can enable the development of an understanding of the meaning people ascribe to their experiences. It can be used in health care research to explore how patients feel about their health and treatment. An understanding of these issues can help those involved in the design and delivery of care to tailor health care to match the individual needs of patients and to develop a concordant relationship. Doing qualitative research is not easy and may require a complete rethink of how research is conducted, particularly if researchers are more familiar with positivist approaches. There are many ways of conducting qualitative research, and this chapter has covered some of the practical issues regarding data collection, analysis and management. Further reading around the subject is essential to truly understand this method of accessing peoples' thoughts and feelings to enable us to tell the participant's story.

We are now going to rejoin Serena and then Rosi to see how qualitative methods might help them to answer their research questions. We will outline how they make the decisions about their research analysis and how they might code and theme their interview transcripts. We will continue with Serena and Rosi in Chapter 17 where they will draw their findings together and present them.

16.5.   CASE STUDY: SERENA

To refresh your memory from Chapter 5 here is a recap of Serena's situation.

Serena Leesi is a 3rd year MPharm student with a Saturday job at her local pharmacy. She really enjoys working with the clients who come into the pharmacy and has got to know many of them who come in regularly. Some of the

older clients seem to come in just for a chat and that's OK with Serena as long as the pharmacy is not too busy. Mrs Olive Trolave is one of the clients that Serena has got to know quite well and they are even on first name terms. Olive is a 56-year woman who has struggled with many health issues, including respiratory disease, high blood pressure and high cholesterol. As she thinks about Olive Serena realises that there are a number of clients like her who struggle with health issues, and what many of them have in common is that they need to quit smoking. Serena is interested in doing something concrete, practical and meaningful to help patients like Olive through the smoking cessation process. The generic tools and approaches she has learned at the university don't seem to be very effective for some reason.

Serena needs to have a look at the evidence for and against different smoking cessation tools and has a lot of planning to do if she is to gain a better understanding of the ones used in pharmacy practice. There are three main strands to her research:

1. Review the methods of smoking cessation that have been used in health care that have a track record of success. This will enable her to decide whether they are tools that actually do help people quit smoking (validity) and that they do so time and time again for a variety of patients (reliability)

2. Identify the smoking cessation methods that might work best for patients like Olive

3. If allowed, Serena could talk to some regular patients who come into the pharmacy about how they feel about quitting smoking.

In Chapter 5 Serena concentrated on looking for evidence of the validity and reliability of the tools that have been used to help people stop smoking, particularly in the community pharmacy setting. She looked at existing research into the use of HRT and found a mixture of results. One thing that Serena learned was that in health care it is important to think ahead to the long-term effects of treatment – particularly where medicines are concerned.

The third strand of Serena's research was to explore the possibility of talking to some regular patients who come into the pharmacy she works in to find out how they feel about smoking and quitting. Serena has to obtain permission from a number of people before she can do this, the first being her project supervisor.

Serena's project supervisor thinks it would be a good idea to do some qualitative work to find out first-hand what smokers feel about quitting. He agrees to guide Serena through the process of obtaining ethics approval to conduct a qualitative study with patients. Below we will outline how Serena might proceed beginning with research ethics approval and study design and ending with the coding and theming of an interview transcript. In Chapter 17 we will follow Serena and Rosi as they draw together their findings and write their project reports. We will give you some examples of what some of their documents might look like as we go along.

16.5.1. Ethics Approval

In Chapter 12, Section 12.3.1 we set out in some detail the principles of qualitative research ethics so we will just briefly recap here the considerations that Serena needs to take into account. First, please remember that the procedures for obtaining research ethics are complex and vary according to the type of research being undertaken. In the United Kingdom the Research Ethics Service comes under the authority of the Health Research Authority and you will find most of the information you require on their webpage at http://www.hra.nhs.uk/. It is essential, however, that you follow your own institution's procedures for obtaining ethics approval and your supervisor will be able to guide you through this process.

Some of the things Serena needs to think about are:
- ensuring the anonymity of individual participants wherever possible
- maintaining the confidentiality of participants
- asking only that which is absolutely necessary
- respecting and honouring the participant's involvement
- making sure participants have the option to withdraw from the research at any time without giving a reason
- giving participants the opportunity to review what they have said and to review any publications that come from the research
- making sure that all data collected in the study are securely stored
- making sure informed consent has been obtained
- making sure that participants are fully aware of and capable of providing consent to their participation in your study
- making sure that a 'safety netting' procedure is in place.

More information about all of these issues may be found in Chapter 12 (Section 12.3.1) and in the Further Reading section at the end of this chapter.

Serena must try to think about how her participants might feel at every stage of her research and if she does so she will help to ensure that their needs are put first. Serena has also written to the boss of the pharmacy in which she works, sending him the information about her research project and asking for his permission to talk to some clients.

16.5.2. Study Design

Serena decides that the most appropriate way of collecting information from her participants is to talk to them face-to-face. Chapter 13 of this textbook is devoted to research interviewing and so you will find much of the information you need about this approach in that chapter. Serena has chosen semi-structured interviews because they will give her some guidance during each interview whilst at the same time allowing her participants to speak freely. Sample interview schedule and topic guide are given in the next section.

16.5.3. Study Materials

Serena needs to ensure that her potential participants have all the information they need to enable them to make a decision about whether or not they want to take part. The most usual way of doing this is to provide them with a participant information sheet (PIS) which sets out in detail what they need to know. We have not given an example of a PIS here because they can be quite lengthy. However, if your research is based in the United Kingdom please follow this link and you will find lots of resources on the HRA website: http://www.hra.nhs.uk/resources/before-you-apply/consent-and-participation/consent-and-participant-information/.

You will also find information on the HRA website about what it means to give consent to take part in research and some examples of consent forms.

Serena will need an interview schedule to help guide her through her interviews with participants. You will find the rationale for using a schedule or 'topic guide' in Chapter 13 and in Box 16.2 we provide you with an example of what Serena's schedule might look like.

16.5 4. Identifying and Recruiting Potential Participants

Serena has received permission from the pharmacy boss to carry out the interviews.

Having worked in a community pharmacy for 2 years now Serena has got to know a number of the customers quite well including Mrs Truelove who has already said she would be happy to talk to Serena. Serena asks her pharmacist who else she might approach and how. The pharmacist suggests that rather than singling out individuals Serena puts a notice in the pharmacy telling people about the research and how they can get more information by asking her for an information sheet. That way no one is made to feel uncomfortable if they don't want to take part. Serena's supervisor agrees that this is the best way to recruit people to a research project and is in line with university and HRA guidelines.

16.5.5. Setting up the Interviews

Serena designs an eye-catching poster to place in the pharmacy. Instead of telling people they can ask for more information at the counter she decides to make up some packs with a letter and information sheet, and place these

BOX 16.2   Serena's Interview Schedule

Project Researcher
Serena Leesi
e-mail:

University of Fazakarly

Lead Researcher
Professor A.N.
    Other

**School of Pharmacy I Faculty of
Science I University of
Fazakarly**
*Exploring the Views of Smokers
About Smoking Cessation
Semi-Structured Interview
Schedule*

e-mail:

Introduction
The aim of today is to learn more about your experiences of smoking and your views on trying to give up. I have some questions to start us off but please feel free to tell me anything you think might be useful to help me understand how to help people quit smoking.
1. How long have you smoked for?
Prompts:
  • What made you start smoking?
  • How many cigarettes do you smoke?
  • Do other members of your family smoke?

2. Have you ever tried to give up?
  • If 'Yes' how did that go?
  • What made you relapse?
  • Is there anything that might have helped you more?
  • If 'No' would you like to give up?
  • How does the thought of giving up smoking make you feel?
4. If you have tried to give up what do you think might help you try again?
Prompts:
  • Help from other people
  • Which people helped the most?
  • Smoking cessation aids, e.g. chewing gum
5. If you have never tried to give up, what do you think would help?
Prompts:
  • Help from other people
  • Which people helped the most?
  • Smoking cessation aids, e.g. chewing gum
6. Is there anything else you would like to tell me?
  Thank you for taking part in my research.

---

next to the poster so that if anyone is interested they can just help themselves. This way people don't have to go to the counter to ask and so it makes the whole process far more discrete. In the information sheet Serena gives details about how people can contact her directly if they would like to take part. This is by email or by telephone to her supervisor's work number so that Serena doesn't have to give out her mobile number.

Serena is please that five people say they would like to be interviewed and they have given her their contact details so that she can make arrangements to do the interviews. She has already said in her information sheet that the interviews will take place in the consulting room at the pharmacy. This is a convenient place for the participants and also a safe place for Serena to meet people as there will always as be either a pharmacist or a counter assistant around if she needs help.

16.5.6.   Conducting the Interviews

The consulting room at the pharmacy is large enough to seat two people comfortably. There is also space for a small table in between them on which to place the recording device. There are toilet facilities and Serena can offer light refreshments, e.g. water, tea, coffee and biscuits. Serena gets the room set up well in advance to make sure that she is well prepared when her first participant arrives. She has prepared two copies of the consent form and she will ask each participant if they have read the information sheet and if they have any questions about the research. When the first participant arrives (Mrs Truelove) Serena greets her and shows her into the consulting room. She checks that Mrs Truelove is happy to continue with the interview and to have it audio-recorded. Mrs Truelove then signs the two copies of the consent form – one for her to keep and one for Serena's records.

Serena begins the interview as per her schedule and is very pleased she asked Mrs Truelove to be the first participant because she knows her quite well. The interview goes really well and Serena is looking forward to listening to the recording. When Mrs Truelove has left, Serena makes some additional notes (for more about field notes – see Chapter 13) about how the interview went – these will help her to make sense of her transcription. Serena has fixed the next interview for a week's time to give herself time to transcribe the first one so that she can follow-up any interesting topics in subsequent interviews.

BOX 16.3   Serena's Transcript of the Interview With Mrs Truelove

1   Hello Olive, thank you very much for agreeing to help me with my research.
2   *That's all right dear, anything that helps people like me give up is worth it.*
3   I'd like to start with a few questions if that's OK?
4   *Yes, of course – go ahead.*
5   How long have you smoked for?
6   *Ooh dear – now let me think. Well let me think …..[pause]….Well I'm 56 now and I started smoking when I was*
7   *about 15 or 16 so that's around 40 years now. Everyone smoked when I was a lass and so you didn't really fit*
8   *in if you didn't smoke. They all used to go to the pub too – but that's another story [laughs]. Didn't smoke very*
9   *much in those days, my mum would have been really angry if she knew so I had to be a bit careful.*
10   How many cigarettes do you smoke now?
11   *Well I have tried to cut it down since I had all these problems – Doctor XX said I should and I know she's right*
12   *but it's not as easy as just saying it. Especially when you've smoked as long as I have – it sort of becomes part*
13   *of your life.*
14   Does anyone else in your family smoke?
15   *My husband did smoke but he gave up years ago. Said we couldn't afford for both of us to smoke and I couldn't*
16   *face trying to give up then what with all the problems with our boy. Ooh he was a terror … [pause] … always*
17   *getting into trouble at school, if he ever went that is. I was working full time then and it was a real struggle to*
18   *cope. The thing I looked forward to most of all when I got home was a quiet sit down with a cuppa and a ciggie*
19   *for two.*
20   Have you ever tried to give up?
21   *Can't say I have to be honest. There was always a reason why I couldn't – I think we make excuses don't we?*
22   *That's why I've ended up in this state what with all these health problems – they're all to do with smoking you*
23   *know and it does make me feel guilty. Especially when my husband badgers me to stop… .*

16.5.7. Transcribing

Serena has been told that it can take a long time to transcribe an interview and that turns out to be quite right. The interview had lasted for nearly an hour and it takes her almost the rest of the week to finish the transcribing in between her lectures and other work. She finally has what she feels is an accurate account of what was said during the interview and listens to the recording one last time whilst going through the transcription. She adds in any pauses and notes about when they happened using her field notes. In Box 16.3 you will find an extract from Serena's transcript of the interview with Mrs Truelove.

16.5.8. Coding

As Serena looks through the extract a number of things that Mrs Truelove said seem really important. The main thing that hits Serena is that Mrs Truelove knows that most of her health problems have been either caused or made worse by the smoking but she hasn't been able to give up. Serena begins to write down her thoughts in the margins of the extract and you can see these in the box below (Fig. 16.1). As Serena codes the extract she realises that she missed the fact that Mrs Truelove didn't answer the question about how much she smoked. She makes a note to be more careful about following things like that up in the future.

TABLE 16.1   Emerging Themes

Influence of Family and Friends	Reasons for Smoking	Feelings About Smoking
Fitting in	Smoking part of	Making excuses
Everyone smoked	her life	for carrying on
Going against	Problems with	smoking
Mum	son	Feeling guilty
	Relieves stress	about health

16.5.9. Theming

As Serena continues she sees that there are some patterns emerging just from this short extract. She begins to enter the codes into a table and gives the 'clusters' of codes a theme (Table 16.1).

Even in this short extract we think you can see some patterns emerging and the things that Mrs Truelove says seem to fit into groups of phrases that have some similarities in meaning. In Chapter 17 we will look at how Serena might draw these themes together with some of the data from her other interviews and present them as part of her project report.

1   **Hello Olive, thank you very much for agreeing to help me with my research.**

2   *That's all right dear, anything that helps people like me give up is worth it.*

3   **I'd like to start with a few questions if that's OK?**

4   *Yes, of course – go ahead.*

5   **How long have you smoked for?**

Fitting in

6   *Ooh dear – now let me think. Well let me think .....[pause]....Well I'm 56 now and I started smoking*

7   *when I was about 15 or 16 so that's around 40 years now. Everyone smoked when I was a lass*   *Everyone smoked*

8   *and so you didn't really fit in if you didn't smoke. They all used to go to the pub too – but that's*

9   *another story [laughs]. Didn't smoke very much in those days, my mum would have been really*

10   *angry if she knew so I had to be a bit careful.*   *Going against Mum*

11   **How many cigarettes do you smoke now?**

Doesn't answer question

12   *Well I have tried to cut it down since I had all these problems - Doctor XX said I should and I know*   *Smoking part of life*

13   *she's right but it's not as easy as just saying it. Especially when you've smoked as long as I have*

14   *– it sort of becomes part of your life.*

15   **Does anyone else in your family smoke?**

Reasons for smoking

16   *My husband did smoke but he gave up years ago. Said we couldn't afford for both of us to smoke*

17   *and I couldn't face trying to give up then what with all the problems with our boy. Ooh he was a*

18   *terror ...[pause]... always getting into trouble at school, if he ever went that is. I was working full*   *reliever stress*

19   *time then and it was a real struggle to cope. The thing I looked forward to most of all when I got*

20   *home was a quiet sit down with a cuppa and a ciggie for two.*

21   **Have you ever tried to give up?**

22   *Can't say I have to be honest. There was always a reason why I couldn't – I think we make*   *making excuses*

23   *excuses don't we? That's why I've ended up in this state what with all these health problems –*

feeling guilty about health

24   *they're all to do with smoking you know and it does make me feel guilty. Especially when my*

25   *husband badgers me to stop....*

FIGURE 16.1 Coded extract.

CHAPTER SUMMARY

- This chapter has introduced qualitative data management.
- It has described the importance of being authentic to your participants' stories.

- It gives some examples of how to code and interpret data using Serena's research.
- It describes how to bring your data together into a coherent whole in a research report.

REFERENCE

Smith, J. A. (1996). Beyond the divide between cognition and discourse. *Psychology & Health, 11*, 261–271.

FURTHER READING

Pharmacy Practice Research
Farrell, B., Pottie, K., Woodend, K., et al. (2010). Shifts in expectations: evaluating physicians' perceptions as pharmacists integrated into family practice. *Journal of Interprofessional Care, 24*(1), 80–89.

Gregory, P., & Austin, Z. (2014). Postgraduation employment experiences of new pharmacists in Ontario in 2012–2013. *Canadian Pharmacy Journal, 147*(5), 290–299.

Marks, P. Z., Jennnings, B., Farrell, B., et al. (2014). "I gained a skill and a change in attitude": a case study describing how an online continuing professional education course for pharmacists supported achievement of its transfer to practice outcomes. *Canadian Journal of University Continuing Education, 40*(2), 1–18.

Nair, K. M., Dolovich, L., Brazil, K., & Raina, P. (2008). It's all about relationships: a qualitative study of health researchers' perspectives on interdisciplinary research. *BMC Health Services Research, 8*, 110.

Pojskic, N., MacKeigan, L., Boon, H., & Austin, Z. (2014). Initial perceptions of key stakeholders in Ontario regarding independent prescriptive authority for pharmacists. *Research into Social and Administrative Pharmacy, 10*(2), 341–354.

Grounded Theory
Strauss, A. L., & Corbin, J. (1998). *Basics of qualitative research: grounded theory procedures and techniques.* Thousand Oaks (CA: Sage Publications.

Constructivist Grounded Theory
Charmaz, K. (2000). Grounded theory: objectivist and constructivist methods. In N. Denzin & Y. Lincoln (Eds.), *Handbook of qualitative research* (2nd ed., pp. 509–535). Thousand Oaks (CA: Sage Publications.

Thurston, W. E., Coupal, S., Jones, C. A., et al. (2014). Discordant indigenous and provider frames explain challenges in improving access to arthritis care: a qualitative study using constructivist grounded theory. *International Journal of Equity in Health, 13*, 46.

Qualitative Data Collection
Arksey, H., & Knight, P. (1999). *Interviewing for social scientists: an introductory resource with examples.* Thousand Oaks (CA: Sage Publications.

Guest, G., Namey, E. E., & Mitchel, M. L. (2013). *Collecting qualitative data: a field manual for applied research.* Thousand Oaks (CA: Sage Publications.

Social Constructivist Theory
Social Constructivism. Berkeley (CA): University of California, Berkeley, Berkeley Graduate Division, Graduate Student Instruction Teaching & Resource Center; [Available from: http://gsi.berkeley.edu/gsi-guide-contents/learning-theory-research/social-constructivism/.

Transcription Editing Software
Rosenfelder, R. A. (2011). *Short introduction to transcribing with ELAN.* Philadelphia (PA): University of Pennsylvania Linguistics Laboratory. Available from: http://fave.ling.upenn.edu/downloads/ELAN_Introduction.pdfTitle.

Group Dynamics
Farnsworth, J., & Boon, B. (2010). Analysing group dynamics within the focus group. *Qualitative Research, 10*(5), 605–624.

Naturalistic Inquiry
Lincoln, Y. S., & Guba, E. G. (1985). *Naturalistic inquiry.* Thousand Oaks (CA: Sage Publications.

Presentation of Qualitative Findings
Latif, A., Boardman, H. F., & Pollock, K. (2013). A qualitative study exploring the impact and consequence of the medicines use review service on pharmacy support-staff. *Pharmacy Practice, 11*(2), 118–124.

Miles, M. B., & Huberman, A. M. (1994). *Qualitative data analysis.* Thousand Oaks: Sage.

Research Ethics
Oliver, P. (2010). *The student's guide to research ethics (Open up study skills).* Oxford, England: Open University Press.

Data Synthesis and Presentation of Findings

After reading this chapter you should be able to:
- understand the meaning of data synthesis
- describe the different types of authenticity
- understand the constant-comparative method

- define verification and give examples

17.1 INTRODUCTION

Qualitative research – regardless of technique used – typically generates a large volume of data that can be challenging to store, manage and analyse. While most frequently these data are in the form of words (for example, transcripts from interviews or focus group discussions), on occasion these data may be artefacts (e.g. a photograph, a video or a tangible object produced by an individual or group). In Chapter 16 we discussed ways of analysing qualitative data. Analysis involves reducing or breaking down data into its constituent components to facilitate comparisons and contrasts. This is a crucial step in the qualitative research process as it allows the researcher to manage the complexity inherent in human interactions and communications and focus on specific components. The desired end result is to be able to re-tell the participants' stories in such a way that the meanings of their actions or feelings can be better understood by others.

Analysis is also the necessary precursor to synthesis, an equally important step in the qualitative research process. **Synthesis** is usually described as the process of combining disparate components in order to construct something new. Within qualitative research, data synthesis is sometimes explained as 'turning data into insights': it is a creative process that allows the researcher (who has been immersed in the data and the research context) to *communicate* findings, sense and meaning to diverse audiences who are not as connected to data and context.

While data analysis can be a somewhat technical and proceduralised step in the qualitative research process,

synthesis is by definition, a highly creative process that relies equally on rigour and intuition. Though creativity is required, this is not to say that it is pure invention: instead skilled qualitative researchers can bridge the distance between participants and audiences, between subjects of research and broader communities, by speaking both languages in a respectful and constructive way. In this chapter, we will review formal and informal mechanisms for data synthesis and techniques for presenting qualitative research findings in meaningful ways to diverse audiences. The process of synthesis begins with an honest appraisal of the data by the researcher – in being true to ourselves we stand a better chance of being true to our participants. We need to ask ourselves when our memory and interpretation of what was said is indeed correct. In the next section we outline one of the key processes researchers can use to ensure they recognise their participants' meanings.

17.1.1. Authenticity

As you will have realised by now the researcher him/herself plays a central role in qualitative research. As has been highlighted in previous chapters, qualitative researchers must work diligently to ensure reflexivity is built-in to their research processes and activities. There is no attempt in qualitative research to pretend objectivity exists; instead, the researcher works to surface and articulate her/his subjectivities (biases, assumptions) and positions, most frequently through regular maintenance of and consultation with a reflexivity diary.

The objective of this is to support the authenticity of the research process. In this context **authenticity** refers to the extent to which the actual research process and its communication to others is respectful, accurate, genuine and trustworthy with respect to the participants who were involved in the work. Put more simply, authenticity is about being true to our participants' stories. Equally important for authenticity is the recognition that the findings of any research have implications that are both political and social. While quantitative research is frequently concerned with issues of reliability and validity, qualitative research recognises that these narrow psychometric dimensions do not adequately capture the spirit of authenticity.

Authenticity in qualitative research is generally described in terms of five core attributes or criteria that were developed by Guba and Lincoln in 1989:

a. Fairness: Authentic qualitative researchers are constantly reflecting on the fairness of their work. In this context, fairness relates to the opportunity for participants to co-create the research, rather than simply respond passively to questions. It means, for example, developing research questions in conjunction with the participants, or having participants integrally involved in data analysis through member checking processes. Fairness is key to authentic research because it recognises that the participants – not the researcher – are the centrepoint of the research work, and must be respected as equals in the process, not interchangeable widgets that can be discarded once questions have been answered.

b. Ontological authenticity: The effects of research on participants themselves must be considered as part of the research process. Qualitative research is typically filled with conversations and dialogue, and in this way, participants are exposed and vulnerable throughout the process. Being 'on display', or 'opening your heart' as a participant in research has a real effect on participants and not only must this be respected but it also must be honoured. Authenticity in this context requires a quid pro quo: while the researcher benefits from the participant's willingness to disclose or be observed, what benefit is conferred on the participant? Ontological authenticity suggests that the process of qualitative research (whether through interview, focus group, observation or other method) should help each participant engage in self-reflection and building of self-awareness. Participants need to feel good and proud about their contributions to the research. We must never lead participants to say things that they are not ready to say – this is the antithesis of ontological authenticity.

c. Educative authenticity: the interaction between researcher and participant is a mutually beneficial relationship, not a one-way benefit. Authenticity in this context means that the process of gathering information has an educational quality to it, allowing both the researcher and the participant to learn and develop in the process. A participant leaving an interview with a researcher should feel they have actually learned something as a small reward for being willing to disclose and be vulnerable.

d. Catalytic authenticity: qualitative research may produce a wide variety of intended and unintended outcomes, particularly from the perspective of participants. Catalytic authenticity refers to the ways in which the participants respond by taking some action or step to change after the interaction with the researcher. For example, through the process of responding to a researcher's questions, the participant may engage in self-reflection and deliberation and as a result may actually do things differently. The extent to which the research process itself triggers change in the participant is an expression of catalytic authenticity.

e. Tactical authenticity: the disclosure and exposure that is inherent in most qualitative research may produce the desire for change on the part of participants, but circumstances and environment may frustrate participants' intentions to change. At this point, what is the responsibility of the researcher to support, empower or enable change? Tactical authenticity suggests qualitative researchers are not simply passive outsiders who swoop in, gather data, and quietly exit stage left. Instead, by virtue of engaging in qualitative research and in respect of the relationship that forms between researcher and participant, there is an obligation on the part of the researcher to engage with the participant in constructing change.

For some health care professionals, these layers of authenticity may appear daunting: they may say, 'we are researchers, not social workers!'. For others, there may be a belief that, 'this is just all too much and not necessary – my goal is to understand, not to change!'. The extent to which these various authenticities are prominent or play out in research is of course a function of context, environment and the researcher's own psyche. At the core, authenticity is focussed on honouring the participant and not simply treating them as an incidental prop to further the researcher's own interests and ambitions. It is important to remember that we are all changed in some way by our everyday experiences, so just think how much more our lives are changed if we divulge personal information in a qualitative interview. For Further Reading about authenticity please see the work of Guba and Lincoln referenced at the end of this chapter.

17.1.2. The Participant's Voice, the Participant's Story

Authenticity reminds us of the fundamental proposition that is central to all qualitative inquiry: the researcher is simply a vehicle to amplify the participants' voices and facilitate the telling of the participants' stories. The stories are not about the researcher but about the participants. For example, in telling the story of the impact of systemic discrimination in the southern United States, the classic story of *To Kill a Mockingbird* is sometimes criticised for – yet again – selecting upper middle class white voices as the vehicle by which the story is told. While, of course, systemic discrimination had effects on these upper middle class white individuals, is this REALLY the story that is of most importance or interest? Why was this story told from the perspective of Scout Finch and not from the perspective of Boo Radley? Or from the perspective of Calpurnia, the Finch family's maid? Some may say that, as a southern white woman, the author (Harper Lee) wisely decided she could ONLY respectfully tell the story from the perspective of a white upper middle class child, for she had once been that person. She had never 'been' an African-American maid, or a developmentally challenged young man, so to 'tell' the story from those perspectives would have betrayed authenticity.

This is clearly a complicated and highly sensitive issue: can a white person – no matter how outraged by injustice and unfairness – 'tell' a story of racism? Can a straight person – no matter how open-minded – 'tell' a story of homophobia? Can a man – no matter how well intentioned and supportive – actually 'tell' a story of sexism? And if they cannot – or should not – what are the implications for building awareness, respect and understanding? Can a researcher who has never experienced cancer 'tell' a story of what it is like to live with cancer?

There is no clear consensus on these issues within the qualitative research communities: some researchers firmly and passionately believe that 'outsiders' cannot and should not be involved in research in worlds they know little about. To do so is to appropriate or steal stories from others for the benefit of the researcher, not the participant. Others believe there is great value in qualitative researchers acting as intermediaries between and amongst diverse communities. *To Kill a Mockingbird* is one of the greatest, most enduring classics of American literature, read and beloved by generations of people the world over, and for many, it is one of the most searing indictments of racism and intolerance ever written – precisely because it was written by a white woman for a predominantly white audience.

As a qualitative researcher, sensitivity to the participant's voice and respect in its reporting is crucial for your credibility, success and conscience. Does this mean that you can only perform qualitative research with people who are 'just like you'? And if so what might be lost – or gained – from such a specific perspective? The integrity of your research – and in fact of qualitative research in general – is intimately connected to the participants who must not only recognise

and accept but actually value the interpretation of sense and meaning the researcher imparts to the data.

There are safeguards that can be developed to support the authenticity described above. We can facilitate the engagement and involvement of participants throughout the research process to the very best of our ability, and they can tell us when and if we deviate from their stories. However, the full engagement and involvement of participants may not be feasible during the process of data synthesis, the point in the research process where researchers are '…turning data into insights'. What researchers can do at this stage is hold the participants' voices in their minds as they are working, as a constant reminder to be authentic.

17.2 SYNTHESIS OF FINDINGS IN QUALITATIVE RESEARCH

The novice qualitative researcher can be forgiven for second-guessing their initial decision to undertake research using a qualitative method. Typically, the data generated during qualitative research can turn into an avalanche of transcript snippets, word counts, coding structures and theme titles. The attempt to reduce the complexity of the raw data set through analysis – cutting back and cutting down into smaller constituent components – may frequently give the appearance of actually increasing complications and complexity.

It isn't easy to articulate what something actually 'means' to different stakeholders to get across to them why it matters, why it is important, what we should do – after we have made 'sense' of it – understood it and explained it.

A central challenge in the process is the recognition that, with the exception of an in-depth case study method (covered in Chapter 18), most qualitative research methods generate data from different, unique, individuals. Each individual is a product of their unique environment, circumstances and context. Even though, in many cases, qualitative research attempts to focus on a community of individuals who share a specific demographic characteristic (for example, in Sandy's research, 'young' people with diabetes), the reality is that sharing one specific demographic characteristic does not mean that the individual has anything in common with anyone else. A young person with diabetes who is poor may have more in common with an older non-diabetic person who is poor than with another young person with diabetes who is rich – or perhaps not. It is simply not possible to rely upon defining demographic characteristics (which are typically the starting point for most research in health care) to ensure consistency amongst participants.

In synthesising findings in qualitative research, a central dilemma then becomes how to find commonalities where they exist whilst simultaneously respecting and expressing the differences within the community studied.

Beyond this complexity lies the further challenge of then presenting both similarities and differences in a way that is meaningful, authentic and respectful to both participants and to the diverse audiences that will be consumers of the research.

One key technique for synthesis utilised widely in qualitative research is the constant-comparative method.

17.3.   THE CONSTANT-COMPARATIVE METHOD

Though frequently described as an analytical method (particularly in the context of grounded theory (see Chapter 18)), the constant-comparative method can be extended as a vehicle for actually synthesising findings, when used in conjunction with other methods to enhance trustworthiness such as member checking and triangulation (see Chapters 12 and 16).

Constant comparative synthesis involves building an understanding of the participants' experiences by making sense of their words and then finding meaning from this sense. The term 'constant comparative' captures the process itself as the researcher is constantly comparing (i.e. regularly checking) earlier ideas, concepts and themes as the research evolves step by step. For example, the researcher may know little about the subject but will interview the first participant; during this process, and after consulting field notes and undertaking initial analysis he/she will move to the second participant. During the interview with the second participant, the researcher continuously reflects back upon and compares the first participant's responses and behaviours with what is occurring in the second interview. Experienced interviewers are able to flexibly use terms, language and words from the first interview during the second interview as a technique of validating or establishing the credibility of these terms. After the second interview has been transcribed and field notes reviewed, this new data are compared reflexively with the first interview to establish sense and meaning from what both participants have said. This process continues throughout the data-gathering process and in essence, analysis and synthesis are occurring simultaneously and in tandem with data gathering through this recurrent and constant process of comparison.

17.3.1.   Case Study: Sandy

Let's go back to our pharmacist Sandy who you'll remember is interested in learning about his young patient's lives, experiences and choices, particularly with respect to food, since he knows this is a major issue with young diabetic patients. We will show how Sandy can begin to synthesise the narratives from one participant to the next. The first person he interviews says this:

Participant: *Yeah, well, you know my dad isn't around much, right? So it's only my mum and my three sisters and me. Money's tight, we haven't got a lot of cash, so I know she is trying but sometimes no one gets around to the shop to buy food or groceries so we do the best we can with the McDonalds and whatever else is close by.*

Interviewer: What about lunch, at school? Do you bring your own lunch?

Participant: *Nah, we ain't got no time for that. Sometimes, I'll bum a sandwich or something off one of my mates, sometimes, there's the caf, right and they have good chips or whatever. Sometimes you just go without, you know?*

In the above extract the interviewer begins to pick up that there might be a connection between money (or socioeconomic status), dietary habits and health related to diabetes. Since Sandy himself grew up in a conventional family structure with two middle class parents, he is struck by how uncomfortable he feels when a child in his community who looks, acts and sounds like he did when he was a teenager, can be so matter-of-fact about sometimes not having enough money for food. He notes that 'chips' seem to be this child's default food and why not? They are cheap, filling and plentiful even if they are not healthy. In the second interview, the next participant says this:

Participant: *I'm from a very strict family, right? We're Jains, do you know about that? We have all these really strict rules about what you can eat and what you can't eat. Even stricter than vegetarians, right? It's impossible to eat anything. Sometimes I'll cheat, you know when I'm with my mates or whatever but, well, I don't like to do that too much if I can help it. Makes me feel bad really, like I'm disappointing my parents.*

Interviewer: What about lunch, at school? Do you bring your own lunch? Would you be able to afford to buy lunch there if you needed to?

Participant: *No choice really is there? Can't eat anything they serve in the caf, it's all chips and crap that's either meat or made with lard or animal parts or whatever. I can't eat that stuff. My mum is like super organised about this food stuff, she has to be, so I get a lunch made every day. It's funny, I'm one of the only kids I know like that. But I like it – always good and saves me money.*

This interview raises new ideas for Sandy, about the role of ethnicity and culture in dietary choices and behaviours. Sandy has never heard of these 'Jains' before but is intrigued by how well organised this family must be to maintain such strict dietary controls on their children. In his community there are many families that seem to have dietary restrictions and Sandy admits he always found this irritating and off-putting – why can't they just fit in like everyone else? Now he wonders if he needs to be less judgmental. It also echoes an emerging idea from the first interview about family structure and parental influence and how all of this may affect food choices and ultimately diabetic control. Again the issue of 'chips' as a food choice came up, but this time the participant's culture and heritage appear to be protecting him somewhat from making bad choices. In the third interview, the participant says:

Participant: *I get 5 quid every day to buy lunch, so do my brothers and sisters. Dad just gives it to us in the morning. Sometimes I eat at the caf – love the chips there – or sometimes me and my mates go down the road to a shop that serves dead good pizza. Never go hungry if you know what I mean. But I know it's kinda crap food – I've had all the lectures already from everyone about it but, well it's just too easy right?*

Interviewer: So you have enough money to buy a good lunch at school, but you don't? Why not?

Participant: *I dunno.*

Interviewer: Do they serve healthy food, could you buy it there or close by?

Participant: *Yeah for sure but who wants that? Like salads and things like that. Ugh. My mum used to try to pack me like fruit and veg but I'd just throw it out every day anyway so she gave up and now they give me the fiver every morning.*

After this interview, the researcher is struck by how similar the end behaviour is of the first and third participants with respect to dietary choices, despite the obvious socioeconomic and family structure differences. Despite having a comfortable socioeconomic status and a conventional family, this participant is making similar choices to the first participant – and again those 'chips' keep coming up as an issue. The second participant's cultural background may have an important influence that needs to be followed-up in subsequent interviews.

17.3.2. Data Analysis and Synthesis

As can be seen in this example, data synthesis is occurring simultaneously and in real time along with data analysis as the interviews are progressing. Interviewing is not simply a robotic data gathering exercise in which the researcher reads off a prepared script of questions and carefully documents responses. Instead, interviewing gives the researcher an opportunity to play around with emerging ideas and themes, test certain assumptions (e.g. Sandy initially thought lack of money equated with bad food choices but after the third interview he's not so sure), and start to build some mental models and theories around the behaviours being observed.

All the participants in Sandy's – or any researcher's – study are unique human beings with distinct stories to tell. The art and science of qualitative data synthesis involves a variety of skills related to listening, thinking, analysis, open-mindedness, deductive reasoning inductive reasoning, and ultimately

insight without judgment about the choices people make. It is impossible for us to provide you with a roadmap of how to undertake synthesis in qualitative research – it is a process that must be customised to each individual situation, taking into account your own reflexivity and environment.

Novice researchers are encouraged to consider working closely with more experienced qualitative researchers through an initial set of interviews or focus groups or observations, so they can learn through role modelling how this process works best. While it may be tempting to assume anyone who can talk can interview and anyone who can think can analyse and synthesise, the reality is much more nuanced that this. If you are new to research you can benefit immensely from a qualitative methods teaching strategy known as 'talk-aloud', in which the learner literally says out loud what she/he is thinking through the analysis stage and the mentor/teacher poses reflective questions back to push the learner higher towards synthesis.

17.3.3. Field Notes Again

While the 'art' of data synthesis may be clearer to you now, the 'science' of it is also important to keep in mind. An important feature of the constant-comparative method is careful note-taking and documentation, in field notes, reflexivity logs, and transcripts. In the above example involving Sandy, all three of these participants arrived independently at a discussion or mention of 'chips'. If this trend persists across future interviews (and there is no reason to believe it wouldn't) careful documentation in field notes and methodical review of transcripts would highlight this word in Sandy's consciousness. The frequency with which certain words, phrases or terms are mentioned (or in some cases studiously and deliberately avoided! Think back to Serena's interview with Mrs Truelove, where she avoided telling Serena how many cigarettes she smoked – without documentation as part of the scientific approach to this process, the researcher would overlook or forget such patterns. As this word 'chips' rises in frequency, the context within which the word is used will allow Sandy to start to make sense of what 'chips' mean to teenagers. Fast, cheap, convenient, social bonding, social signal of fitting in with one's mates, taboo prohibited by religion/culture, etc.

For most researchers, the process of data analysis and synthesis through the constant-comparative method is amongst the most exhilarating and stimulating parts of the qualitative research process. There is a puzzle to be solved and clues abound, only if the researcher is adept enough to find them and clever enough to connect the dots.

The analysis and synthesis of qualitative data are ultimately interpretive and therefore subjective processes; different researchers may consequently interpret the same data set in different ways. For example, in the above example with Sandy's participants, a researcher may reasonably decide that the real issue isn't culture, money or family structure – it's simply availability of chips in the school cafeteria. Get rid of the chips – get rid of the problem! Most researchers (and virtually all teenagers) would scoff at such a simplistic synthesis, knowing full well that prohibition of chips in the cafeteria will simply lead to a clever entrepreneur opening a 'chippy' two doors down from the school. The issue here is not one of right or wrong synthesis, but instead of the credibility of the synthesis that can potentially be enhanced through verification activities.

17.4. VERIFICATION

In the qualitative literature, there is significant debate as to the need or value in having analyses and syntheses verified or validated by external parties. On the one hand it is argued that this can make the process more rigorous and robust, emulating in some ways the reliability or reproducibility checks that are common in quantitative research. On the other hand, some purists believe that since no claims to generalisability exist for research of this sort, verification is a meaningless bureaucratic exercise that will inhibit rather than promote effective scholarship.

The most common forms of validation are respondent validation (sometimes called 'member checking') and peer review (sometimes called 'peer debrief').

17.4.1. Respondent Validation (Member-Checking)

This generally involves returning to participants and asking them to carefully read through their (and sometimes other participants') interview transcripts and compiled field notes and/or compiled analyses or syntheses documents. In this way, participants actually get to see how their own words were interpreted, analysed, used and synthesised by the researcher – with the important safeguard of having some control and potentially a veto on what was done. This significantly enhances the authenticity of the research as it allows participants to engage as co-creators of the synthesis itself. As might be imagined this can be an incredibly time-consuming, contentious, and sometimes ultimately futile process when no agreement or consensus can be reached amongst disparate participants and the researcher. Further, if this process does not occur relatively soon after data collection, participants' views and opinions may evolve and change over time, and sometimes simply by virtue of having participated in the study in the first place (see Section 17.1.1. for the value of this evolutionary process in terms of authenticity). In some cases, participants may actually want or insist on a re-write because having seen their own words on paper they may exhibit a social desirability bias and want

to restate, reframe, or simply change entirely what was initially said, so they feel they do not come across in a certain, negative way. Despite these potential threats and challenges to the process, member checking continues to be one of the most recognised and respected validation processes available for data synthesis.

17.4.2. Peer Review (Peer Debrief)

This involves collaboration with at least one other suitably qualified and experienced researcher who will independently review, analyse and synthesise all data, transcripts, etc., from the research process. The key feature of this process is independence. Asking two similarly qualified individuals with access to the same data to undertake separate processes, and comparing final results, can be an important safeguard against lone researcher bias, and can help to provide additional insights that can meaningfully contribute to synthesis. There are some useful tools available designed by Lincoln and Guba that use a questionnaire to assess researcher bias (see Further Reading). There is, of course, a risk that the two independent researchers may reach completely different conclusions, which can make life a little difficult. One solution to this is to obtain a third review as a sort of tie-breaker; although this can lead to a continuous spiral where no-one agrees with anyone else. An alternative is to have the two independent researchers meet to discuss differences and come to a compromise – a process that may be easier to suggest in a textbook such as this than to arrange in reality! Conceptually both approaches are flawed: if both researchers' perspectives are grounded in and supported by the data, how can anyone (most of all, qualitative researchers grounded in the post-positivist tradition) say one is 'right' or more valid than the other?

There is no clear consensus in the literature about the value, need or best process for validation of analysis and synthesis. A further process that may be used to address this issue is triangulation, the process of using alternative, complementary sources of data to confirm or refute themes, analysis and synthesis.

17.4.3. Triangulation

As the term suggests, 'triangulation' means taking multiple (generally three) perspectives on the same issue, the idea being that when the same object is observed from three different places, its truest nature will become apparent. In qualitative synthesis terms, this can mean asking different people to comment on the same situation, topic or individual, then examining their responses in a constant comparative manner to define commonalities. It can also mean using different types of data: for example, triangulation can occur through an interview, observing video footage of students purchasing chips in a school cafeteria, and examining potato consumption logs kept in the school kitchen. The point of triangulation is not to claim there is a singular truth, rather it is to support the notion that different perspectives contribute different faces or aspects of the truth and seeing a situation from these multiple perspectives provides the researcher with a robust method for verification.

At first read, this process of data synthesis in qualitative research may appear overwhelming and impenetrable. While it is complex, and as much art as it is science, it is a process that can be learned, and when practiced and refined, can be an invaluable tool for researchers. It is not a process that is undertaken trivially or lightly; when undertaken in an amateurish manner, the results will lack credibility and will be dismissed by your audience. Learning the process under the guidance of a teacher or mentor, through the actual act of doing qualitative research in a rigorous manner, is frequently the best mechanism for honing skills and developing confidence. Once you get hooked on doing qualitative research it really is an exciting and enriching process!

17.5. REPORT PLANNING AND WRITING

The presentation of qualitative research to diverse audiences is as important as the synthesis of the data itself. Finding the balance between your voice as a researcher immersed in the data itself and the voices of your participants (which admittedly at times may be a cacophony of disagreement and contradiction) can be a challenge. There are two general approaches that are used in the presentation of findings of qualitative research.

The first involves somewhat straightforward narrative reporting, in which key findings under each main theme or category are presented and supported using relevant and appropriate verbatim quotations from the transcripts themselves to illustrate each point. This approach has the advantage of placing the participants' voices front and centre and minimising the voice of the researcher. It also allows the reader of the research the opportunity to understand the thinking behind the analysis and to determine for him/herself whether the themes are indeed appropriate and adequate. In many ways, this approach transfers some of the burden for synthesis onto the reader, leaving the researcher to assume responsibility for the analysis (which of course can still be refuted by the reader). The advantage of this approach is that it does not lead or force the reader to a preconceived conclusion and therefore can be seen as minimising the risks associated with researcher subjectivity or bias. Ultimately, the reader decides if she/he agrees with the analysis (since proof or evidence for each theme is provided in the form of transcript excerpts). If in agreement, the reader then formulates a large part of the synthesis him/herself.

Alternatively, it is possible to present findings in the form of a discussion, in which the researcher's voice dominates and is supported by selected transcript excerpts along the way. This discussion approach highlights and presents the researcher's synthesis and provides quotations not for the purpose of verification or evidence but instead to simply be illustrative. The risk of this approach is of course that the researcher's voice overwhelms the participants, and the true story may be lost. Further, this approach requires readers to have significant trust in the researcher's abilities and motives. For many readers, however, there is a significant advantage to this approach, particularly when the researcher is considered a trusted expert in an area: the distillation of complexity through such an expert is indeed exactly what some readers will want, not the 'opportunity' to double-check the researcher's themes and synthesise them for themselves. In the next section we will rejoin Serena as she draws her findings together using a combination of the two methods.

One very helpful resource to consult when both developing a qualitative research protocol and generating a report that flows from data synthesis is the Equator Network (Enhancing the QUAlity and Transparency Of health Research: www.equator-network.org). This group has published consolidated criteria for reporting qualitative research (COREQ), a 32-item checklist for those using interviews and focus groups. This checklist can be used both proactively in the design and implementation of research and retrospectively when publications, posters, or abstracts are being developed.

Like so much in this chapter, there is no clear consensus in the literature or in the qualitative research community in terms of what is best or most beneficial. It will depend on the individual context and circumstance of both reader and researcher.

17.5.1. Publishing Qualitative Work

Historically there have been concerns expressed by researchers using qualitative methods that their work may not garner interest and support from the broader health sciences community, due to the erroneous perception that qualitative work may lack scientific rigour. Today, this is no longer the case. All major, high-impact journals will publish high-quality work rooted in qualitative methods, and in fact many major journals in the health sciences have even commissioned and published primers and guidelines to support the production of high-quality qualitative research. Using qualitative methods and methodologies is not a barrier to publication in the top-ranked journals, provided sufficient attention is payed to quality.

Beyond publication of articles, there are other methods for disseminating qualitative research including the following:

a. Posters: Poster presentations are an important vehicle for dissemination as they allow novice researchers and those who are just commencing their work to start to share observations and findings with a broader community. In some cases, posters may be 'presented', usually in the format of a brief oral presentation to introduce the poster to conference attendees followed by an opportunity for those attendees to review the poster and speak with the presenter directly. Alternatively, some posters may not be formally presented but the researcher is still available, standing beside the poster during the session, to interact informally with interested readers.

b. Abstracts: Where possible, submitting your work in a way that is adjudicated (or peer reviewed) will heighten both the credibility and impact of your research. Abstracts are summaries of the work designed to provide a high-level summation to a busy audience who may then choose to follow-up in more depth. In many cases, conferences that peer-review posters will also publish abstracts for accepted posters which can then be searched using tools such as MedLine or International Pharmacy Abstracts (IPA). This will allow your work to be accessed by many more people than only those who attended the conference itself.

c. Podium presentations: Many conferences offer opportunities for oral presentations to a diverse audience. In most cases, these presentations are peer reviewed and abstracts will be published. Podium presentations are considered somewhat more prestigious than posters as the oral component of the presentation presents unique opportunities for in-depth discussions.

d. Invited or keynote presentations: As your research career and experience progress, invitations to present your work at local, national or international meetings and conferences may flow. These are considered amongst the highest form of praise and acceptance; invitations from peers to present or lead a keynote lecture provide unprecedented opportunities to reach diverse audiences. Increasingly, qualitative researchers are being recognised on par with quantitative colleagues at such meetings and qualitative work is being incorporated within many seemingly quantitative research keynote lectures.

17.6. CASE STUDY: SERENA

In Chapter 16 we looked at how we might approach the coding and analysis of qualitative data. We ended that chapter with a table showing how Serena had begun to theme her coding, and this is reproduced in Table 17.1.

The themes shown in Table 17.1 were those that emerged from one interview only, so as Serena continued her

TABLE 17.1 Emerging Themes

Influence of Family and Friends	Reasons for Smoking	Feelings About Smoking
Fitting in Everyone smoked Going against Mum	Smoking part of her life Problems with son Relieves stress	Making excuses for carrying on smoking Feeling guilty about health

interviews she included some questions about the things her first participant had said.

What particularly interested Serena is that however much her first participant wanted to quit smoking there were things going on in her life that prevented her from doing so. It is almost as if smoking is a crutch that helps people get by – rather like over eating or drinking too much alcohol.

In the next interview Serena asks her participant about whether they have ever tried to give up smoking:

Serena: So have you ever tried to give up smoking?

Participant 2: *Oh, have I ever. I can't remember how many times I've either said I'm going to give it up or actually tried. Never last more than a few days though.*

Serena: What sort of things make you start again?

Participant 2: *Oh, mostly work stuff. I've got a really rotten boss who just expects everything yesterday and I really can't cope without a fag….*

Serena: How does relapsing make you feel?

Participant 2: *To be honest, love, I feel like a complete and utter failure – the fact that I can't cope with life without those weeds at my age… .*

Serena is beginning to see two things that seem to be associated with giving up smoking. One is that it seems to help people cope with life and the second is they feel guilty about not giving up. The first two participants are older (in their 50s) but the next participant is younger (23 years), so Serena asks the same questions to see whether the length of time people have been smoking makes a difference.

Serena: So have you ever tried to give up smoking?

Participant 3: *Well I have but it makes a real difference when I go out with my mates. They all smoke and it's really hard to resist – they're always saying 'Go on, have a fag'. Also, I've been out of a job for ages and that makes me really stressed. Every time I go for a job someone else has got there before me – I suppose I get bored too….*

Serena: Do cigarettes make you feel less stressed?

Participant 3: *Oh yeh, you know, as soon as I have a fag I feel better but then when I haven't got any that's stressful too.*

Serena: How would you feel about trying to give up?

TABLE 17.2 Adding Codes and Themes

Influence of Family and Friends	Reasons for Smoking	Feelings About Smoking	Cost
Fitting in (P1)	Smoking part of her life (P1)	Making excuses for carrying on smoking (P1)	Damage to health (P1)
Everyone smoked (P1)	Problems with son (P1)		Cigarettes are expensive (P3)
Going against Mum (P1)	Relieves stress (P1)	Feeling guilty about health (P1)	
Peer-group pressure (P3)	Stress at work (P2)	Feeling a failure (P2)	
	Stress from not having a job (P3)	Can't cope with life without a fag (P2)	

Participant 3: *I'd really like to give it a go. Apart from anything else it's so expensive – almost all my unemployment money goes on fags... .*

Now Serena has conducted some more interviews she can begin to add codes and themes to her table. She names her participants by number in the order she interviewed them so that she can both refer to them without using their names, and find the quotes she will need to write up her findings. In the table you will see that the first participant becomes 'P1' and so on. Serena has found that other participants talked about feeling a failure and not being able to cope. But now she thinks there is something more. There are costs involved in smoking, for P1 these are damage to her health and for P3 it is monetary cost. Serena adds 'Cost' to her table as a theme.

We have enough information in Table 17.2 to begin to write up Serena's findings. Remember that there is more than one way of presenting qualitative findings and you should choose the one that enables you to depict the participants' stories in the way you feel most exemplifies their narratives. Serena has already written up her literature review and described the method she used in collecting her data (see Chapter 2). She now adds her findings to her report. Please note that we are writing up the data from three participants, which would be quite acceptable in qualitative research because we are not trying to generalise across a population as we would be if we were doing quantitative research. You will notice that in some places we indent the quotation and in others it forms part of the text. This is because the rule of thumb for writing up qualitative research is that quotes of under 40 words go in the text, but please check with your supervisor or the publisher you are writing for before proceeding.

FINDINGS FROM INTERVIEWS

The coding from the interview transcripts of three participants was drawn together and four themes emerged that helped the researcher to develop a picture of how the people interviewed felt about giving up smoking. The themes are 'Influence of family and friends', 'Reasons for smoking', 'Feelings about smoking' and 'Cost'. The findings are written around the participants own words and these are shown in italics in the text. Each participant's unique identifier is shown at the end of each quotation and their words have been changed as little as possible to retain the authenticity of their stories. Participants are referred to as 'they' in the text, rather than 'he' or 'she' to maintain their confidentiality.

Influence of Family and Friends

Other people appear to play a big role in whether someone starts smoking in the first place and whether they continue to smoke. The participant below talked about how they started to smoke at an early age because it was something that everyone did:

'Well I'm 56 now and I started smoking when I was about 15 or 16 so that's around 40 years now. Everyone smoked when I was a lass and so you didn't really fit in if you didn't smoke. They all used to go to the pub too – but that's another story [laughs].' (P1 – see Chapter 16).

Participant 3 also spoke about peer group pressure saying, *'Well I have but it makes a real difference when I go out with my mates. They all smoke and it's really hard to resist – they're always saying "Go on, have a fag"...'* (P3). This quotation shows that the influence of others has an effect at different points in a smoker's life. For the first it was at the beginning of smoking and for the second it

Continued

FINDINGS FROM INTERVIEWS—CONT'D

was when they were trying to give up. The second participant was younger and seemed to find it difficult to withstand the pressure from friends. With no job and very little money it is possible that keeping their friends was more important than quitting smoking. Influences of others also came from other places and had an effect for different reasons. Participant 2 spoke about their boss saying '*I've got a really rotten boss who just expects everything yesterday and I really can't cope without a fag...*' (P2). The fact that this participant cannot cope without a cigarette suggests that reasons for smoking are complex and they vary from person to person.

Reasons for Smoking

Reasons for smoking varied as did reasons for continuing to smoke. Participant 1 said '*When you've smoked as long as I have – it sort of becomes part of your life.*' (P1 – see Chapter 16). However they went on to say that family problems had played a big part in continuing to smoke:

> '*I couldn't face trying to give up then what with all the problems with our boy. Ooh he was a terror ... [pause] ... always getting into trouble at school, if he ever went that is. I was working full time then and it was a real struggle to cope. The thing I looked forward to most of all when I got home was a quiet sit down with a cuppa and a ciggie for two.*' (P1)

This participant talks about the cigarettes at the end of the day as if they were almost a reward for getting through it and both of the other participants talked about relief from stress when they gave their reasons for smoking. Participant 3 said, '*Oh yeh, you know, as soon as I have a fag I feel better but then when I haven't got any that's stressful too.*' (P3). In this case having a cigarette made the participant feel better but then they felt worse again if they ran out. This indicates that the effect of nicotine on the body is quite profound if its withdrawal can cause

symptoms so quickly. In the summary at the end of these findings we will draw on the literature about smoking cessation to identify some of the withdrawal symptoms and how they might be alleviated.

Feelings About Smoking

Feelings about smoking itself were mixed with participant 1 saying they felt guilty about smoking, '*That's why I've ended up in this state what with all these health problems – they're all to do with smoking you know and it does make me feel guilty. Especially when my husband badgers me to stop...*' (P1). The feeling of failure was expressed by participant 2 as they felt they should be able to give up at their age saying '*To be honest, love, I feel like a complete and utter failure – the fact that I can't cope with life without those weeds at my age.*' (P2). The issue of coping came up in each interview. Participants talked of not being able to cope without cigarettes for different reasons – for participant 1 (as we heard earlier) cigarettes helping to cope with their son's behaviour. On the other hand participant 2 said that it helped them to cope with their 'rotten boss'.

Cost

In each of the narratives participants referred to some form of cost that was involved in smoking. For participant 1 smoking had resulted in a succession of health problems and they had been advised to give up by their GP. '*Well I have tried to cut it down since I had all these [health] problems - Doctor XX said I should and I know she's right but it's not as easy as just saying it...*' (P1). As we heard earlier, participant 1 said they felt guilty about not being able to give up and it must be very hard to know that a lifestyle has resulted in ill health. Participant 1 had started smoking many years before when 'everyone smoked' and had used it as a crutch ever since. It might be suggested that these sorts of feelings are taken into account in a non-judgemental way when designing smoking-cessation programmes.

Hopefully, you will have felt you were part of the participants' stories as you read through Serena's findings. Lending her voice to theirs enabled her to show sympathy and understanding and to point to ways of making smoking-cessation programmes more effective.

Finally, as you will have gathered from this chapter, qualitative data synthesis is a complex and challenging process, but it is essential to high-quality, rigorous qualitative

research. A balance of idealism and pragmatism will ultimately guide your decisions as a researcher. As outlined in this chapter, there are many different and controversial practices that have been proposed, and there is no clear consensus on which are considered best practices. As a result, we cannot provide you with a clear roadmap of how best to synthesise data. Each situation, circumstance, researcher, participant and reader will have unique concerns and issues that will factor into the final decision. In this complex environment, it is advisable for novice researchers to consider working closely with more experienced qualitative researchers to learn-through-doing. Simply being able to talk and read does not qualify anyone to undertake qualitative research; while this may be obvious, it is striking how many well-intentioned but inexperienced clinicians suddenly and without background or training launch into qualitative work because it appears 'easier' than quantitative research. There is inherent rigour, discipline and a strong scientific tradition to qualitative research: when employed effectively, the results can be most impactful.

CHAPTER SUMMARY

- This chapter has defined data synthesis.
- It has described how to present research findings and how to get them published.
- It has used the research of our case study student, Serena, to illustrate this.

FURTHER READING

Data Synthesis

Quinn Patton, M. (2015). *Qualitative Research and Evaluation Methods: Integrating theory and practice* (4th ed.). Thousand Oaks: Sage.

Trustworthiness

Lincoln, Y. S., & Guba, E. G. (1985). *Naturalistic inquiry*. Thousand Oaks (CA): Sage Publications.

18

Other Qualitative Methods

LEARNING OBJECTIVES

After reading this chapter you should be able to:
- describe some of the other ways of doing qualitative research including participant-observer research, action research, grounded theory and case study research
- understand the complexities of such research
- understand the place of reflexivity in qualitative research
- define some of the ethics issues that accompany the different forms of research

18.1. INTRODUCTION

It has been said that qualitative measurement methods are mainly limited by the creativity of the researcher. While the primary data-gathering methods discussed in previous chapters related to interviews, focus groups and observational methods are most widely used, there is a diverse and proliferating array of other techniques that may be applicable in different situations. Regardless of the method selected, qualitative researchers must be mindful of the need for rigour in the work they perform. While creativity is an important tool for the qualitative researcher, this must not be interpreted as giving license to simply inventing data corresponding to a pre-existing belief or assumption. Quantitative constructs such as 'reliability' and 'representative sampling' are important safeguards to ensure consumers of research can believe in the work that is produced. While these terms do not necessarily transplant directly into qualitative research, the analogous terms 'trustworthiness' and 'indicativeness' highlight the central importance of a systematic and defensible process for generating questions, gathering data and analysing results.

18.2. OTHER QUALITATIVE METHODS

While one-to-one interviews, focus groups, and observational/ethnographic research techniques are most frequently used by qualitative researchers (especially novice ones), there are additional methods that may be useful in different contexts. These methods are typically used by more experienced researchers, but it is still valuable for all researchers to be aware of these techniques and to understand their appropriate application. In Chapter 15 we outlined some observational techniques (including participant observation) and showed how Dorothy might use them in her research. In this chapter, we provide an overview of four techniques that may be of interest or value: participant-observer research, action research, grounded theory and the case study method.

18.3. PARTICIPANT-OBSERVER RESEARCH

A popular method amongst **cultural anthropologists**, **sociologists** and **social psychologists**, participant observation research relies upon the notion that the invisible wall between researcher and subject diminishes both individual's abilities to truly engage in any meaningful research. We have included more about this type of research in this chapter because learning how to observe is a key skill researchers should develop. Historically, the positivist orientation of scientific inquiry has valued the separation of the scientist from that which is being examined, in the name of preventing bias, subjectivity or undue influence of baseline assumptions. Within this positivist paradigm, there is a strong belief that researchers not only can, but actually must withhold subjective judgments and assessments and remain objective throughout the process so as to not bias findings and analyses. Within the qualitative tradition, this belief is frequently questioned; to many such researchers there is no point in even pretending any human being can be objective and disinterested. We all have biases and motives that drive our work, and rather than pretend they don't exist, or develop well-intentioned but ultimately unsuccessful safeguards (such as **randomisation** or **blinding**) to prevent these biases and motives from influencing our work, we should instead simply articulate our positions clearly and honestly, whilst maintaining a reflexive and self-aware approach to all stages of the research process.

18.3.1. Reflexivity

It is out of the reflexive tradition that participant-observer research initially emerged. Early ethnographers, examining cultures of indigenous peoples, quickly learned that simply observing individuals in their local cultures without interacting directly with them resulted in unsatisfactory and incomplete understanding. Anthropologists such as Cushing and Malinowski (see Further Reading at the end of this chapter) highlighted the significant value of cultivating personal relationships with those individuals who were being studied as a way gaining deeper understanding of what was being observed. At the time, such an approach was frequently labelled unscientific or subjective. By breaking down the wall between researcher and 'subject' and getting to know 'subjects' as 'people' rather than simple participants in a research project, significant challenges and opportunities emerged. Increasingly, many researchers recognised the value of going beyond simple cultivation of personal relationships to actively participating in the day-to-day social life of the group being studied, or being a fully fledged member of that group.

Participant-observer research begins with the belief that only those who have lived experiences as part of a group can truly recognise and understand the myriad hidden symbols, meanings, language and behaviour clues, and codes of that culture. There is no attempt to claim participant-observation research is better than or superior to more traditional observational research that attempts to maintain objectivity and separation between researcher and participant; instead, participant-observer research suggests a very different and meaningful picture of a culture, an organisation or process can be developed when those actually from the culture, organisation or process are the ones doing the research.

As human beings, we have all had the experience of being participant-observer researchers. This is the foundation for social learning, particularly during the teenage years. Teenage cultures around the world are typically associated with significant stress, tension, emotion and volatility. Well-intentioned parents and teachers (who may have been teenagers decades earlier and consequently not subject to the contemporary environmental stresses shaping today's teenage culture) may believe they 'understand' or 'get' what the problems facing teenagers today are, and may use this observational research to implement well-intentioned but

spectacularly misguided supports and interventions designed to help. Teenagers themselves – those who currently live in an environment of economic scarcity, precarious employment, technologies producing vulnerabilities, and completely new words and acts such as 'sexting' – will have a very different understanding of the problems they face. In such situations, the seeming objectivity and distance of the well-intentioned adult may in fact generate data that are not only unhelpful, but completely wrong from the perspective of those being studied. Being an active member of the group, organisation, culture or process being studied affords important and unique insights into the tacit or secret practices of the group, and participant-observer research is uniquely well suited to this purpose.

18.3.2. How Do You Conduct Participant-Observer Research?

Simply being a member of a group does not immediately confer the ability to claim one is doing participant-observer research. There are a series of well-defined techniques and data sources that are used in conjunction with one another to permit triangulation and confirmation of findings and themes in the research. Such methods include informal interviews with key members of the group, ongoing direct observation of other group members, reflections upon active participation in the day-to-day activities of the group, collective discussions, review of **artefacts** produced by the group, etc. A key feature of participant-observer research is its **longitudinal** quality – by being 'embedded' or part of the group itself over a period of time, the true story of the culture can naturally evolve in a more detailed and accurate manner. Specific hidden details (such as taboo behaviours) are frequently very challenging to identify using other research methods.

A key strength of this approach is the ability to bring out differences between what participants say (and perhaps even actually believe) and what happens in reality. This is sometimes referred to as the difference between the 'formal system' and the 'real system'. Other research techniques such as surveys or interviews can only gather data from the formal system, one in which participants may be on their best behaviour! Participant-observer research, because of its longitudinal nature and the embedded relationships between researcher and participant, is better suited to root out these potential unconscious inconsistencies.

18.3.3. Stages of Participant-Observer Research

While a variety of stages may be used in the participant-observer research process, there are generally four critical stages:

a. Establishing rapport: Whether one is naturally a part of the group being studied or not, it is crucial that the researcher establishes mutually reinforcing friendly relationships with the participants so she/he is perceived to be part of the group. Simply being tolerated as an outsider to the group will not yield the rich data that is possible using this technique. Instead being fully accepted and embraced as a true member of the group will help break down barriers between the researcher and the participant to allow for honest and authentic interactions that are the foundation of participant-observer research.

b. Walking the walk: Being embedded within the group being studied will, of necessity, require the researcher to fully participate in the day-to-day activities of the group. In some cases, this may produce certain tensions and feelings of discomfort. For example, if one is undertaking participant-observer research around illicit drug-taking behaviours in high-risk youth populations, it may be impossible to be accepted in the group without participating in the behaviour that unifies that group. It is essential that researchers recognise this potential tension: participant-observer research may not be ethical, legal, moral or possible in all situations, and the researcher must be very clear in terms of personal limits and boundaries. Fortunately, in many other less-dramatic cases, participant-observer research will come naturally to the researcher who is already part of the group. For example, as we saw in Chapter 15, if Dorothy is interested in understanding the inter-professional dynamics involved in the communication of antibiotic stewardship, she (as a pharmacist) is already a member of the group and can use her previous life history and experience as not only an entry ticket to the team dynamic, but as a unique lens through which data can be analysed.

c. Data capture: The main sources of data in participant-observer research are conversations and observations. As in other forms of qualitative research, participant-observer researchers are well advised to maintain, constantly update and studiously reflect upon a reflexivity journal (see Chapter 12). This is particularly crucial in this type of research because researchers should have no misconceptions that they are objective, outside of, independent of, or somehow not connected to the group being studied – this connection is of course the essential element of this method. It is, however, important for the researcher to honestly document in the reflexivity journal how being a member of the group being studied does not mean she/he is exactly the same as everyone else, and how these differences may play out in interpretation and understanding of conversations and observations. **Field notes** are usually maintained on a daily if not more frequent basis. Many participant-observer researchers use an audio or video taping device to capture both content and the emotion surrounding the content being delivered in personal field notes, then transcribe the content into a written format later. The emotional context within which initial field notes are recorded is an important source of information in participant-observer research that is difficult to capture if one immediately writes or types field notes in a paper format.

d. Data analysis: As with other forms of qualitative research, captured data must be stored, managed and analysed appropriately. Two dominant forms of data analysis are most frequently used: thematic analysis, which involves organising data according to recurrent common ideas found in the data and narrative analysis, which involves categorising the information gathered, finding/identifying common themes, then using these themes to construct a coherent story from the data. Further details regarding data analysis using qualitative research outputs can be found in Chapters 16 and 17.

18.3.4. Knowing Our Boundaries

Researchers involved in this type of work must determine how active they wish to be and can be (especially where ethical, moral, or legal boundaries may be an issue) in the group itself. Failure to be able to participate in the life of the group renders this form of research pointless. Even passive participation involving mainly observation as a bystander, severely limits the researcher's ability to establish the rapport necessary to support data capture using this method. In both cases, participant-observer research is possibly not a viable or meaningful method. In most cases, somewhat active participation in key elements of the group's day-to-day life is the aim for most participant-observer researchers, providing a healthy balance between maintaining sufficient involvement with the group to generate rich data and keeping sufficient distance to ensure that some measure of critical analysis is possible.

Within the qualitative research literature there is some controversy as to the impact of the **observer-expectancy effect**; that is the influence a known researcher has on the participants' behaviour, even when she/he is an embedded and accepted part of the group. A useful technique for managing this issue can be triangulation (the use of multiple different data sources to confirm a finding or theme) and member checking (actively eliciting the participants' feedback and response to the researcher's findings and analysis). For more about these techniques see Chapter 16.

18.3.5. Ethical Considerations

Like many forms of research, ethical considerations must be carefully identified when using participant-observer research. There are situations where this type of research is completely inappropriate due to legal or moral issues as discussed previously. Conversely, there are times when researchers using this method may inadvertently be co-opted by the group itself. For example, during the Gulf War in the early 2000s, many journalists were embedded within army or marine units and (while not actually involved directly in combat missions) lived side-by-side with soldiers in difficult conditions for months at a time, creating strong positive relationships between these individuals. Subsequent analysis of these journalistic reports suggested that such embedding may have adversely affected the quality and trustworthiness of the reporting that came out of this experience, which in turn may have had an adverse influence on the political and military policies and decisions that occurred based upon these news reports.

If undertaking this form of research, it is usually advisable to consult with a relevant ethics review board to determine the type of approval that is most appropriate for the specific circumstance of the research. Simply being a member of a group already does not automatically exempt participant-observer researchers from seeking and obtaining informed consent pursuant to an approved ethics review.

18.4. ACTION RESEARCH

For many health professionals, the ultimate objective of research is to solve a real-world problem using data and systematic processes. The kinds of real-world problems faced by health professionals are frequently messy, involving complex interpersonal, communication, ethical and legal dimensions that must be balanced. In this environment, action research has emerged as a potentially useful technique when a 'right answer' may not be possible and instead a 'least-worst alternative' is the main objective.

At its core, action research relies heavily upon groups of interested and involved individuals, constantly reflecting through a process of progressive problem solving as a way to address pressing issues. Crucial to the process is the explicit focus on the feedback loops that connect individuals, the systems they work in, the organisations that manage them, and the broader culture within which all of these operate. Action research is a spiral of steps that involves planning, action, fact-finding and reflection.

18.4.1. The Plan-Do-Study-Act Cycle

One of the most common forms of action research for health professionals is the PDSA cycle (Plan-Do-Study-Act). Whilst this is by no means the only or even best example of action research, it is for health professionals one of the most practical applications of action research methods in a clinical context, specifically focussed on quality improvement.

Most frequently depicted as continuous wheel, the PDSA cycle is sometimes referred to as the Deming Wheel, in honour of the person who developed this approach:

P(lanning): While the cycle is a never-ending, constantly repeated spiral, the initial point of entry to the process involves specific planning. During this stage, a group of people needs to identify and articulate a goal or purpose of function. It need not be overly detailed or specific at the outset. A key strength of this form of action research is its iterative nature which, over time, will take general or vague questions or problems and refine them down to something more concrete and solvable over subsequent cycles. During the P step, the group needs to actually determine what problem they want to solve and why this is a problem worth solving, and generate a hypothesis or theory as to what might solve the problem. As part of the process of planning, starting to generate a series of success metrics – those quantitative or qualitative indicators that the problem you are trying to solve has indeed been solved – is essential. Based on all of this, the group develops a plan – a concrete series of steps to simply try something to address this issue.

D(o): The second stage of this process is to attempt to solve the problem identified in the planning step, building upon the initial hunches and hypotheses of the group. A key feature of action research is the need for some kind of concrete action. In this 'Do' step, the emphasis is on simply trying to solve an old problem in a new way. At this stage, success is less important than trying: one does not wait for a perfect, watertight solution when dealing with difficult or complex problems. Instead, there is value to simply trying something and seeing how it works. The 'something' should be as well thought through as possible under the circumstances.

S(tudy): A key feature of action research, and the PDSA cycle in particular, is the importance of monitoring and measuring outcomes and comparing these outcomes to initial hunches, hypotheses and suppositions. Having tried something new as an intervention, there is now an opportunity to measure or determine (either quantitatively or qualitatively) what actually happened – and how close or far from your initial hunch you ended up. A diverse array of different methods can be used in this study phase, including traditional quantitative measurement (time/motion studies, output measurement, surveys) and qualitative methods (interviews, focus groups, observations). The goal is to triangulate and use different sources of data to define how close – or far – from 'success' this intervention actually was, having defined success metrics in the 'Plan' stage. Most importantly in action research of this sort, there is no expectation that, on the first attempt or first PDSA cycle, one will have achieved all one hoped to achieve. Instead, there will be small, incremental gains, perhaps two steps forward-one step backward, and this sets the foundation for the next stage of the process.

A(ct): The objective of this stage of the process is to integrate the learning generated across the entire process, which can then be used to adjust the initial goal/remit of the project, try an alternative method, or perhaps reformulate a hypothesis. Acting upon the qualitative and quantitative data gathered from trying to implement something new requires reflection and a willingness to change pre-existing assumptions and beliefs. In this phase, new theories and ideas are generated, new questions are formulated and old ideas may be discarded, as a step to recommencing the next PDSA cycle.

18.4.2.   Using Plan-Do-Study-Act Cycles in Health Care

Clinician-researchers are used to making 'educated best guesses' when clear evidence is unavailable and when a decision needs to be made. The PDSA cycle is – in essence – a series of small-scale trial-and-error learning experiments run over time as repeated cycles, with each cycle contributing incrementally to a greater objective. PDSA cycles function best when action researchers compare predictions (based on theory, **hypothesis** and hunches) with actual results (data generated qualitatively and quantitatively from the implementation). Forcing yourself to make such predictions and articulate the reasoning behind them will support better and more effective implementation in the 'Do' and 'Study' phase. Those new to action research frequently underestimate the time required to 'Plan' and instead may want to rush ahead to 'Do'. Without a carefully constructed plan – including the hypothesis, the expected outcomes, the measurements that will be taken, etc., the rest of the cycle may not function as effectively as hoped. In particular, paying careful attention to defining metrics for success – using both quantitative and qualitative methods – facilitates the 'Study' part of the cycle and so spending the necessary time and effort to define this as clearly as possible at the outset, is generally time well spent.

It is sometimes easy to become discouraged after the second or third PDSA cycle does not succeed as hoped, but remember that action research is an incremental process in which each cycle contributes a little bit more to the broader understanding of a problem and its solutions. There is no prescribed or magical number of PDSA cycles necessary to 'solve' a problem using this method – each situation is different, and patience with this form of action research is required to generate a satisfactory outcome.

PDSA cycles are most frequently used in the context of quality improvement projects in health care, where innovations in processes are desired. For example, Dorothy may hypothesise that one of the main reasons why inappropriate

prescribing for antibiotics continues to occur in her setting is that prescribers are unaware of current prescribing guidelines. As a PDSA cycle, she may first:

P(lan): Having generated her hypothesis, it becomes clear that a knowledge-based intervention may be a good first step to address the problem. If this solution is successful, she should find that the incidence of inappropriate prescribing will decrease. How can this be measured? Since ultimately 'appropriate' prescribing has both subjective and objective elements, a combination of qualitative and quantitative indicators may be required. As a measurement, she may want to take a random sample of recent antibiotic prescriptions and perform a drug utilisation review audit, comparing clinical indication, culture+sensitivity reports, and antibiotic selected to the guideline she develops, and report a percentage rate of adherence to the guidelines. She is hopeful there will be a 50% reduction in inappropriate prescribing from current levels. In addition, she may want to undertake some interviews with prescribers to determine their experience with the guidelines and the process and how that influenced their prescribing behaviour, hypothesising that the existence of guidelines might increase prescribers' confidence in making the right decision.

D(o): Dorothy develops the antibiotic guidelines and has them validated by experts in the field. She provides prescribers with copies, along with a brief training programme on what she is trying to accomplish and how to use the guidelines. She makes herself available to answer questions and troubleshoot during the implementation pilot period, which she has set arbitrarily as 2 weeks.

S(tudy): After 2 weeks, Dorothy takes a random sample of 10% of all antibiotic prescriptions written. This is turning into a lot of work for her, so she recruits an MPharm student on a research placement with her to help. The student undertakes a clinical audit of those 10% of prescriptions, retrieving clinical indication, relevant laboratory parameters, culture+sensitivity findings, and prescription written and generates a spreadsheet with this information. The student also interviews several of the prescribers involved for the implementation and elicits their opinions regarding the process and what can be improved.

A(ct): It turns out that the prescribing guidance document Dorothy developed had a font that was too small for some of the prescribers. They liked the idea and really wanted to use the document but when they tried to read the algorithms, it was too confusing and too small. So, they simply lost interest and reverted back to their historic practices. As a result, there was only a 5% change in inappropriate prescribing during the 2-week period studied, much less than expected. Through this process, Dorothy learns her idea was strong and generally accepted – but the format of the guidelines themselves was an unexpected but fixable barrier. For the next iteration of PDSA she will work with the student to develop a more user-friendly document, and start the PDSA all over again to determine what the next change to make is to enhance the value of this process, and to reduce inappropriate prescribing by 50% as she initially hoped.

PDSA cycles are an important example of action research that will be commonly seen in health care settings. The strength of this approach is the incremental focus on quality improvement – a step-by-step approach that allows for constant refinement of ideas. Action research, with its strong focus on practical problem solving using real-world situations and data in a rigorous and informed manner, is a valuable tool for clinicians in diverse settings.

18.5. GROUNDED THEORY

The term grounded theory is sometimes – erroneously – used interchangeably with the term qualitative research. Grounded theory is a very specific and rigorous methodology that supports the generation of a theory through the analysis of data, sometimes resulting in the expression 'let the data speak'. For some researchers more inclined to the **positivist tradition**, grounded theory seems to be a reverse-engineering process. When using grounded theory, the researcher does not begin with a hypothesis, a theory or, in some cases, even a specific or refined research question: instead, the researcher simply collects qualitative data and through an analytical process begins to identify recurring ideas that emerge from the data. As more and more data are assembled, these ideas can be gathered into codes, clusters, and eventually into categories. The researcher can then weave these categories into a new theory that can subsequently be researched in a more 'traditional' way. In this way, grounded theory is very different from not only traditional quantitative research, but also most forms of qualitative research, which begin a priori with a theoretical framework, hypothesis and specific research question. In grounded theory, it is the results of the research itself that help a researcher generate a theoretical framework, hypothesis or specific research question, which can subsequently be tested using traditional qualitative and quantitative methods.

This method was pioneered by sociologists Glaser and Strauss (see Further Reading at the end of this chapter) as they examined how patients experienced the process of dying and death in hospitals. Over time, they and others refined an analytical process that allows raw qualitative data generated by interviews, observations, focus groups or other techniques to be transformed ultimately into theory.

The following basic steps are found in almost all grounded theory work:

Step 1 – Codes: The attempt to generate a theory from data starts from the very first piece of data collected. The process of coding involves selection, identification and naming of key, recurring and relevant points of data, for example specific words or phrases used by the participant to describe an experience. These anchor codes provide the researcher with a first opportunity to start to identify commonalities and differences in the way individual participants and participants in general describe, name and experience a situation. There are different models for coding:

- Open coding involves systematically breaking down, comparing and contrasting data using the researcher's intuition and experience as the main guide.
- Axial coding involves reassembling of data in new ways, after open coding is completed, by explicitly finding connections between codes.
- Selective coding involves the identification and selection of a core, central, or primary focus and then relating all other codes back to this core and examining how relationships between these codes work.

Step 2 – Concepts: A careful re-reading of data and codes will allow the researcher to start to detect patterns or similarities amongst codes which can then be grouped together as a concept. Concepts provide a higher level of analysis because they require the researcher to encapsulate/summarise or use his/her own words to distill the essential meaning from these similar codes. The process of defining concepts helps the researcher to engage with the data at a higher level, looking at making sense of the codes and communicating it in a way that can be understood and appreciated by those who are not as immersed in the data.

Step 3 – Categories: Categories involve the clustering of concepts that are similar or aligned into broader named and defined segments. Categories help the researcher move beyond simply making sense of codes to finding meaning in them. 'Meaning' is a complex concept: frequently, individuals may say one thing but mean something different. They may want to please the researcher or not use certain terms or phrases they know will make them seem intolerant or bigoted or uneducated. As categories surface through the analysis process, both sense and true meaning will emerge. In some cases the true meaning may be completely at odds with the specific words used. For example, in some cases an individual who says 'I'm not homophobic, no not at all, but I just don't think same-sex marriage is a good idea' is saying several different, potentially contradictory things. The individual is self-categorising as non-homophobic, though the stance on same-sex marriage may raise suspicions as to the truth of this self-categorisation. The self-declaration regarding the label of 'homophobic' makes sense: most homophobic (or racist or sexist or otherwise biased individuals) recognise the social stigma generally given to the terms and would prefer not to be labelled as such. In this analytical process, one would never trust a single statement such as this to generate any kind of theory or hypothesis about a single participant or participants in general. As with all forms of qualitative inquiry, triangulation and member checking are valuable tools to confirm the trustworthiness of the analysis. In grounded theory work, the researcher must look for other codes and concepts that might contribute further evidence to support the case for categorising.

Step 4 – Grounded theory: During the process of analysis, when codes, concepts and categories are being built, grounded theory highlights the value of memoing. Memoing is the process of keeping running notes of concepts that are identified and the actual thinking/analytical process that results in categorisation. It is often easy to forget the underlying thought process that results in categories forming, but it is this underlying thinking that is actually the beginning of a theory. Memoing provides a real-time running commentary of your thoughts and insights and is an invaluable parallel source of data for theorising.

Throughout this process, grounded theory relies heavily on the technique of the constant-comparative method (see Chapter 16). Constant-comparative analysis requires the researcher to continuously examine new data from the perspective of previously analysed data and to continuously reconfirm initial codes, concepts and categories as additional data becomes available.

For most clinical researchers, grounded theory may sound intriguing but may require additional education or support from an experienced researcher. Though it may be intuitively appealing and seem particularly helpful in situations where little or nothing is known about a phenomenon and where no pre-existing theory, literature or hypotheses exist, grounded theory can be a very time consuming, laborious and frustrating process. There is a great deal of discipline and rigour involved when grounded theory is used: the simple act of memoing, or using constant-comparative analysis properly, requires training. For these reasons this is not a form of research that one generally stumbles into or uses on a trial-and-error basis. When implemented effectively, grounded theory is an important qualitative method to support greater understanding, and theory generation, in areas and topics where little or no literature or theory currently exists.

18.6.   CASE STUDIES

The case study method is amongst the most frequently used research methods favoured by clinicians. Initially pioneered in the discipline of psychiatry by Sigmund Freud, case studies allow researchers to examine individuals, groups or situations over a period of time. The longitudinal nature of the case study – following the subject of interest over a period of time, across different settings and contexts – is one of its greatest strengths. It is a naturalistic research method closely aligned with observational research techniques that generally suggest a level of detachment (or lack of direct interaction/involvement) between researcher and participant. Unlike participant-observer or action research, the researcher remains somewhat outside the actual arena of the subject and instead observes, documents and analyses.

The power of a case study is its depth; as a result, great care must be taken in supposing that the findings of a case study can be generalised beyond the specific case or cases studied. The relevance and applicability of a case study must be carefully detailed: in most cases, a case study only applies to those involved, and care should be taken in assuming findings can apply in different cases or contexts.

18.6.1.   Selection of Cases

A crucial decision for use of case study methods relates to selection of the specific cases themselves. Two broad categories of cases exist: key (or indicative) and outlier:

- Key (or indicative) cases are generally selected because the researcher believes this particular case is, in a broad and general way, somehow representative of others. While this may be an explicit objective of a key case, the reality of course is that no one individual actually is indicative or representative of everyone else; still, it may be useful as a starting point for subsequent research to select key cases as a way of building understanding that eventually may become more generalisable.
- Outlier cases are frequently selected specifically because they are outside the norm or expectations for individuals, situations, or process. Frequently, we can learn a great deal about what is 'typical' by examining situations that are atypical; outlier cases can provide a unique perspective using this approach, but again caution must be exercised in trying to generalise beyond the specific conditions of the specific case at hand.

Case studies may be undertaken for a variety of reasons:

- Illustrative case studies are primarily descriptive, and typically use one or two examples as a way of building interest in or awareness about a topic.
- Exploratory case studies are frequently used as a way of gaining a deeper understanding of topic, process or event

and begining experimenting with different models of analysis.

- Cumulative case studies (sometimes called case series) involve aggregation of different individual case studies with the purpose of finding commonalities that may facilitate broader generalisations.
- Critical instance case studies are useful for examining a significant moment in time (for example a landmark decision or a plane crash) and examining what happened before and after that critical moment in time.

Case studies provide an organisational framework within which different qualitative and quantitative data collection and analysis methods may be used. There is no single way a case study should be constructed and each case study will be unique in its approach, based on the context of the case itself. The experience of performing case study research is frequently transformational for the researcher as it allows the researcher both the opportunity to gain in-depth knowledge of and connection to the subject of the research as well as see the subject from diverse perspectives and through different lenses. The ability to 'walk around the subject' and see the situation or case from these multiple perspectives helps facilitate a level of sophisticated analysis that is difficult to achieve using any one single research method or technique. Case studies allow researchers to assemble diverse methods and data gathering techniques, customised to the unique context of the particular case, and this is its unique strength.

Case studies are sometimes framed as 'n-of-1 studies' to highlight the fact that each case is unique and consequently one must be cautious in any attempt to generalise. Each 'n' is unique and while over multiple cases it may be possible to start to identify common features, such common features do not necessarily equate with generalisability (see Further Reading for more about doing case studies).

18.7.   THE DELPHI METHOD

One important research method that is increasingly used by qualitative researchers is the Delphi method. It is generally described as a structured communication technique, one that is most frequently used when trying to elicit input from a group of experts or individuals who are either too busy or geographically dispersed to meet face to face for an interview, focus group or observational research method. In some cases, Delphi is used to generate consensus through the use of anonymised summary reports undertaken through a series of rounds. The Delphi is based on the belief that decisions that emerge from groups facilitated in a structured manner will be more accurate and of better quality than those from individuals or using unstructured groups; in

other words, that group judgements are better and more valid than individual ones.

While there are many variations of the Delphi method, there are several principles that are generally adhered to when using this approach:

a. Anonymity of participants: Protecting the identity of the participants serves multiple purposes in the Delphi. First, it will sometimes free the participant to be more truthful and honest if they know others will not associate their comments with his/her name. Second, it also prevents the reputation or personality of some participants from dominating the discussion or process, minimising the 'bandwagon effect'. In this way both honest discussion and more empowered participants result from the process.

b. Highly structured information flow: The Delphi facilitator (sometimes called the 'panel director', usually in an online format) controls the flow of information amongst participants. All information flows through the panel director who can edit, redirect or refocus content to ensure it is relevant and appropriate. While this may appear overly controlling to some qualitative researchers, it has the advantage of maintaining order in the proceedings and solving certain group dynamics problems when a free-for-all focus group devolves into pandemonium.

c. Ongoing feedback provided to participants: Through the Delphi process, and moderated by the panel director, participants are provided with perspectives, data and feedback from all other participants throughout the process. In this way, individual participants are able to recalibrate their thinking and restate their thoughts as necessary. As there is anonymity throughout the process, there is no need for participants to 'save face' by sticking tenaciously to an opinion that the rest of the group has clearly discounted.

The Delphi method is most frequently used in order to achieve a consensus on a question or problem. In such a situation, the panel leader may send out an initial questionnaire/survey then feed the results back to the participants once the initial data have been analysed (this is called round one). Having seen the initial analysis, a second round is usually convened: in many cases, it might be the exact same survey/questionnaire that is redistributed; now, having seen how the rest of the group have responded, individual participants may begin to reconsider their initial responses. In some cases the second round may use a modified survey/questionnaire (for example, if 100% of participants strongly agreed to an item, there may be no need to include it again in round two). Data from round two are compiled and again distributed back to the panel for their review and consideration. If there is still disagreement or areas of contention, additional rounds following a similar process may be undertaken. If, after two rounds, there is sufficient convergence (as defined by the panel leader), a final, more qualitative round may be convened, in which participants are invited to submit their free-form text thoughts and opinions about what the data actually mean. These text notes can be analysed using traditional qualitative methods to identify categories, codes and themes, and can help contextualise quantitative findings.

It is important to note that the track record of the Delphi method – particularly in the context of making predictions, and particularly in the political/democratic setting – is quite mixed. There have been some spectacular examples of failures of Delphi method to make accurate predictions (for example, in predicting who will win an election or a referendum). In part, this may be due to the method itself: it relies heavily on experts, and is structured to force consensus through a wisdom-of-the-crowd approach. Recognising that it is – like all research – an imperfect method should allow researchers to consider its strengths (e.g. useful for busy participants who are geographically dispersed and would otherwise not be able to participate in a focus group or interview, and allows for individual participants to refine their views and opinions based on on-going data feedback) and potential limitations prior to use.

CHAPTER SUMMARY

- This chapter has reviewed a variety of different qualitative research methods.
- It highlights that the choice of research method must align with methodology, which turn must align with research questions and objectives.
- It demonstrates the diverse array of potential techniques that are available to qualitative researchers.
- It shows some of the ways of approaching complex problems with research.

FURTHER READING

Participant-observer Research

De-Walk, K. M., & De-Walt, B. R. (2011). *Participant Observation: A guide for fieldworkers* (2nd ed.). Plymouth, UK: AltaMira Press.

Anthropology

Bronislaw Malinowski published widely during the first half of the 20th Century. Most of his work is now out of print but information about him and his work and that of Frank Hamilton Cushing can be found in:

Tetlock, M. (1991). From participant observation to the observation of participation: the emergence of narrative ethnography. *Journal of Anthropological Research, 47*(1), 69–94.

Action Research

Reason, P., & Bradbury-Huang, H. (Eds.), (2007). *Handbook of Action Research: Participative Inquiry and Practice*. London: Sage.

Grounded Theory

Glaser, B., & Strauss, A. (1967). *The Discovery of Grounded Theory*. Chicago: Aldine.

Strauss, A., & Corbin, J. (1998). *Basics of Qualitative Research: Techniques and Procedures for Developing Grounded Theory*. Thousand Oaks: Sage.

Case Study Research

Yin, R. K. (2003). *Case Study Research: Design and Methods* (3rd ed.). Thousand Oaks: Sage.

Delphi Method

http://www.rand.org/topics/delphi-method.html provides access to research that has used the Delphi Method.

19

Multimethod or 'Mixed-Methods' Research

LEARNING OBJECTIVES

After reading this chapter you should be able to:
- understand the concept of multimethod or mixed-methods research
- describe how quantitative and qualitative methods might be used in one research project
- understand why there are some objections to the mixing of research methods
- describe the CIPP Model for programme evaluation and the Kirkpatrick model

19.1. INTRODUCTION

Clinical and health services research is by nature an extremely complex subject because there are so many issues to be taken into account. In most cases, the kind of research problem that is the focus of the work involves a diverse array of components: health system factors, interpersonal and inter-professional communication issues, as well as some kind of financial, resource or capacity constraint. Such complex problems are of course one of the reasons why research is so important: without data and evidence, it is tempting to think we can solve such problems using our own experiences and emotional responses alone. Generating evidence – both in sufficient amounts and of appropriate quality to facilitate decision-making – is sometimes supported through the use of multimethod, or mixed-method research.

The term **multimethod research** was coined in the 1980s as a way of describing research that uses more than one method of data collection through a set of interdependent and related studies. Strictly speaking, the term '**mixed methods**' research is reserved for situations where both qualitative and quantitative research paradigms, methodologies and methods are used to achieve the same research goals. The underlying philosophy of this approach is based upon the principle of **triangulation**: multiple lenses focussed on the same problem will provide different and complementary results, that, when taken together, can perhaps come closest to approximating the reality of a situation. Interestingly, triangulation is a principle that is relevant to both the qualitative and quantitative traditions: regardless of methodological preference or selection of specific method, researchers are generally encouraged to not be satisfied with single measurements or overreliance on a single measurement technique, as no single method or measurement is without flaw. Mixed-methods research extends this thought to the entire paradigm of qualitative and quantitative research and suggests that the blending of these two traditions provides researchers and consumers of research with the best possible quality evidence upon which to base decision-making.

19.1.1. Models of Multimethod Research

There are three predominant models of multimethod research:
1. Quantitatively driven mixed-methods research: In this approach, the research plan is more strongly rooted in a quantitative tradition (e.g. using survey methods) but qualitative research may be used to help provide a context to interpret and understand findings.
2. Qualitatively driven mixed-methods research: In this approach, the research plan is more strongly rooted in a qualitative tradition (e.g. using interviews or focus groups), but a quantitative method (e.g. surveys) may be developed from the findings of the qualitative research, as a way of quantifying or scaling the magnitude of findings.
3. Equal status designs: Research of this nature frequently takes an iterative approach in which qualitative and quantitative methods are used in roughly equal proportions and in which findings from one method inform the

next step in the evolution of the project using another method.

In most cases, multimethod research is considered valuable as researchers try to balance the competing issues of **reliability**, **validity**, **indicativeness** and **trustworthiness**.

19.1.2. Mixing Research Paradigms

As we have shown in previous chapters in this book, these terms have different connotations to different researchers, using different paradigms and methodological traditions. Traditionally, the terms reliability and validity are more frequently associated with the quantitative methods and speak to issues of reproducibility and veracity of findings. Even within the quantitative traditions, it is accepted that there are many layers of validity that must be considered: face validity, content validity, predictive validity, concurrent validity and construct validity (see Chapter 5). As one moves up this validity chain, it becomes clear that 'validation' in many cases has a qualitative element. For example, the definition of **'face validity'** is the extent to which a measurement is viewed as covering the concept it purports to measure, or the relevance of a measurement to its audience. This is the most frequently discussed type of validity – yet it is of course inherently subjective as it is all about perceptions of a diverse audience. At the other end of the spectrum is construct validity, which is defined as the extent to which a measurement instrument (e.g. a survey) does, in fact, measure what it claims to be measuring. For example, do IQ tests really measure innate intelligence, or do they measure the test-takers test-taking skills? Or English language comprehension? Or knowledge of contemporary society? Again, the idea of a 'construct' has a strong subjective component – how can an idea like 'intelligence' be quantitatively or objectively defined as it has multiple meanings in different situations?

On the other hand, the qualitative traditions value similar ideas but framed in a different way. 'Trustworthiness' is an important facet of any researcher's work, but the term itself has a somewhat positivist connotation. It is defined as the ability to be relied upon to do or provide what is right, in a black-and-white sort of way. How do qualitative researchers reconcile concepts like 'right' and 'trustworthy' with a **constructivist** paradigm that suggests multiple truths may simultaneously co-exist?

Arguably, the epistemological and ontological shortcomings of both the qualitative and quantitative traditions may be somewhat mitigated by simply blending them in a coherent, problem-focussed manner, which coincidentally, will also offer as an additional benefit, the opportunity for triangulation. As a result, multimethod research is now amongst the most common types of research in the health sciences and is rapidly emerging as a standard best practice

in research. The modern world – and in particular, that slice of it concerned with people and their health – is so complex that narrow views and perspectives of it will inevitably be misleading or incomplete. Approaching complexity from different perspectives – or paradigms – provides us with the best opportunity to gain a holistic view. Ultimately, this is a highly pragmatic approach to research that recognises the limitations of methodological or methods-based singlemindedness.

19.1.3. How Realistic Is This Approach?

While there is intuitive appeal to the idea of taking a number of different approaches in one research study, there are some practical issues to consider. First, the reality is that, at their core, positivist and constructivist paradigms are mutually contradictory. The former supports the worldview that there are singular unchanging truths awaiting discovery, while the latter believes all truths are contextual, socially negotiated and ever-changing. Within research circles, there is the **incompatibility thesis**, which states that mixing of qualitative and quantitative research paradigms, methodologies and methods is not only counterintuitive, it is actually inherently wrong, since the foundations of each worldview are so contradictory that it becomes the equivalent of trying to mix oil and water. With that in mind how can researchers simultaneously adopt and accept both of these standpoints?

The answer is that human beings who are not researchers must struggle with this contradiction in their day-to-day life and health care research has at its foundation the health of human beings. There are some positive truths that most people accept (e.g. 2+2=4, no matter where you are in the world or who you are) and there are some constructivist truths (e.g. the differences in the role of women in Western societies compared to their role in other societies). However, even within our own Western liberal-democratic-capitalist societies, there are enormous disagreements that cannot be reconciled (e.g. can a family have two mothers instead of mother and father? How many genders are there – two or many more?) While it can be an advantage to see multiple sides of an issue, multimethod research can sometimes force researchers into intellectual stretches that they simply cannot accept. Other limitations to multimethod research are the abilities and biases of the researchers themselves: some of us are simply more inclined to either qualitative OR quantitative ways of viewing the world, and find it very challenging to assume another mindset no matter how hard we try. For example, for some people mathematics is quite a daunting subject and formulae are terrifying, for others it is exciting and stimulating. The reality for some researchers is that they will simply lack the knowledge and experience or even cognitive ability to perform both types of research and will thus naturally gravitate preferentially to one form over another. Often we feel more comfortable with a type of research because we have used it previously in our studies and so we tend to stick with that. Lastly – and particularly in the health sciences and professions – there may be a cultural bias towards quantitative research as it somehow more naturally conforms to a stereotyped view of what 'science' is supposed to be.

Despite these criticisms – many of which are, to a greater or lesser degree, reasonable and valid – the reality is that multimethod research is gaining increasing popularity and that comfort with both qualitative and quantitative methodologies and methods is increasingly a prerequisite for any researcher, even if she/he has a preference for one over the other. A crucial method for managing these tensions and contradictions is to be ever mindful (or '**reflexive**'") and to be careful and deliberative in how, when, and why specific methods are being mixed within the context of one particular research project. Finally, we must always acknowledge the limitations of our research methodologies and methods, and recognising the incompatibility thesis will be one such limitation.

19.2.   PROGRAMME EVALUATION AS A MODEL OF MULTIMETHOD RESEARCH

One of the best ways to learn about multimethod research is to consider a prominent example that is highly relevant in the context of health sciences and health services research. In many cases, clinician researchers have fairly good reasons for undertaking research related to specific activities or events in their own day-to-day practice with patients. In these cases, clinicians are frequently trying to answer the question 'Did my changes make a difference to the health and lives of my patients' (or some variation of this question).

Much of the day-to-day work of clinicians involves some measure of trial-and-error. The nature of clinical work is highly focussed on interventions: clinicians actually DO something, perform an activity or intervene in a process in a specific way. This can involve everything ranging from providing education, to prescribing a medication, to suggesting a treatment or to implementing a new policy. One of the most relevant forms of research for clinicians – and for those whom they serve – is **programme evaluation research** (PE).

PE is usually described as a systematic method for identifying, collecting, analysing, interpreting and drawing conclusions from relevant data to answer questions about interventions, whether they are at the patient-specific (**micro**), groups of patients or organisational (**meso**) or societal, or governmental (**macro**) level. One of the central goals of PE is to determine if the intended effects of the intervention were achieved, to identify and determine the

consequences or unintended consequences of the intervention, and to assess the effectiveness and efficiency of the intervention itself. In short to determine if the intervention was 'worthwhile' or if it 'worked'.

This seemingly simple question – 'Did my intervention work?' – is of course an incredibly important and difficult one to answer, one that lends itself particularly well to multimethod research, given the complexity of issues that need to be considered. In particular, the importance of capturing 'unintended consequences' as part of PE means that researchers must use every tool in their research toolkit. This can help to identify such consequences and the reasons for their occurrence. To this end, programme evaluators must use a diverse array of qualitative and quantitative research methods and techniques to undertake their work.

A number of different PE models have been proposed and successfully used, and virtually all of them support or require the use of multimethod research. As we continue in this chapter, we will highlight two of the most widely used PE models: CIPP and the Kirkpatrick model. You will also find more information about these models in the Further Reading section at the end of this chapter.

19.3.   THE CIPP MODEL FOR PROGRAMME EVALUATION

CIPP is an acronym for Context, Input, Process and Product; this model was first developed in the 1960s and variations of it continue to be used extensively, particularly in the manufacturing and service sectors, where decision makers require a foundation of evidence in order to make resource allocation decisions, and for quality improvement purposes. It is very much focussed on providing decision makers with data, evidence and insights to support making difficult decisions (e.g. Do we continue to fund/support this intervention? Should we continue to do this work?).

Though various types of CIPP models exist, most of them are focussed on providing answers to the following critical questions:

a. **Context: What should we be doing?** This is an important initial question in PE and helps us to determine the specific goals, objectives and priorities for the intervention. Other questions associated with this are the following:
   • Who is the intended audience for the intervention?
   • What evidence exists to support the fact that they actually need, want and will respond positively to the intervention?
   • Why do we believe our intervention is both necessary and has a reasonable likelihood of success before we even embark upon it?

- What is the actual problem we are trying to solve with the intervention?

These are crucial questions that are sometimes overlooked, particularly because many clinicians (and politicians!) feel the need to be seen to be doing something – anything – even if there is no clear rationale for what the intervention actually is.

b. ***Input: How should we be doing this?*** The actual planning and implementation of an intervention is crucial to success: too often, interventions may be done in a well-intentioned 'wing-and-prayer' manner with little attention paid to efficiency, effectiveness or organisation. Questions associated with how we do our intervention are the following:
  - What are the actual step-by-step processes that will be used?
  - What are the resources (human, fiscal, environmental) that will be consumed?
  - Are there ways of repurposing resources so they can serve double-duty and therefore save time and money?
  - Are there more efficient ways of providing the intervention?

Paying attention to the process of implementation – not simply the intervention itself – is an important step to ensuring the intervention works as expected and is financially viable and sustainable.

c. *Process:* ***Did we actually implement the intervention as we'd hoped and planned?*** It is sometimes said that 'a great idea and two dollars (or pounds) buys you a cup of coffee': by this, it is meant that great ideas are easy to come up with and really not worth much more than a cup of coffee. In the real world, what determines success of an intervention most frequently is not the 'greatness' of the idea but the strength of the implementation process. A mediocre idea that is properly executed has more impact than a great idea championed by disorganised people. This question in the CIPP model really focusses attention on the process of translating a great idea into action and, in particular, issues related to the time, resources, attention and money that was consumed in order to bring an idea to life.

d. ***Product: Did the programme work?*** In this phase of the PE, expected and desired outcomes are compared with actual outcomes and unintended consequences. Results from this phase of the research can help decision makers determine how best to support the intervention (if at all) going forward, and can be used for quality-improvement processes.

As can be seen from these four questions of the CIPP process, there are ample opportunities for multimethod research. For example, in establishing the context and determining what we should be doing, both quantitative

(e.g. a survey of intervention preferences expressed by the target audience) and qualitative (e.g. interviews with members of the target audience to determine what they think are the best interventions to support their needs) can provide important but complementary information. Only doing a survey or only doing interviews will likely result in an incomplete picture of the needs. For time and logistics reasons, we can only perform so many interviews and thus not everyone in the target audience can be involved in the process of identifying needs. Conversely, if the researcher him/herself generates a survey of options without first consulting with members of the target audience through interviews, the survey may be incomplete as the target audience itself may have many more ideas than any researcher or clinician could generate.

The key with multimethod research is to use different methods in a complementary way and to recognise the strengths and limitations of each specific method. Where little is known about a subject (e.g. needs of a specific audience), qualitative research methods can be used to pave the way and highlight content that can then be turned into a survey, which in turn can reach far more people than an interview process could by itself. On the other hand, when surveys have been completed and initial quantitative results have been compiled, interviews with a select number of research participants can help the researcher contextualise and make sense of what the numbers in the survey are saying. This iterative approach to research is a significant strength and hallmark of multimethod research using the CIPP process.

19.4.   THE KIRKPATRICK PROGRAMME EVALUATION MODEL

'Does it work?' is a key component of the CIPP model, and in essence, the key question PE research seeks to answer. The Kirkpatrick PE model is a widely used system, particularly in the context of educational programmes. A major insight of this model is that the question 'does it work?" is multi-dimensional in nature and requires both qualitative and quantitative perspectives in order to fully determine the value of an intervention.

The Kirkpatrick model is conceptualised as a sequence of different ways of answering the question 'does it work?'. The step-wise approach highlights increasingly specific and refined perspectives on what 'success' in an intervention means. In general, one progresses up the ladder from Level 1 to Level 4 of the Kirkpatrick model rather than moving randomly across different levels. Within the PE there is an ongoing debate as to whether or not this sequential approach is required or even desired: many experienced individuals suggest it is best to 'start with the end in mind' and consequently begin their evaluation at Level 4.

The four levels of Kirkpatrick's Evaluation model are the following:

Level 1 – Reaction: Participants' subjective, emotional, unfiltered thoughts and feelings about, and experiences of, the intervention are important sources of data and critical components of establishing an answer to the question: 'did it work?' Reaction – or satisfaction – is amongst the most frequently used tool for determining the success or failure of an intervention. The belief behind this approach is that subjective, emotional connection and engagement with the intervention is a necessary precondition for higher level, cognitive outcomes. Consider, for example, your own experience as a student in a university class. If you 'like' a course, a subject or a teacher, you are more likely to be interested in paying attention to the content, doing the homework and trying to apply what was learned. 'Liking' the course is your way of reacting (subjectively and emotionally) to the intervention. In Level 1 – Reaction – the objective is to simply measure (either qualitatively or quantitatively) what these subjective emotional responses to the intervention actually are. The most common form of quantitative measurement involves surveys using Likert-type scales (see Chapter 6) and statements such as 'I found this course to be valuable' or 'I would recommend another student take this course'. This quantitative approach allows the researcher to determine the magnitude of reaction, and its extent across the audience of interest, but does not allow for in-depth exploration into questions of why the student liked the course – and why he/she did not. In this case, qualitative methods can be used to complement the quantitative measurement and in this way magnitude, extent, and reasons can all be determined using multimethod research.

Level 2 – Learning: Liking an intervention (such as a lecture) is meant to support uptake of new learning and development of new skills. However, as we all know from our own experiences of being students, sometimes we may 'like' a lecture but not really learn anything from it – we simply found it diversionary or entertaining for a period of time. Conversely, there may be many things that we subjectively and emotionally do not like (for example, memorising multiplication tables) that we go ahead and learn anyway. In Level 2 – Learning – the aim is to characterise (qualitatively and quantitatively) what increase in knowledge and skills, or change in attitudes, occurred directly as a result of the intervention. Quantitative methods for measuring learning typically involve pre- and post-testing methods. For example, for an educational intervention, a 5-question quiz may be administered to participants before they take the class: let's say the group average is 60%. After the educational intervention, the same 5-question quiz is administered and this time the group average is 90%. This represents a 50% increase in knowledge, which is suggestive of learning. To follow-up on this quantitative measurement, it may be useful to host a focus group with learners to describe what SPECIFICALLY was learned – and what was not learned. The numbers provide us with a sense of the magnitude of the change but not the specifics of what was learned; in this way, qualitative and quantitative methods can complement one another in measurement of this level of the PE.

Level 3 – Behaviour: Within the context of an educational intervention in the health care context, the goal of teaching is not to simply change thinking, but generally to actually change a behaviour. For example, if a pharmacist spends 45 minutes educating a patient on reasons to quit smoking, options for quitting smoking, then how to actually use a specific method such as nicotine patches to support quitting smoking, what the pharmacist is most interested in is that the patient indeed has quit smoking! The pharmacist of course wants the patient to like the education (Level 1 – response) and to actually have learned something new about smoking cessation options (Level 2 – learning), but if this learning does not translate into actual action (i.e. behavioural change that involves quitting smoking), the pharmacist would not consider his/her work to be successful. Remember that Serena used qualitative interviews in Chapter 16 to find out more about why people smoke and what might help them quit. Once again, both qualitative and quantitative methods can be used to determine behavioural change: questionnaires can be developed asking participants simple yes/no questions about their behaviour (i.e. 'Did you quit smoking') or more nuanced questions involving ranged answers (e.g. 'Prior to being counselled by the pharmacist, how many cigarettes did you smoke in a day: 0–5, 6–10, 11–15, 16–20+?' and 'After being counselled by the pharmacist, how many cigarettes did you smoke in a day: 0–5, 6–10, 11–15, 16–20+?'). In either case, traditional descriptive statistical methods can be used to describe behavioural change that flowed from the intervention. Again, these quantitative data are useful but incomplete – a qualitative component to this study could help the pharmacist understand what particular parts of the counselling session may have been more or less impactful, and that could be used to further refine the intervention itself. Level 3 – Behaviour focusses the PE on the desired outcome of interest.

Level 4 – Results: Particularly with respect to meso- and macro-level interventions that affect groups of patients/ organisations or society as a whole, the specific behavioural changes made by individual patients (Level 3

– Behaviour) are of interest but not necessarily the most significant issue. Instead, what may be of greater significance is the outcome (expected and unintended) and impact of the intervention. For instance, while the pharmacist might consider it a success when his/her patient quits smoking following a counselling session, the result of interest to a regional health authority, an employer or a professional association may be something broader; for example, prevention of hospitalisations or reduction in workplace absenteeism. These real-world results are of interest in understanding why the intervention was needed in the first place. In many cases, there is pressure to convert Level 4 – Results – into a monetary quantity: how much money was saved (or spent) because of the intervention? This quantitative approach, however, frequently requires some qualitative groundwork to help the researcher better understand the monetary value of '**absenteeism**' to a workplace.

Each of these four levels of the Kirkpatrick PE model contributes important and meaningful evidence about the overall success of an intervention, and each level benefits significantly from use of multimethod research. As illustrated, the value of this approach relates to the way it helps you to answer the question: 'did this work?' The complexity of this question, particularly within the context of a health care system is immense. The four levels of this model help to clarify what is meant by 'work' and using complementary qualitative and quantitative research methods to address the issue will support the generation of better data and evidence with which to make informed decisions. So, we are back to evidence-based practice again!

19.5. BRINGING MULTIMETHOD RESEARCH TOGETHER: CASE STUDY (ROSI)

To see how multimethod research methods can work and be operationalised, and how best to weave together data from different sources using different methods we will return to our case study MPharm student, Rosi Magruder. Rosi has been given some literature on using a mixed- or multimethod approach and finds this very useful. You will find the references to this work by Creswell in the Further Reading section at the end of this chapter. We will also look at how the principles of the Kirkpatrick PE model relate to the research project.

As we first met Rosi much earlier on in this textbook and haven't looked at her research since Chapter 4, we will recap who she is and what her research interests are.

Rosi is an MPharm student at the University of Fazakarly. She is in the fourth and final year of her studies and for her research project her supervisor has suggested that she and her project group (four other MPharm students) explore whether

there is a need and demand for an on-campus pharmacy to provide a service for the 22,000 students and staff that come to the institution each day, as well as those in neighbouring communities. Rosi herself has often wondered why there is no 'model pharmacy' that would allow students like her to be able to practice pharmacy in a way that they have been taught. She and her team wonder if university students and staff – who they assume to be generally healthy – actually need, want and would use a campus-based pharmacy offering the highest quality pharmaceutical care available. Rosi and her team are exploring a situation that occurs at many universities, and she wants to explore people's views rather than fixing a potential health problem that she has already identified. Although Rosi is part of a team we follow the research from her perspective.

For the MPharm project, Rosi needs to determine the optimal method of gathering these data and analysing and interpreting them. In the following section you will find the research protocol that Rosi and her team have written. In real life such a protocol would begin with a literature review that would result in a rationale for the research being conducted. As we have limited space in a textbook like this we ask that you assume that this has been done and join Rosi as she defines the aims and objectives of the project

Survey data will be analysed using descriptive statistics (please see the Data Analysis section). Focus group data will be analysed using Interpretative Phenomenological Analysis (IPA) (Smith & Etough 2006). IPA is a method of collecting and analysing qualitative data which is based on the idea that individuals are constantly trying to make sense of the world around them. They do this by interpreting events and experiences. This method will enable the researchers to make a closer examination of the use of and need for pharmacy services than could be gained from survey data alone. The process of doing IPA is a dynamic one that allows the researcher's own knowledge of the subject to be included in the interpretation.

19.5.1. Collecting Further Information

Rosi can collect information about who works and studies on campus from the university website which will provide the number of students and staff. If there is time she could also talk to someone in the university who makes decisions about what services are provided on campus. This would help to gain a fuller picture about the provision of a pharmacy and the challenges that might be faced. She could also collect information from other universities to see if any of them has an on-campus pharmacy and how that works.

19.5.2. Data Treatment

You will remember from Chapter 4 that the term 'data treatment' refers to what we are going to do with our data

1. Aims and Objectives

The primary aims and objectives of the research focus on finding out from stakeholders whether there is a need and/or demand for an on-campus pharmacy.

Aims

- To identify whether there is a need for an on-campus pharmacy
- To identify whether there is a demand for an online pharmacy
- To explore stakeholders' attitudes towards the provision of a pharmacy service

Objectives

- To describe who is on campus, e.g. job, department, age, sex, whether they have any health conditions requiring medication
- To describe what prescription medication they take including over-the-counter products
- To describe how often they visit a pharmacy off-campus and why
- To explore the views of people on campus regarding the provision of a pharmacy

2. Method

2.1. Ethical Approval

Approval for the study was received from the University of Fazakarly Faculty of Medicine and Health Sciences Research Ethics Committee on 15th April 2016 reference number: 123456A.

2.2. Introduction

A mixed-method approach (Creswell et al. 2003) will be undertaken to provide an account of the need and demand for an on-campus pharmacy. Data collection will be carried out in two phases (please see below for details of the two phases).

Quantitative and qualitative data will be collected and analysed separately. However, during the focus groups, participants will be invited to discuss some of the anonymised results from the questionnaire and provide further context and explanation of how these findings related to their experiences using a pharmacy as part of their health care. Following the analyses, the two sets of data will be triangulated before interpretation of the findings in relation to the original aims and objectives of the research. Equal priority will be given to the qualitative and quantitative data.

2.3. Phase 1: Online Survey

A quantitative online survey of the views of people who work, live and visit the university will be administered through the online survey software SurveyMonkey™.

2.3.1. Participants

We will aim to recruit up to 100 people on campus to complete the online survey. We hoped to recruit an even range of people who study, work, live and visit the university.

2.3.2. Recruitment

Permission has been sought and received from Head of Departments for the research team to place posters on their noticeboards. These will give information about the research and how to contact the research team if they are interested in finding out more. As if people contact the researchers they will be sent an email at the end of which will be a link to the SurveyMonkey™ website page. The website will open at the participant information sheet. At the end of the information sheet the potential participants will be asked if, having read the information, they would like to continue and participate in the survey. If they click 'yes' they will be taken to the beginning of the survey. If they click 'no', they were told that they could return to the participant information sheet at any time. Once participants completed the survey, final consent to take part in the study was implied if participants clicked the submit button on the online survey.

2.3.3. Withdrawal From the Study

Potential participants were told that it was up to them to decide whether or not they wanted to take part in this research. If they decided to take part, they were still free to change their mind later without giving a reason, provided this was before they submitted their response. They were told in the information sheet that their decision to participate or not would not affect their roles at the university in any way.

2.3.4. Questionnaire

An online survey will be administered using a questionnaire especially designed for the purpose. The questions in the questionnaire will be devised in consultation with the project supervisor and members of staff and students in the Department of Pharmacy. Once the draft of the questionnaire is ready three members of staff and three

Continued

students will be asked to complete the questionnaire. This pilot work will help to make sure that the right questions are asked and also establish how long the questionnaire takes to complete so that this can be indicated in the participant information.

The questionnaire used for the survey aimed to explore the following:

- Information about who is on campus, e.g. job, department, age, sex, whether they have any health conditions requiring medication
- What prescription medication they take
- What over-the-counter products they use
- How often they visit a pharmacy off-campus
- What they visit their pharmacy for
- Whether they think it would be a good idea to have a pharmacy on campus
- Why they think it would be a good idea or not

2.4. Phase 2: Focus Groups

A qualitative study will be conducted, where people who completed the survey questionnaire will be invited to participate in a focus group with others who have also completed the survey and two members of the project team. The focus groups will be conducted to further explore some of the issues associated with the provision of a pharmacy on campus that could not be gained from a questionnaire alone. Asking people to discuss some of the issues arising from the questionnaire provided a greater richness of data to inform the outcomes of the research.

2.4.1. Participants

Participants for the focus groups were selected from people who submitted a response to the online survey and expressed a wish to take part in a focus group.

2.4.2. Recruitment

At the end of the online survey questionnaire, there will be a final section inviting people to take part in a focus group. They will be asked to express their interest in finding out more about the focus groups by clicking on a link to another SurveyMonkey™ webpage where they find a

Participant Information Sheet. At the end of the information sheet they will be asked to provide their names and preferred method of contact. On receipt of the contact details of potential participants, the researchers will send each one a paper copy of the Participant Information Sheet. Participants who agree to take part in a focus group will be asked to sign a consent form immediately prior to the start of the focus group. It is planned that two focus groups will be held on campus. Each focus group would have six to eight participants so a total of between 12 and 16 people will be included. The focus groups will be held in a private room with refreshment and toilet facilities available. Purposive sampling of focus group participants will be used to ensure that the focus groups included people who were students, staff and visitors to the university. Participants' travel expenses will be reimbursed if they have to travel to and from the focus group and they will also be given a £10 shopping voucher as an expression of thanks for taking part.

2.4.5. Topics for Focus Groups

A broad list of topics to be covered in the focus groups will be developed. However, it is important that the focus group participants have the freedom to pursue areas of interest to them so the list below is a guide only:

- Tell us about what you do at the university:
  How often are you on campus?
  - How long do you spend on campus each day?
- Tell us about your current use of a pharmacy:
  How often do you go to a pharmacy?
  - Do you use the same one each time?
  - What do you use the pharmacy for?
  - How many prescriptions do you collect a month?
  - What do you buy at the pharmacy?
- Would you find it convenient if there was a pharmacy on-campus?
  - If 'Yes', why?
  - If 'No', why not?

Other topics that emerge from the survey results will also be explored.

---

once they are compiled. Rosi and her team will need to make some decisions about data analysis as early as when they are reviewing the literature concerning the topic of interest to them. Data analysis is part of the data-treatment process and how the data are analysed will depend on how they were collected in the first place. For example, if we used a questionnaire to collect data we would need to think about how the questions were asked to provide answers that

we could enter on a database. In Chapter 6 we looked in detail at how to design a questionnaire, and the specific methods used to deal with data collected in different ways can be found in Chapters 9 to 11.

It is also important to think through the statistical analyses we want to perform so that when we design the database we will use to manage the responses to say, a questionnaire, our database 'works'. This involves understanding what sort of data we have and in Chapter 4 you will find detail on how we categorise the things we want to measure to provide us with answers to our research question.

19.6. APPLYING THE KIRKPATRICK PROGRAMME EVALUATION MODEL

Rosi's research does not involve an intervention, but it is a research project that is a compulsory part of Rosi's education. For this reason we are going to shift the focus and show you how the Kirkpatrick PE model can be used to evaluate Rosi and her teammates' project as an educational experience for them:

Level 1 – Reaction: As we said earlier, participants' subjective, emotional, unfiltered thoughts, feelings and experiences about the intervention are an important source of data and a critical component of establishing the answer to the question: 'did it work?' Reaction – or satisfaction – is amongst the most frequently used tools for determining the success or failure of an intervention. Rosi and her fellow students could provide feedback to their supervisor on what the experience of doing the project was like for them. They may have formed a bond with their supervisor and liked the way he/she encouraged their learning. That emotional connection may have helped them to engage with the project's cognitive outcomes. In Level 1 – Reaction – the objective is to simply measure (either qualitatively or quantitatively) what the subjective emotional responses to the project experience (intervention) actually are. If you re-read the outline of the Kirkpatrick model in Section 19.4 you will recall that Rosi's supervisor could use a series of Likert-type scales (see Chapter 6) and statements such as 'I found this project to be valuable' or 'I would recommend another student do this research project'. Here you can see that the quantitative approach allows the supervisor to determine the strength of Rosi's reaction to the project experience, and its extent across the rest of the group but does not allow for in-depth exploration into questions of why Rosi and her colleagues liked the project – and why they did not. In this case, the supervisor could use qualitative methods to complement the quantitative measurement, for example by interviewing Rosi and her group members individually or together and in this way magnitude, extent, and reasons could all be determined using multimethod research.

Level 2 – Learning: Liking an intervention (such as a research project) is meant to support uptake of new learning and development of new skills. In Level 2 – Learning – the aim for Rosi's supervisor would be to characterise (qualitatively and quantitatively) what increase in knowledge and skills, or change in attitudes, occurred directly as a result of doing the research project. The supervisor administers a quiz to Rosi and her teammates before and after the project to see whether there was any change in their level of knowledge and understanding of research. To follow-up on this quantitative measurement, it may be useful to meet with Rosi and her teammates so that they can describe what was learned – and what was not learned and why. Again, the numbers provide us with a sense of the magnitude of the change but not the specifics of what was learned; in this way, qualitative and quantitative methods can complement one another in measurement of this level of the educational experience.

Level 3 – Behaviour: The desired behaviour in the case of Rosi would be that she went on to obtain a distinction in her project and once qualified became an excellent clinical researcher. In this case Rosi's project report results are easy enough to quantify but as to her behaviour as a researcher in the future – only time will tell. However, Rosi's supervisor could contact Rosi in a couple of years' time and ask her if she has used and/or extended the skills that she learned during the project experience. This application of knowledge could be regarded as *Level 4 – Results* – as the real-life outcome of teaching research skills to undergraduate pharmacy students becomes evident.

Multimethod research is a valuable tool for health sciences researchers and for decision makers who rely upon the evidence and insights produced through the research process. The example of PE research used in this chapter highlights the ways in which qualitative and quantitative research can complement one another. It also further reinforces the need for individual researchers to develop a broad repertoire of research skills and competencies, to allow them to function comfortably and effectively use different methods, methodologies, and paradigms. When well planned and effectively implemented, multimethod research is one of the most powerful tools available to support evidence-informed decision-making, and one of the best mechanisms for triangulation.

CHAPTER SUMMARY

- This chapter has shown that it is possible to combine different research methods in one study.
- It demonstrates the power of taking a multimethod approach.
- It has used the example of programme evaluation research to show that quantitative and qualitative methods can complement each other.

- It uses the example of our case study student, Rosi, to show how such research might be planned.

FURTHER READING

Programme Evaluation Research

Centres for Disease Control and Prevention. *Introduction to program evaluation for public health programs.* https://www.cdc.gov/eval/guide/introduction/

Mixed-Methods Research

Creswell, J. W., Fetters, M. D., & Ivankova, N. V. (2004). Designing a mixed methods study in primary care. *Annals of Family Medicine, 2*, 7–12.

Creswell, J. W., Plano Clark, V. L., Guttman, M., & Hanson, W. (2003). Advanced mixed methods research designs. In A. Tashakkori & C. Teddlie (Eds.), *Handbook on mixed methods in the behavioral and social sciences* (pp. 209–240). Thousand Oaks CA: Sage.

Research Outputs and Knowledge Translation

20.1 INTRODUCTION

For most researchers, health care or otherwise, there is a sensible and realistic (pragmatic) reason to undertake a research project. There is a problem to be solved, an improvement to be made, or an efficiency to be found, and through the application of qualitative and/or quantitative research methods, there is the expectation that the findings of research will help to make things better.

The pragmatic drive behind research is a source of considerable strength for clinician-led research, as it frequently grounds the work in a real-world, practical context that is relevant to many others. Unlike more theoretical or abstract forms of research, clinician-led research is generally focussed on immediate application. In some cases, this can lead the clinician-researcher to believe his/her work may not be as 'important' as the work of other types of researchers. Nothing could be further from the truth!

Knowledge translation is a wide-ranging term that emphasises the movement of research out of the laboratory/clinic/university/hospital – or pharmacy – and into the hands and day-to-day practice of people in other organisations who can put it to practical use. The Canadian Institutes for Health Research (CIHR) has defined knowledge translation (KT) as '*the dynamic and iterative process that includes synthesis, dissemination, exchange, and ethically-sound application of knowledge to improve the health of (the population), provide more effective health services and products, and strengthen the health care system*'. Increasingly, it is recognised that KT is just as relevant and important to clinician-researchers as it is to traditional laboratory-based researchers, and that considering what you are going to do with your research outputs is an important consideration even before you have begun your research. Indeed, it may be the reason for doing the research in the first place.

20.2. WHAT ARE 'RESEARCH OUTPUTS'?

As we have seen throughout this book, there are diverse methods for undertaking research, each of which will have context-specific advantages and disadvantages. There are also many others that we don't have space to talk about but we have provided you with plenty of Further Reading throughout this textbook. Each of these methods we have chosen for this textbook will result in production of different types of outputs, ranging from the more quantitative (e.g. descriptive statistics used to present a numerical profile of a sub-population) to the more qualitative (e.g. narratives or life histories produced through an ethnography that can be used to gain in-depth appreciation of individual's stories). Ultimately of course, the research output must be relevant to the research in order to achieve initial project goals and objectives. Importantly – especially for clinician-researchers working in health care settings – these initial project goals and objectives are likely to be fairly similar at other institutions and organisations and, consequently, the findings in one context may have applicability somewhere else. The question then becomes, what are the best ways for clinician-researchers to frame their research outputs in a manner that will be both accessible and relevant to others in different contexts?

To answer this question about research outputs, it is helpful to develop a dissemination plan for what we want to achieve from our research in tandem with other aspects of research project planning. While your research focus may be on solving your own, immediate problem, being mindful of applicability beyond the four walls of your setting can allow you to structure a dissemination plan that will support further uptake of your work by others. Four key questions should be considered as part of this dissemination strategy:

1. *What is your goal?* Why are you interested in disseminating or spreading the findings of your research? In some cases it may be altruistic, a way of giving back to your professional community, or helping to ensure others don't struggle with similar issues as you have been. In other cases, it may be more self-interested – some workplaces may reward successful research either financially or through promotions and other status enhancement. For some, the goal of disseminating research is to reorient their career in a different manner. For others, the goal may be to try to establish a broad national or international network of others with similar interests. All of these goals are legitimate and important, but the dissemination strategy for one type of goal may be different from that for another. Being clear in your own mind as to what your true goal or goals is/are is critical. For example, if your objective is to give back to your professional community you may wish to present your work at a local or national conference to peer professionals. This may not carry the same status as, for example, publishing your findings in a prestigious, high-impact, peer-reviewed journal, which may not actually be read by members of your own profession, but will be seen as impressive by your bosses and managers. Fitting your dissemination strategy to your goal – whatever that may be – requires you to first know why you want to disseminate your research.

2. *Who is your audience?* Clinician-researchers may frequently underestimate the interest others might have in their work. For most researchers exploring clinical issues, the most obvious audience for dissemination of findings is usually thought to be other clinicians or other clinician-researchers in the same profession. While this is true, it may be unnecessarily limiting, so it is worth asking yourself if other clinicians in different professions might be interested in your work. For example, it may be of interest to administrators responsible for managing clinicians. Perhaps health system authorities who oversee large and complex geographic regions of health care settings could apply your work broadly. Is your audience more local, national or international? In general, the broader and wider an audience for your work, the more impact it will have. In defining the audience for your work it is important to balance realism with idealism. Everyone wants their research to be highly respected by a diverse international audience, but the reality is that differences in language, culture, health system structure and professional context mean that it can be challenging to generalise research outputs too broadly.

3. *What's your medium?* As a researcher, it is important to recognise your own strengths and interests with respect to dissemination of your research outputs. Some individuals are very comfortable presenting verbally in front of a large audience with only PowerPoint slides to guide them. Others are more comfortable writing in an academic style. Some may prefer the systematic, orderly structure of the peer-review manuscript process, while others wish to go straight to the media (newspaper, TV). Having a clear roadmap for yourself of where you would like to target your dissemination strategy can help you to shape it in a way that is most effective for you and plays to your strengths. The other advantage of disseminating research according to your skills is that the more confident you are, the more compelling your research output will be to your audience.

4. *How are you going to do this?* A reality check for the questions listed above, it is important to realise that dissemination requires time, energy, work and a bit of talent. Manuscripts don't write themselves, presentations don't magically appear, and many others are competing for scarce airtime with the media. Balancing ambition for the spread of your work with these realities is important. Conversely, don't allow these realities to lead you to a path of least resistance in which you assume no one else will be interested and it is just all too much work anyway. In answering questions 1–3 above, you will start to achieve some clarity that will allow you to focus on the execution and implementation of your dissemination plan.

20.3. DISSEMINATING YOUR WORK IN WRITING

The most common – and in some cases the most prestigious – form of dissemination of research findings is through some form of written communication such as a formal report, a research manuscript suitable for publication, a thesis, or an article for a professional journal. Some clinician-researchers are hesitant to embark on writing-up their research outputs for a variety of reasons. In some cases, clinician-researchers don't think of themselves as writers, or find the process of writing slow and painful. In other cases, there may be a perfectionist tendency that paralyses us and prevents us from committing to our work in a public format through writing – what if we are wrong, or made an error and somebody catches on? In other cases, we may simply struggle with format and the 'culture' of publication, having never done this before.

Some tips for disseminating your work in writing include the following:

a. Know your audience: Be responsive and write in the style your target audience expects. For example, if you decide you are going to submit an article to a professional journal, use the language and jargon of the profession, not of the scientific community. Conversely, if you aim to write for a prestigious peer-reviewed journal, it may require you to 'up your game' with respect to the formal tone and vocabulary you use. It is very helpful to be familiar with the journal to which you will submit your work in advance. Read a few articles to understand the tone and structure of papers they have already accepted and published. Also, read the 'Instructions for Authors' which are usually to be found on the websites of journals. In some cases if you don't adhere to these your article will be rejected.

b. Be concise: There are very few circumstances where researchers get 'paid by the word'. Regardless of the prestige or status of a journal, it is useful to note that, from the editor's perspective, each additional unnecessary word in an article costs them money to publish. Consequently, learning to be concise and clear in your writing is essential. Many less-experienced writers may mistakenly believe using big words and jargon increases their credibility with readers (note: that preceding sentence could have been written as 'Many novice writers erroneously believe florid and pedantic writing enhances stature within the scientific community' – which sentence is clearer to you as a reader?). Get to the point with as few, well-chosen words as possible.

c. Be interesting: As the researcher, perhaps everything you have found is fascinating and important to you. Honestly, this is rarely the case! Still, it is important to recognise that not everything you have found is relevant to your audience. Finding a way to turn your findings into a compelling story which highlights important and interesting insights is essential. Don't turn your writing into a storage tank for all forms of trivia and factoids that no one else will care about. It is important to be ruthlessly self-critical and recognise that what interests you may not interest your audience. Typically, your audience will want a story that has a clear beginning, middle and end, not a random assortment of details.

d. Pay attention to formatting of your key points: Use bullet points, numbered lists or other formatting techniques that draw attention to the key points you are trying to raise. Avoid putting everything into text – readers will tend to skim large sections of text and instead focus on concise bullet points that are clearly written.

e. Pay attention to your own logic: As one who is immersed in the research and writing, it is frequently easy to forget that, for your readers, this may be the first time they have ever heard of you, learned about your work, or even thought about the issues you have raised. As a result, it is important you walk them through the process in sufficient detail so they understand the importance of your work and what you are trying to achieve. Don't assume readers have the same level of knowledge and insight as you do. Instead, highlight for them, in a logical and systematic way what you have done, why you have done it, and why it matters. It frequently helps to ask a friend or colleague who is not interested in your work but who is generally representative of your target audience, to read your work and give you feedback, to ensure logical missteps are avoided.

f. Be useful in the conclusions and recommendations you make: Help the reader know what to make of your work, in a way that is not only useful but defensible. Do not overstate the impact of your work. Overblown conclusions not only raise suspicions with readers but will result in your work being discounted by others. Be practical and clear in providing readers with the guidance they need to apply your findings in their contexts.

g. Remember, pictures are worth a thousand words! Don't overlook the value of graphic design. Using tables and figures, rather than text, to depict complex ideas or raw data can be very effective and more engaging to an audience. While, in some cases, graphics may be expensive (particularly if you must commission someone to produce them for you), this is usually an expense worth budgeting for in terms of uptake of your research by others.

Writing is by far the most common vehicle by which research outputs are disseminated. Learning to become comfortable and efficient in writing is as important a skill for researchers as any method or methodology.

20.4. VEHICLES FOR DISSEMINATING RESEARCH OUTPUTS

As we have said previously, there are a number of ways to get your research out into the public domain. Here are just a few:

20.4.1. Research Summary

In many cases, if your research is funded by an external agency, there will be a requirement to report to the funder to ensure compliance with stated initial objectives. A research summary document is frequently used as part of this report, and is simply a way of clearly and concisely summarising the key findings of a study. Typically, these are presented in the form of a three to five bullet point list for each major research objective, though this can be modified based on specific needs. The summary is also often paired with a 'Fact Sheet' or other document that helps readers understand the rationale, context and importance of the study as well as the methodology and methods that were used. In total, the fact sheet generally should not exceed one page, and it is usually preferable if graphics/visuals can be incorporated to enhance the reader's interest and impact of the work.

20.4.2.   Research Brief

A research brief is a somewhat more elaborate and detailed version of the research summary, usually aimed at professional colleagues who are likely to have more interest and more exposure to you, your work and your general area of research interest. Research briefs might be structured along the lines of a manuscript for publication, though the detail/content in each section would be considerably shortened. Typical research briefs include the following sections:

- Background/Introduction
- Literature Review/Context
- Methodology/Methods
- Findings and Discussion, and Conclusion.

   Depending upon the complexity of the project, research briefs are typically two to four pages long (single spaced) and also replete with graphics and visuals where possible to the enhance reader's interest.

20.4.3.   Study Newsletter

Particularly relevant in studies involving participants over a period of time, or in studies that have produced interest within your community, a study newsletter is a convenient way of periodically updating stakeholders on your progress, right up until the time findings and conclusions have been made. Study newsletters are useful communication vehicles and can be also used to recruit participants through the study itself. This is a particularly valuable medium where there is a need to maintain and nurture a community of researchers, participants, stakeholders, or others and keep them connected to you and to one another. The newsletter format is generally informal and closely aligned with the audience's level of scientific literacy, need, and interest. The newsletter can also be developed as part of online materials, e.g. a website associated with the research project (see Section 20.4.11).

20.4.4.   Poster

Posters are emerging as one of the most important initial vehicles by which novice researchers disseminate their work.

Posters are large-scale (e.g. typically 60" x 48") documents that are presented at conferences and meetings. The idea behind the poster is that it provides an opportunity to engage passers-by with your research. The researcher typically stands beside the poster, hands out miniature versions or abstracts, and is available to engage in informal conversation with other individuals. Depending upon the specific discipline, profession, or conference, there may be different requirements for formatting and submitting posters. In most cases, poster acceptance is an adjudicated process. Researchers submit outlines or brief abstracts of their work and, if selected, then proceed to generate the poster. Commercial software such as PowerPoint can be used to create the poster and, as most individuals don't have printing/production facilities in-house to actually print off a 60" x 48" poster, commercial printers will usually accept electronic files. It is important on posters to acknowledge funding sources and/or potential conflicts of interest, as well as the names and primary appointments/locations of collaborators and co-authors.

20.4.5.   Abstracts

Abstracts are an important tool in modern research which many researchers rely heavily on during the literature review phase, to identify potentially valuable background sources of information. Most frequently, abstracts connect directly with and are part of another form of scholarly dissemination (i.e. a poster, a paper or a presentation). However, in some cases, stand-alone abstracts can also be produced. In general, there are two formats for abstracts: structured and unstructured:

- Structured abstracts typically provide an outline of topic headings, and the researcher is expected to populate each heading with text, up to a maximum number of allowable words (usually 250–500 words). Topic headings usually include Background, Research Objective(s), Methods, Findings, Discussion and Conclusion. Depending upon the organisation, point form may be acceptable in some abstracts.
- Unstructured abstracts usually prescribe a word count and little more. It is up to the researcher to determine the best story to tell (in the number of words allowed) and what to emphasise.

   An important feature of both types of abstracts is the use of key words and phrases. Using the correct words in your abstract will facilitate others finding your work when they are using online searching tools such as Google Scholar or Medline. Each discipline, profession and journal may have standardised key word lists to reduce ambiguity and enhance 'searchability' and where these are available, they should be used in order to enhance the likelihood that your work will be retrieved when people undertake electronic searches of the literature.

20.4.6. Publications for Professional Journals

Each health profession maintains a series of journals that are aimed at practitioners in the field. Larger professions such as pharmacy have sub-specialty journals (i.e. journals aimed at niche clinicians such as hospital pharmacists or primary care pharmacists). An important route of dissemination for clinician-researchers will be their peers, the readers of these professional journals. Typically, professional journals are interested in scientific rigour and practical application, but may not be to the same high level of impact as more established peer-reviewed scientific journals. In most cases, when considering any publication, it is usually best to consider the journal with the highest impact and highest value that is a feasible option for your work as your first choice. While professional journals may be an attractive option because they are 'comfortable' to clinician-researchers, they may not have sufficient breadth and impact for some researchers who aspire to a more diverse audience. Each professional journal will publish its own 'Guidelines for Authors' which are usually accessible through the journal web page. Follow these directions closely, especially with respect to referencing and authorship requirements. It is most helpful to familiarise yourself with the most recent few editions of the journal you are interested in before you even start writing your manuscript. Most professional journals today utilise online submission systems which require you to generate an electronic account and submit your work electronically. Wherever possible, even for professional journals, consider a journal that has some form of peer-review process to enhance both the quality of your work and to establish your credibility as a researcher. Be prepared, however, for the inevitable comments and suggestions that will come from the peer-review process.

20.4.7. Publications for Scientific and Scholarly Journals

Journals that are associated with a discipline (i.e. psychology, economics) rather than a profession (i.e. pharmacy, nursing) tend to have higher impacts and more diverse audiences. Clinician-researchers will frequently dismiss the option of publication in a scientific or scholarly journal, believing they are underqualified to report in such prestigious places. This is a mistake: such journals are frequently very keen to receive high-quality work from clinician-researchers, provided of course the work is rigorous, well written and developed in a way that makes the links to the relevant discipline clear and appropriate. These journals function in a manner that is very similar to professional journals, though they may require many more peer reviews prior to acceptance, and the acceptance rate is often much lower in these journals.

Still, the benefit of publication in such journals can be significant from an impact, prestige and future opportunities perspective. These journals are usually international in their reach and will introduce your work to a highly diverse, highly skilled group of individuals, which in turn can foster development of important professional and research networks in the future.

In most cases, journals now maintain an online presence, meaning your work is accessible in a non-print format. More importantly, this online presence facilitates easy searching and finding through diverse search engines. In some cases, open-source journals place no restrictions on who may access them. In other cases, a journal subscription is required to access both print and online versions. In yet other cases, journals will require a publication fee to support costs of copy-editing and type-setting. Every journal has a different specification, and prior to submitting to a specific journal it is useful to know what they may expect from you in terms of not only your manuscript, but also additional processes and fees. Avoid the temptation of believing that all publications and all journals are good, or better than nothing. Choosing a less than reputable journal that charges you money to publish your work may be simply a way of making money, one that may not result in anyone eventually seeing your work. In particular, be cautious of unsolicited email invitations to submit your work to a journal that breathlessly trumpets its importance in the scientific world. In most cases, these journals may be more about business than about science.

20.4.8. Oral Presentations

Many conferences – both profession-specific and scientific-scholarly – provide opportunities for researchers to make oral presentations about their work. There is a wide variety of formats available for these presentations, ranging from podium presentations (in which PowerPoint slides are presented in a lecture-style format with limited audience interaction), to workshop-style presentations (highly interactive, usually focussed on acquisition of a new skill rather than simply knowledge), to panel-type discussions moderated by an expert in the field to debates. Increasingly, conference planners recognise the importance of using different, creative structures for oral presentations as a way of keeping audiences engaged and researchers involved. In most cases, a 'call for proposals' is issued several months prior to a conference, and researchers are invited to provide an outline of what they would like to do in the presentation, which in turn will be reviewed by an advisory committee before an acceptance decision is issued. Conferences represent a unique and invaluable opportunity to network with peers and learn what is on the cutting edge in your field; being successful in the competitive process of gaining acceptance to deliver an oral presentation of some sort is quite prestigious. Often, the conference will publish abstracts of oral presentations which can then be searched and retrieved by those who were not actually in attendance at the presentation itself. Increasingly, conference planners may also request your permission to videotape and archive your presentation so non-attendees can have access to it. Ensure you are clear on the intellectual property rights issues associated with agreeing to this so you retain control over your work, your research and your video depiction.

20.4.9.   Keynote Invitation Presentation

Amongst the most prestigious dissemination vehicles, an invitation to deliver a keynote lecture at a conference is considered a career highlight for many experienced researchers. The keynote is usually a highlight of any conference and one of the few opportunities during a conference where all delegates are gathered together in the same room simultaneously. Keynote presentations are often used to encourage people to actually attend a conference, and there is usually much buzz and interest in the keynote speaker. Typically, the stature of keynote speakers means that they have relatively free reign to present on whatever they wish. In some cases keynote speakers may be given additional direction but there is general recognition that by the time one gets to the stage of receiving keynote invitations, there is an established body of work and a track record of success that commands respect and admiration.

20.4.10.   Books

Books are a somewhat underutilised and forgotten type of dissemination strategy, given the significant amount of time and effort they require and the generally limited financial returns that are generated. Still, despite the advent of the 'Internet Era', books continue to be a highly prestigious and important medium for sharing your work. Typically, single research studies, or even a research programme will not provide sufficient content for an entire book; instead, a general topic area replete with both your work and the work of others in your field is necessary. In many cases, individual researchers can, however, contribute chapters to textbooks and other types of books. Such edited volumes will usually be coordinated by a senior, respected researcher in the field who will issue invitations to others to participate. The process of writing a book or a chapter can be simultaneously energising and challenging; working closely with your editor to ensure tone, content and approach are appropriate is essential. If considering writing a book, it is essential to work closely with a commissioning agent from a reputable publishing house in the field; the temptation to self-publish may be high, but the quality and reach of your final product is likely to be compromised.

20.4.11.   Web-Based/Internet-Based Dissemination

A significant vehicle for dissemination of research today involves bypassing traditional channels described above with a direct-to-consumer approach that allows anyone in the world to access your research through bespoke websites. Most researchers today have established their own web-presence which allows them to keep followers 'in the loop' of what they are doing. Technologies such as Twitter and Instagram, or self-produced webinars aimed at the public or other stakeholders, can be useful in promoting your studies to followers and building awareness of and interest in your work. While there is a legitimate place for such activities within scientific work, one must be cautious that this does not necessarily give the appearance of self-aggrandising marketing that can be quite off-putting to many potential audience members.

20.4.12.   Commissioned Policy Briefs

As you research career progresses and your research becomes better known and accepted, governmental agencies may be interested in the work. Commissioned policy briefs, in which a researcher is tasked with supporting policy and decision makers through a specifically prescribed series of research questions or tasks, are a highly impactful way of disseminating your work. These are most typically the purview of senior level, established researchers.

20.4.13.   Letter of Thanks to Study Participants and Other Stakeholders

One of the most overlooked but important dissemination strategies for your research is actually mainly about simply being polite. A short, personalised and sincere note to individuals who contributed to your research is one of the best ways to build goodwill with diverse audiences and help build interest in your work. More importantly, it is a necessary and important activity to maintain your reputation as an ethical, courteous and professional researcher.

The thirteen techniques described above don't represent a comprehensive list; researchers are becoming more and more innovative in developing and implementing creative dissemination plans that balance the need to be scientific and professional and the reality that, in today's world, marketing and some measure of restrained self-promotion are important. It is generally most useful to simply stay attuned to what researchers in your own circles appear to be doing, and what techniques appear to be most successful, and use this as a starting point for your own efforts and activities.

20.5 FROM DISSEMINATION TO KNOWLEDGE TRANSLATION

As a clinician-researcher, you are not only interested in using research to solve the day-to-day problems or issues in your practice, but in sharing your work with others in similar situations who may benefit from your work and insights. There are various barriers and facilitators to the uptake of research by others. Being mindful of knowledge translation principles and incorporating them in your dissemination plan can make it easier for other individuals to overcome some of these barriers and actually apply your work in their settings.

20.5.1 Barriers to Uptake of Research

a. Perceptions of other practitioners: Trustworthiness is crucial – arguably the single most crucial – aspect of research. There will be no uptake of any research findings unless there is implicit trust in the credibility of the researchers and what they have done. Indeed, why should someone who doesn't even know you actually trust that you did what you said you did? In part, this issue of trustworthiness can be addressed through selection of the best dissemination vehicles possible: a prestigious peer-reviewed journal, or an established international conference are some ways in which this trust issue can be mitigated substantially. Beyond these options, there are other ways to enhance trustworthiness, most of which have to do with the rigour, transparency and appropriateness of the research design itself. Clarity in strengths, limitations and generalisability of findings enhances trustworthiness.

b. Organisational culture: Most clinicians work in an organisational culture, even if that culture is that of a sole practitioner. Every culture prescribes different rules for how the work of others is perceived. In disseminating your findings, it is important to be mindful of the fact that there are diverse audiences and readers, but equally they work in diverse cultures and contexts. Clarity and specificity in how your work is relevant to these cultures and contexts will help encourage uptake of your work.

c. Lack of ability to analyse and interpret research: Overly complicated methods, findings or analysis may turn potential readers off of your work. Conversely, overly simplistic descriptions of your work may raise suspicions as to your trustworthiness. Finding the right balance is essential, and begins with clarity in the mind of the researcher as to who – exactly – the intended audience of the work should be. Generalisations (e.g. 'health care workers in England') are not helpful: instead having a specific audience in mind (e.g. 'pharmacy technicians in mid-sized non-academic hospitals') may be very helpful

in allowing you to calibrate the delivery of your research in a way that will support its uptake.

d. Information overload: One of the most significant barriers to knowledge translation is the fact that we are all bombarded with information all the time. Finding cognitive space to pay attention to one new study – your study – will be a stretch for most individuals (particularly those who have never heard of you before). Finding engaging ways to present your research (e.g. rely more on graphics and visuals rather than text or establish a context for the importance of your research to your audience from the very first paragraph) is crucial in supporting knowledge translation.

20.5.2. Facilitators to Uptake of Research

a. Ensure your research connects to the existing evidence base: Most clinicians have a belief in incremental change and development, rather than abrupt discontinuities in knowledge. Clearly establishing where your research and findings 'fit' into the existing knowledge base – rather than suggesting or implying that everything that came before you is wrong or incomplete – will increase the willingness of readers to engage with your work.

b. Strengthen the capacity of readers to understand your work: Know your audience and their needs. Don't assume they have the same level of interest, understanding or skill to interpret research as you do. Through engaging with your work, readers should learn not only about your findings and insights, but also something new and valuable about the process of research itself.

c. Collaboration: Working with other clinicians and researchers in a collaborative project is not only an important way of establishing credibility and diversifying the audiences that may be interested in your work, but also a strong social signal to consumers of your research that what you are doing is more important than a one-person shop. Collaborating across geographic regions, different practice settings, and different professions can heighten interest in your work by illustrating how the work is generalisable. Collaboration also enhances the trustworthiness of work by providing a built-in series of peer-review mechanisms throughout the research process itself.

d. Create targeted messages and dissemination strategies: Frequently, researchers may believe their dissemination and knowledge translation work is done once a paper has been published or a conference presentation has been delivered. The reality is that, once these are done, there are abundant opportunities to customise your findings for specific audience's needs. Helping specific audiences to understand how their unique situations can apply to your findings is a job best accomplished by you, the researcher. If consumers of research have to work too hard to determine how to apply your work to their needs, they are more likely to simply disconnect and walk away. If instead, you can help them with this through short communications or letters to the editor of targeted niche journals, you may build interest in your work and support knowledge translation.

e. Personal contacts: Depending on how interested you are in actually facilitating knowledge translation of your work, one of the most valuable techniques available is personal contact. Engaging one-on-one or in small group discussions with interested audiences and building personal, trusting relationships has a highly impactful effect on uptake and knowledge translation: as potential audience members get to know you, your research will take on significant new relevance for them.

20.6. EVALUATING DISSEMINATION EFFORTS

An important part of the dissemination and knowledge translation processes involves a plan to critically evaluate the success and areas for improvement of your work. As highlighted in this chapter, deliberate and strategic planning of your efforts is necessary, but it is often helpful to have some clarity around what your ultimate goal in the dissemination of your work actually is. One guiding question that may be helpful to keep firmly in mind for this evaluation is: 'What will actually change if my dissemination/knowledge translation activities are completely successful?' While complete success in this rarely (if ever) happens, having specific, measureable, relevant, timely objectives in mind to guide your evaluation will be helpful.

Ultimately, most researchers do not simply want to get their findings 'out there' and into the public domain. Rather, they are interested in having specific audiences who need their work actually act on the findings/recommendations that are made: what, then, are the kinds of actions and changes that will equate with success?

One tool that can be helpful for this is the 'Impact Log': this is an informal document that allows the researcher to actually track what has changed as a result of his/her research. Sources of information for this log can include informal observations that are made within and across the profession and practice sites, articles or papers that quote or cite the researcher's work, or email requests for information made by different audiences. Such a log is frequently a fascinating story of unintended consequences: in many cases, researchers are actually surprised by what aspects of their work gain the most traction with others and have the most impact. An impact log is a useful tool to prompt reflection about processes and methods, and can be invaluable to you as you start to plan your next research project.

20.7. A FINAL LOOK AT OUR CASE STUDIES

This is the last time we will meet our case study researchers Serena, Rosi, Dorothy and Sandy. To round off their contribution to this textbook let's have a look at how they might disseminate the findings of their research.

Serena: MPharm Student

Serena's research stemmed from her experiences of working in a community pharmacy. She became interested in smoking cessation and how some people respond well and manage to give up, whereas others just can't kick the habit. Serena's interest in this was sparked by one particular client – Mrs Olive Truelove – who had been coming into the pharmacy for years and whose health had gradually deteriorated. Some of her problems were as a direct result of smoking but she had never succeeded in giving up.

In Chapter 5 we followed Serena as she reviewed the methods of smoking cessation that have been used in health care that had a track-record of success. This enabled her to decide whether they are tools that actually have some validity – they do help people quit smoking and reliability – that they do so time and time again for a variety of patients. Out of these methods Serena thought she might be able to identify the smoking cessation methods that might work best for patients like Olive.

In Chapters 16 and 17 we followed Serena as she planned and conducted a qualitative study that involved talking to some of the pharmacy clients who smoked to find out reasons for smoking and what might help or hinder them giving up.

In Chapter 17 we gave an example of how Serena might write up the findings from interviews with three participants but she managed to interview another four and has the findings from these analysed and ready to write up.

Dissemination

Serena discusses the different ways she might get her research findings into the public domain with her supervisor and the pharmacist she works for. They realise that the

Continued

findings from Serena's interviews make really interesting reading, and might be of interest to other pharmacists involved in smoking cessation. For this reason, they decide to write an article to be submitted to a professional journal of pharmacy practice. Serena would like her work to reach people in pharmacy who would really benefit from understanding more of the reasons people find it difficult to quit smoking. More than that, if other researchers read her findings they might be able to conduct a larger-scale research project that could inform practice.

Rosi: MPharm Student

Rosi is also an MPharm student who worked on a research project with a group of other students. The project formed part of her final year assessments and was carried out under the guidance of a lecturer in pharmacy practice. The project focussed on whether there was a need or demand for a pharmacy on-campus.

In Chapter 4 we followed Rosi as she tried to set out the design of her project and as she began some of her priorities were to:

- collect information about who is on campus, e.g. job, department, age, sex and whether they have any health conditions requiring medication
- find out what prescription medication they take and what over-the-counter products they use
- explore how often people visit a pharmacy off-campus and what for
- find out if people thought it would be a good idea to have a pharmacy on-campus and whether they would use it (a key question).

We rejoined Rosi in Chapter 19 we gave an example of how she might begin to write her research protocol and set out the design of her research using a mixed-methods approach.

Rosi's research is in two phases. In the first she and her teammates designed a questionnaire which they sent out to staff, students and visitors on-campus. They then set up focus groups with some of the people who completed the questionnaire to try to find out more about their thoughts on a campus pharmacy (see Chapter 19 for full details).

Dissemination

After discussions with her project team and supervisor it is decided that the best way to get the results of their research into the public domain is to send in an abstract for a poster presentation at one of the top conferences in the United Kingdom for research in pharmacy.

The reason they chose a poster is because they can use it for part of their assessment and refine it for the conference. If the poster is accepted, their supervisor has told them that they would get funding from their department to attend the conference. This would be a great opportunity for them and look good on their CVs.

Sandy: Pharmacist Working in a GP Practice

Sandy has featured heavily in this textbook because we wanted to give an example of how a qualified health care professional can use research to further practice, in a variety of ways. The example of Sandy gave us the opportunity to show you how different research techniques combined to provide some of the tools you would need to conduct a piece of research yourself.

When we first met Sandy in Chapter 1 he was working in a GP practice as a pharmacist specialising in the care of patients with diabetes. He gradually comes to realise that the blood sugar control of some of his younger patients might not be as good as it should be, and he sets out to discover whether that is really the case. As we follow Sandy through the textbook (see Chapters 1–5, 7–11, 13 and 14) we see how he develops his rationale for a research project that could make a significant contribution to the body of knowledge about the management of the care of young people with diabetes. We eventually see how Sandy could use quantitative and qualitative methods to achieve his research aims.

Dissemination

Sandy's research turns into a really credible piece of work and reveals some interesting information about young people and not only diabetes, but also the issues involved in living with a chronic condition. Following discussions with his colleagues at the GP practice it is decided that Sandy and the GP he works most closely with will write a paper for an academic journal that specialises in research into issues of interest to those working in GP practices. The reason they choose this means of dissemination is that the journal they have targeted reaches a large number of health care professionals working in primary care. Some of the interventions that Sandy recommends as result of his work could have implications for future practice and ultimately improve care for some young people with diabetes.

Dorothy: Hospital Pharmacist Studying for a Part-Time Msc in Health System Improvement

Dorothy's interest is in the use of antibiotics in secondary care and as part of her role she would really like to

Continued

implement an anti-microbial stewardship programme. This could help save lives and money in her small community hospital. Dorothy knows that she has a big task ahead of her if she is going to win the hearts and minds of all the people involved in antibiotic prescribing and administration. Dorothy's research can be found in Chapters 6, 7, 9, 10, 13 and 15 and we follow her as she plans and revises her research design, which involves both quantitative and qualitative methods. Dorothy's research is going to take place over quite a long period of time and she will not have any results for a while.

Dissemination

The biggest problem for Dorothy has been to get support for her research from the clinicians she works with. Winning hearts and minds really has been one of the most important parts of her research so she decides to set up a website for her research. This will include the progress of the research and plenty of resources on antimicrobial stewardship programmes that are running successfully elsewhere around the world. Sharing knowledge with people in other disciplines and settings can reap rewards for Dorothy as she can find out from sharing with others what works and what doesn't. Dorothy will eventually give the link to the website to everyone at her hospital (and the wider antimicrobial community) so that they can dip in and out of it when they have time. Dorothy also plans to offer a series of presentations to hospital staff to keep them up-to-date with her research and to help maintain their interest. She won't do this too often as she runs the risk of overloading them with information.

Finally, dissemination and knowledge translation activities are an integral part of the research process, but can sometimes be overlooked given other competing demands along the way. A key aspect of this process will be the need to establish the trustworthiness of the researcher/research team, and techniques to help potential audiences for your work recognise the applicability of it to their unique needs and settings. A systematic method for this process begins with clarity around who your intended audiences are and what their specific needs may be – and then how your work can support change and improvements that are needed.

CHAPTER SUMMARY

- This chapter has defined the concept of knowledge translation.
- It has shown that not all research outputs are translated into real-life situations.

- It describes some of the most effective ways of disseminating research findings and shows how our case study students and pharmacists might choose to get their research into the public domain.

FURTHER READING

Grimshaw, J. M., Eccles, M. P., Lavis, J. N., Hill, S. J., & Squires, J. E. (2012). Knowledge translation of research findings. *Implementation Science, 7*, 50.
Open Access: https://implementationscience.biomedcentral.com/articles/10.1186/1748-5908-7-50.

21

Conclusions – For Just Getting Started

21.1. INTRODUCTION

Throughout this book, the research enterprise has been presented as a systematic process for examining a problem, situation or question from diverse perspectives. Health care professionals like pharmacists are comfortable and familiar with the importance of high-quality evidence and good research: it is the foundation of professional practice and clinical decision-making. While all clinicians recognise and respect its value and importance, many of us may feel underqualified and daunted by the prospect that we may actually have the skills to generate evidence, contribute to the literature, and become researchers ourselves. As noted throughout this book, health care professionals are in the best possible position to become researchers. The day-to-day work of any profession is where important and critical questions and problems arise and consequently professional practice itself can be amongst the most fertile grounds imaginable for research to take place and flourish. How can we overcome internal barriers (lack of self-confidence, fear of making errors) and external impediments (time, resources, managerial support) and actually start doing meaningful and valuable research?

This chapter will provide you with some ideas for how to just get started, recognising that in research (as in many facets of professional and personal life), a voyage of a thousand miles must begin with a single step.

21.2. THE FIRST STEP

You already know what the problems are, where the issues lie and why it is important for someone – anyone – to do something about them. As a clinician, a student, a health care professional – your day-to-day world is filled with situations where you will shake your head and say, 'There has to be a better way than this!'. The insights you glean from simply being observant, not ignoring the obvious cues in your environment, and being aware that there is usually something hidden behind the policies, procedures and practices we all take for granted is one of the main reasons why practitioner-led research is gaining credibility within the field. However, it is being increasingly relied upon to solve some of the most important, practical problems facing health systems around the world today.

What is the first step to getting started on your trajectory as a researcher? Simply look around you. Observe how you and your colleagues engage with each other. Take note of how you interact with patients and how they respond (or don't respond) to your suggestions. Consider the way 'we do things around here', and how your bosses and managers – and those for whom you are a boss or manager – respond to the incentives and disincentives in the workplace.

Each health care professional is at the centre of a complex web of interpersonal, inter-professional, technologically rich, procedurally intricate and policy-driven networks. As a person who simultaneously must work within these environments and enforce their rules and cultures, you are uniquely well positioned to know what the problems, issues and questions are, and you have the greatest motivation to think about how things can be improved and enhanced, both for you and for your patients. This first step in the research process is often the most interesting, frustrating and important. In some ways, it might simply be easier for you to ignore it all, just do what you are told, and not rock the boat. Many health care professionals have busy personal lives and interests outside of their work and may look at their professions as simply a way to make a living. They may not have any interest in even thinking about research, and even less interest in thinking about their environments and patients because it may interfere with the rest of their lives. This is unfortunate and as we now know based on several high-profile and catastrophic health system failures in different parts of the world (for example, the Mid Staffordshire scandal in the UK), a disengaged health care workforce that stops being interested in quality improvement and enhancing the experience of patients is the common denominator for error, lapses in judgement and ultimately problems with patient safety.

If you are not interested in your environment and your patients – who else will be? If you are not paying attention

223

to the way things work – who else will? If you are not curious and engaged in your professional practice – who else will be? Front-line practitioners who engage directly with the clinical work of their profession are the glue that holds the health care system together; they are also the first and best source of information, ideas and topics for research.

So look around. Observe, listen and be curious. This is the first most important step in the research activity – simply paying attention to what is going on around you and responding to the statement, 'There has to be a better way than this!'.

21.3.   YOU ARE THE NEXT STEP

It is common today to use the expression 'Big "R" research vs small "r" research' as a way to differentiate different types, qualities and styles of research. In this dichotomy, it is thought that big 'R' research – the sort undertaken by PhD-trained experts working in large institutions like universities or pharmaceutical companies and in interdisciplinary, multinational teams – is the real, valuable and important research that matters. In contrast, small 'r' research undertaken by non-PhD-trained clinicians is somehow less valuable or important.

While the scale of big 'R' and small 'r' research might be different, its impact and value need not be. This dichotomy may often be a form of internalized resistance or self-doubt on the part of clinician-researchers who may worry about their capacity to do research and be concerned about being seen as an imposter if they try.

An important step in your journey as a researcher is to reflect on your own internal barriers to doing research – and then identify how you can manage or overcome these to start a project. Without doubt there is a wide array of internal and external barriers to beginning a research project, many of which you can control, some of which you can't.

21.3.1.   Internal Barriers

Consider first potential internal barriers which you may have some power to manage or control. First and foremost is the question, 'Am I really qualified to do this?'. As we have seen throughout this book, and in the case study examples presented, the answer of course is 'yes'. You are qualified because you are a health care professional who sees there are problems that need to be fixed in an evidence-informed way, and for your environment and unique context, you are in the best position to use appropriate research paradigms, methodologies and methods to respond to the statement, 'There has to be a better way than this!'. While you may not have advanced research training, you have a context and background, a clear understanding of a problem, an incentive to do something about it – and, as a health care professional,

all the intellectual raw material you need to apply research principles in your environment. Along the way, you may identify gaps; for example, you may not feel confident in the application of qualitative methods, or you may doubt your ability to manage complex inferential statistics. The issue in this case is not your qualification per se but instead your capacity to learn an important required skill set in a timely fashion to actually start the research project. You could, of course, go back to your studies, take courses or complete a graduate degree. Or, you could do what real big 'R' researchers do all the time – find a collaborator who has this missing skill set and invite them to join your project. Even the most accomplished and experienced researchers know and understand their own limits and gladly seek out others to work with them when the needs of a project exceed their own capacity. Learning to accept the need for and looking for external expertise to support your project – and recognizing that you need not be a one-man or one-woman band and cannot be an expert at everything – is a crucial way of overcoming this 'Am I really qualified to do this?' internal barrier. This barrier may be amplified if you are a student and not yet a registered clinician. Remember though, your perspectives as a student put you in a unique and invaluable position from which to view problems and issues in practice. Further, as (usually) the youngest members of the profession, you have the greatest incentive to address problems now as you will be likely working for decades to come.

Another important internal barrier to getting started is simply inertia. It's frequently easier to ignore what is going on in your environment and demonstrate selective hearing or seeing so that you don't need to get 'involved' in problems. If inertia is a major barrier for you, it may be the case that starting a research project can be more beneficial than you might know. Consider the following quotation from a clinician-researcher:

'I was never one of those pharmacists who, you know, "drank the Kool-Aid" and thought pharmacy was the greatest thing ever. To me it was always just a job, nothing more. I wasn't excited to start working as a pharmacist – it was just a means to an end in terms of a paycheque. It was actually kinda sad, now that I look back on it. I would shuffle off to work, shuffle around at work, then shuffle home to repeat the next day. Sure, I thought I could do more but I'd convinced myself it wasn't worth it, nothing would ever change, what was the point? At some point though, thinking I could do more changed into thinking I actually should do more. It was after my good friend from school told me she was going back to school to do her PhD because she was bored and wanted something more. I couldn't afford

to do that but I thought – honestly, if she was doing it, I could to. I should. So…well, that was that. It had always bugged me how ineffective the patient counselling we did in the pharmacy was. The pharmacists talked but who knows what the patients heard? So I suggested we try something different, using motivational interviewing I learned at a conference. I thought it was cool, it worked well, but my managers thought it took too much time or was flaky or something. So…long story short… we did a small study, comparing me doing counselling with MI and my manager doing it her way. I used a pre-post quiz, followed up with patients at six weeks and at 3 months – and actually showed my way was better. I presented this at a local pharmacy meeting, lots of people were interested, then a local [pharmaceutical company representative] suggested I could apply to his company for some funding to expand this study, which I did and – well eventually this became a really big thing. You know I've never liked being a pharmacist more! Now I feel I have some control over my work, I've been able to prove something to my manager, I had a presentation accepted at [a national conference], worked with one of my former professors from the uni, working on a publication…wow.'

Inertia can be toxic for both personal and professional reasons. Being bored and disengaged in your job is both symptom and cause of competence drift, and something that can be – as seen in the above narrative – at least partially remedied by taking the initiative and doing something different, like focussing on improving something that has 'bugged' you in your practice.

Another internal barrier that may need to be managed is a single-minded focus on 'the answer'. Particularly in situations where you may feel bored and frustrated by your work, it is tempting to believe you already know what the problem and the solution are, so why bother even doing research? As we have seen throughout this book, the mind of the researcher is his/her most crucial asset, and a closed mind is incompatible with most research success. Willingness to admit new thoughts, ideas or data, and to take an evidence-informed approach to the research itself is crucial. This is true whether you favour qualitative, quantitative or mixed-methods paradigms and methodologies. Genuine curiosity and the ability to see and to hear everything – not just that which already conforms to your prejudgment – are required. As we have seen in this book, different research paradigms frame this in different ways: within the positivist paradigms and many quantitative methodologies, the strong emphasis on managing researcher bias (through controls such as double blinding, placebo control and randomisation) is an attempt to address this issue. Within the constructivist paradigms

and many qualitative methodologies, there is a different understanding: we cannot necessarily control or change our biases and assumptions, but we should articulate them clearly and manage our research reflexively so that consumers of the research understand the positionality of the researcher and its potential influence on questions, methods and findings.

21.3.2.   External Barriers

Beyond these internal barriers, there are the external barriers you need to manage in order to begin research. Interestingly, many of these so-called external barriers may simply be manifestations of internal resistance. Take, for example, one of the most frequently cited external barriers, 'time and money'. Clinicians sometimes say, 'I'm too busy, and besides no one is going to pay me to do this!'. There is no doubt that research takes time. In many cases it may require additional resources that cost money. Where is the novice researcher even supposed to start, given these realities?

As the excerpt above suggested, starting in a small and modest way – even if it involves only one or two participants (one of whom may even be you) – is a way of test-driving research on a small-scale, in a controlled manner that will not consume significant time nor require any additional resources. Of course, you will not be awarded a Nobel Prize for this work, but you may be surprised by the interest others will start to show in your work, and the momentum will start to build. As the pharmacist in the above case noted, after people started hearing about her work, they became interested and financial support became available – and from there a virtuous circle of success building upon success occurred. Time and money are frequently more polite ways of describing inertia and lack of self-confidence – understanding for yourself, truly and honestly, if these are external or internal barriers is essential.

21.4.   GETTING BUY-IN FOR YOUR RESEARCH FROM ABOVE – AND FROM BELOW

As we have seen throughout this book, research is often an organisational, rather than individual, process. Your research occurs within an environment and a context, and usually involves other people directly (e.g. because you interview them or ask them to complete a survey) or indirectly (e.g. because you need access to their medical histories and medication records). As a result, in almost all cases, you will need some form of permission to do your research, whether this involves formal approval from an ethics review board or simple acknowledgement from a manager that you indeed are doing something new and innovative in the practice.

In the vast majority of cases, research is not the sort of thing that is done in a stealthy way resembling espionage. For a variety of reasons related to potential power imbalances between the researcher and the researched, there are strong imperatives to conduct projects that are open, transparent, and clearly understood by all stakeholders. Even before a single datum is collected, there is preparatory work that is required that involves multiple conversations with diverse stakeholders. Whether your research requires formal ethics review approval or not is frequently a question for novice researchers: if you are in doubt, assume the answer is 'yes, I need ethics approval'. An ethics board will cheerfully let you know if they believe you don't require approval; it is generally much easier to get approval BEFORE you start a project (if you need it) than to get approval after you have already collected your data! Collaborating with a more experienced researcher from a local university or academic health sciences centre can be a useful way to manage this issue and gain a broader perspective.

Those who supervise you in your work environment should also be aware and agree to the project you are doing. This is especially important in health care settings where privacy legislation is understandably strict and protection of data is a high priority. Again, consultation with these individuals before any research begins is helpful so you don't end up running afoul of regulations or having to discard collected data because it wasn't appropriately gathered.

In practice-based research, it is sometimes easy to overlook the important contributions of your peers and those whom you supervise (directly or indirectly). Many of these people will be interested in your research and you may want to collaborate with them to facilitate your work and to distribute the workload in a more efficient manner. Remembering that in every practice environment you are actually part of a team reinforces the notion that research is a team sport, not a solitary pursuit. Engaging with your entire team at both ends of the organisational chart will not only help you with workload but will also be a very rich source of ideas that are practical and helpful in structuring your research and interpreting your findings.

As has been discussed previously, there are frequently situations where your lack of experience or expertise may warrant the development of a collaborative research relationship with a more experienced researcher. How is this actually done? In general, one should avoid simply sending an email to an experience researcher or former professor with a general question such as, 'Hey, I wanna do some research, can you help me?'. Instead, you should carefully plan an approach with a potential collaborator in a way that helps that individual answer the question, 'What's in it for me?'. Potential collaborators may be altruistic and want to support the next generation of researchers, but they are also busy people with multiple priorities and despite generosity with their time will still need an incentive. This is particularly true of biostatisticians who are often deluged with requests to provide a consultation, answer a 'quick' question, or run a small analysis, but equally applies to almost anyone acknowledged as a successful researcher.

21.4.1.   Collaboration

When approaching a potential collaborator you should plan your 'pitch' carefully:

a. Email is almost always the best, initial approach. It is less intrusive than a phone call and less time consuming than a face-to-face visit. It also gives a potential collaborator much-needed time to think and reflect upon the request, and avoids putting him/her on the spot. Your initial email should be short, to the point and really designed to pique interest in what you are doing. Simply describe – in very general terms – the problem you are trying to solve and ask for the opportunity to follow-up with a face-to-face or telephone conversation. You may also want to attach a copy of your CV or highlight some professional accomplishments to establish your credibility and trustworthiness.

b. Be informed about your collaborator: just because someone is a 'researcher' or 'professor' doesn't mean they have the skills you actually need for your project. Before contacting a potential collaborator, search them online and read some of their work. Is it actually aligned with your interests and your specific needs? Simply knowing a professor from school and liking them back then doesn't necessarily make this a 'good fit' for both of you; it should be based on complementarity of skills, knowledge and experience.

c. Know what you need – and what you have to offer: A general request such as, 'I need help to do research', is much less likely to be successful than a specific task-oriented request such as, 'I need help using the statistics package "R" to analyse and interpret data I have already collected' or 'I need help converting my observations and ideas into a specific research question before deciding if it is feasible to actually turn this into a project'. It is important to think of this as a reciprocal arrangement: you need the collaborator's help, but what are you offering in return? In some cases, collaborators may genuinely be altruistic or have, as part of their remit, the responsibility for external stakeholder engagement by working with people like you, but this is increasingly rare. Simply because someone works at a university or a research institute that is publicly funded does not mean they 'owe' it to you or the general public to support research projects. Knowing what you need – and what in turn you have to offer – will facilitate the conversation about collaboration and establish a more professional and collegial relationship.

d. Be specific: In many cases, an informal agreement to collaborate can be sufficient to confirm both parties' interests in working together, and what the terms of that collaboration can be. This is usually best transacted through email, if for no other reason than to ensure some sort of paper trail exists. Depending upon your needs and stage of evolution as a researcher, you may or may not need to consider specific issues such as: (i) intellectual property ownership – the ideas that are the core of any research project have value, who owns these and who can use them?; (ii) finances – in the event that there are expenses associated with the research, who pays for these and who accounts for them?; (iii) deliverables – what are you each expecting from one another and how will you know when each have delivered?; (iv) timelines/milestones – what are your respective expectations about the speed at which this work will be done?; and (v) expectations around authorship and credit should your work turn into a presentation, publication, abstract or other form of dissemination. There may be advantages to documenting this more formally, simply to prevent misunderstanding in the future. Further, such a document may actually help you in the event you are moving towards grant applications and external funding.

21.4.2. Making Collaboration Work

Few people enter any kind of collaborative relationship expecting it will turn pear-shaped and fall apart, yet the reality is that for a variety of reasons, this is an unfortunate reality. In some cases, parties may enter a collaborative relationship with all good intentions, but then their 'day jobs' interfere with their best intentions to work together and the relationship simply drifts apart and no research is accomplished. In other cases, fundamental disagreements and arguments may erupt leading to acrimony and discord. While of course it is important to establish a baseline relationship characterised by open communication, trust, mutual consideration and respect, it is important to move beyond words to actual actions. Small things – for example, honouring your commitments, responding to emails/phone calls from your collaborator in a timely fashion, not postponing deadlines, etc. – will send strong signals that you are indeed a collaborator. Conversely, if you notice your collaborator NOT doing these things, it may be important to address this early on and reconfirm his/her ongoing interest in the project rather than muttering under your breath, ignoring it, then acting surprised when the inevitable collapse of the relationship (and your project) occurs. Some key issues to consider in making collaboration work include the following:

a. Don't let small problems become big problems: Ignoring non-verbal signals and clues (such as unanswered phone calls) can be problematic. In many cases, behaviours such as these are a way of one party saying (without words) that they are no longer interested or able to collaborate. Open and honest communication is essential since this will be the foundation of trust that is required to allow research to proceed. Heavy-handed techniques such as a Collaborators' Contract or penalties meted out for lack of performance are rarely successful: for collaboration to work most effectively there must be trust and respect, not punishment and surveillance.

b. Manage authorship and intellectual property issues up front: Credit for your research work is generally expressed as authorship of publications. In most cases the first author is deemed to be the most important. In some research cultures, the last author is deemed to be the most senior, supervising, inspirational author. In all cases, authorship credit must be conferred for actual work completed, not simply because someone was nice to you. The relative contributions in terms of actual work (data management, analysis, writing of manuscripts) and intellectual input (idea for research, methodology or planning) should be weighted carefully to determine sequence of authorship. In most cases, it is most beneficial to assume all authors share 'joint intellectual property', that is all authors can rightfully present on behalf of the team and claim collective credit for the work. In some cases, particularly if the research results in anything that might be patentable or an innovation that is potentially profitable, this becomes much more complicated, and will likely require a lawyer's input to address.

c. Knowing how to disband the collaboration once the research is complete – or if it is simply not working as expected: This can be amongst the most challenging issues, particularly for novice researchers, to manage. Beyond recycling tropes such as, 'be honest' or 'keep open lines of communication', there are few concrete techniques that work in all situations. It is truly challenging to manage dysfunctional collaborative situations (and in many cases a true barrier to research, as many researchers are uncomfortable with this type of interpersonal dynamic). Like any issue, however, it is important to manage it as professionally and efficiently as possible, in a way that can hopefully preserve some future relationship, does not compromise your initial research objectives or ability to undertake collaboration with someone else, and ultimately does not keep you awake at night!

d. If you are working as part of a multidisciplinary team, make sure that you all have shared meanings for the language you are going to use. A meeting early on to discuss what each person means when they refer to X can help prevent problems later on.

21.5.   SOMETIMES, STUFF COSTS MONEY – GETTING FUNDING FOR YOUR RESEARCH WHEN IT IS NEEDED

Money is of course an important part of the research process, particularly when the time of qualified research personnel is needed. While it is possible to do much meaningful research on one's own time with limited need for additional resources, virtually all research consumes some financial resources, and it is important to know how to manage this reality.

21.5.1.   In-kind Contributions

Accountants use the term 'in-kind contributions' to refer to the very real cost of individuals sharing their expertise and time without receiving market-value remuneration or payment for this activity. When you ask a colleague a technical question, or request someone to review an abstract or research protocol, individuals are providing important and valuable support for research without necessarily being paid for their efforts. Most small 'r' research is funded through in-kind contributions whether we acknowledge this or not – colleagues supporting colleagues or experts mentoring novices are an important part of the research process. One way of accounting for in-kind contributions (your own and others), is to simply track the amount of time that is spent on a project, then use a defensible but arbitrary hourly wage rate to convert this into dollars. Incidental research expenses (e.g. photocopying, postage, office supplies) can also be tracked and accounted for. Overhead expenses (e.g. internet access, office space, etc.) can usually be accounted for by applying an arbitrary fixed-rate of 15–20% over and above the sum of all other research costs. Why is it important to monitor and record in-kind contributions? First, for you managers and bosses, it is a valuable way of ascribing a monetary value to work that can sometimes be thought of as invisible. Second, knowing in-kind contribution costs up front can help you to evaluate the sustainability and financial viability of what you are doing, and allows you to undertake cost–benefit analysis to define if the research is 'worth it'. Third, in the event you are considering moving your research ahead by seeking external funding, the in-kind contributions to date are your first and best source of information to start building a budget, which is a required part of any grant application.

21.5.2.   Looking for Funding

When you reach a point where in-kind contributions alone can no longer sustain a research project and other sources of funding must be considered, it is important to be aware of options that are available:

a. Release time: One of the most frequently used sources of funding for practice-based research is release time, the process by which an employer designates some proportion of an employee's time as 'protected' for research-related work. Practically, this usually means that 25–50% of a work week is allocated for research, with the employer determining best ways of backfilling within the organisation to ensure the researcher's other duties continue to be performed. This allows the research work to be done while the employer bears the costs of it through the rest of the organisation.

b. Resource sharing: Particularly in the context of research that actually consumes resources (e.g. photocopying, postage, telephone calls, courier services, etc.), the employer may simply agree to pay for these specific expenses out of day-to-day operating funds, recognising that ultimately research findings may benefit the organisation.

c. Internal funding opportunities: Large health care organisations often will have internal competitions to support promising research ideas. These competitions usually require research to submit a formal proposal that is evaluated in a blinded manner by peers and experts, with the most successful proposals being funded. Organisations such as hospitals, health care trusts and large employer groups may provide internal funding opportunities for research projects modelled upon external grant competitions as a way to spur interest in research and to support promising ideas. Many of these internal opportunities will be open to students in these organisations provided they are collaborating with others in the organisation.

d. External funding opportunities: There are an enormous variety of different private, public and family-run foundations that may be interested in supporting promising researchers and their research, and it can be frequently difficult to know or even find what opportunities may be available. Collaboration with more experienced researchers is often the single best way to learn more about these different agencies and foundations, and what they expect in terms of applications. Simply searching the Web in a strategic way can also help you to identify potential funding opportunities. It can be a challenging process to maintain your knowledge of what external funding opportunities exist and what these agencies expect, and this can frequently discourage novice researchers from even trying to secure funding through these sources. Sources for external funding include: (i) national granting agencies, such as the Medical Research Council of the United Kingdom or the National Institutes for

Health (NIH) in the United States, which use rigorous peer-review adjudication processes to rank applicants – these are highly prestigious, fiercely competitive, and virtually impossible for novice or small 'r' researchers to win due to the large number of highly qualified researchers applying each year; (ii) national or international charitable foundations such as the Easter Seals organisation or the Aga Khan Foundation, which has a specific focus on a target population (in this case, children and adults with physical disabilities) and is interested in funding research focussed on that population – such foundations also typically use rigorous peer-reviewing practices which result in highly competitive application processes; (iii) local or regional foundations, which typically have fewer resources to allocate and consequently attract fewer applicants, and which may have more flexible practices around peer-review adjudication with an emphasis on targeting specific applicants or problems; (iv) corporations (either private sector (e.g. pharmaceutical industry) or public sector (e.g. regulatory bodies) who may have very targeted and specific research questions to address, frequently framed as an RFP or 'Request for Proposal'; and (v) family foundations, which range in scale from the Bill and Melinda Gates Foundation to local philanthropists who may be interested in supporting research. This is by no means a comprehensive inventory as there are considerable variations in potential funders. Unfortunately, each organisation typically operates in a slightly different manner which means for each opportunity a 'new' grant application is required. While this can be time consuming and exhausting, with each iteration it becomes easier to learn how to pitch your research story to the unique interests of each different funder.

Experienced researchers sometimes caution novices to 'be careful what you wish for – the only thing worse than not getting a grant is actually getting one!'. Grants are not simply free money to be used however the researcher chooses; instead there are usually rigorous conditions around spending of money and strong audit and compliance requirements that ensure responsible disbursement of funds. In many ways, successful researchers end up becoming small business people who have to manage budgets, personnel, inventories and all other aspects of any other business. In some cases, this may not be an area of interest or expertise for the researcher – in which case, part of the budget should also involve a project manager/coordinator to oversee these important financial and regulatory requirements.

21.5.3. Learning to Pitch Your Research – At Whoever Might Be Interested!

Increasingly, especially in the context of funding and dissemination of findings, there is a strong element of marketing that is inherent in research. Getting other people interested in your research is not simply about the compelling nature of your questions or the strength of your ideas. Instead, researchers need to demonstrate savvy and insight in finding ways of actually manufacturing and heightening interest in the work they do, by borrowing lessons from the world of marketing. For some, the idea of 'manufacturing' interest or 'marketing' research diminishes the purity, quality and objectivity of the entire process – while this is an understandable sentiment, the reality of course is that there are too many great ideas pursuing too little funding and an ever-decreasing attention span of diverse stakeholders. As a result learning how to present your work – whether for funding or to disseminate findings – in the best possible light for each stakeholder's unique needs and wants is essential.

Some techniques that may be useful in this regard include the following:

a. Establish and maintain a digital identity: An online profile through Twitter or LinkedIn is increasingly a requirement for many researchers as a way of establishing a presence. It may be useful to consider developing a blog as a way of starting to share some of your thoughts and work and, once again, building an online profile.

b. Networking: This is an invaluable technique for novice researchers to start to connect to the broader research community, to learn about funding and dissemination opportunities, to build collaborative relationships, and to remain current in the field. Attending conferences, going to meetings, participating in web-forums and simply being present and engaged in discussions, all help to build other people's awareness of your interests and skills.

c. Share your work online: You may consider setting up your own website which may connect to other online profiles you maintain. Having a venue for dissemination of your findings that you can control may be valuable, though it is important to recognise that to the scientific community the lack of peer review controls on such a website is generally viewed negatively.

d. Seek a mentor – or become a mentor: Ultimately, research is a lifelong process of learning, and one of the best and most rewarding ways of learning is through being or becoming a mentor. The interpersonal dynamic of the mentoring relationship is not only stimulating and transformative it is also a valuable way of initiating and nurturing ideas and discussions that will further support your research.

e. Be resilient: Throughout this chapter, we have presented research as a positive, uplifting and constructive process, and at its best that is exactly what research can be. The reality, of course, is that it is never a straight upward line with a positive slope. Like all activities in life, there are hills and valleys and good days and bad days when you are doing research. Learning to be resilient, to learn from mistakes, to brush-yourself-off-and-pick-yourself-up when rejection letters from journals arrive or things don't go as expected is as critical a competency for researchers as anything else covered in this book. It is always important to take a long view and a broad perspective when doing research: things rarely move in a straight line and opportunities can come from the least expected places. During challenging periods, your social and professional networks will be more important than ever to keep you motivated, keep you grounded and help to keep you positive and looking ahead. It is not easy but the rewards for your tenacity and resilience can be many.

FINAL CONCLUSIONS

It is sometimes said that research is not so much a job as a lifestyle choice. Researchers appear to be forever condemned to always thinking, always looking, always theorising and always wondering what comes next. Researchers play an incredibly important role in society, as arbiters of evidence, knowledge and (for those of a positivist orientation) truth. This is a significant responsibility but also an important opportunity for those who recognise its value.

Often, with research, the first step is the most difficult: overcoming our own internal barriers of self-confidence or inertia is neither simple nor quick. The first step in becoming a researcher is to understand yourself, your environment, and how you are uniquely well positioned to respond to important questions like, 'Surely we can do better than this, can't we?'

Research is simultaneously filled with opportunities and responsibilities, costs and benefits, joys and heartaches, and it can be difficult at times to manage all these contradictions – and to function in new paradigms, work within uncomfortable methodologies, and learn about new methods. Investing in this is investing in yourself and your future. It is an immense learning curve but one that has benefits for you as an individual, the patients you serve, the health care system in which you work and the society in which you live.

Absenteeism   The practice of regularly staying away from work or school without good reason

Adherence   Attachment or commitment to a person, cause or belief. In terms of medicines use this refers to whether or not people take their medicines as directed by a health care professional

Anecdotal   Not necessarily true or reliable, because information is based on personal accounts rather than facts or research

Artefacts   Something observed in a scientific investigation or experiment that is not naturally present but occurs as a result of the preparative or investigative procedure

Assessment tool   Something used to test human behavior, e.g. a questionnaire

Authenticity   The property of being genuine

Bias   Inclination or prejudice for or against one person or group or idea, especially in a way considered to be unfair or incorrect

Binomial theory   A mathematical expression stating that $(a+b)^n$ may be expanded to the sum of products (e.g. $(a+b)^2 = a^2 + 2ab + b^2$)

Bivariate   Two-way

Black sheep effect   In psychology, the black sheep effect refers to the tendency of group members to judge likeable ingroup members more positively and deviant ingroup member more negatively than comparable outgroup members

Blinding   The process of ensuring that participants, practitioners or researchers do not know which participants have been assigned to experimental conditions

Cascading   Flowing from one thing or person to another

Cerebro-vascular accident (CVA)   Stroke

Compliance   The extent to which a patient sticks to the instructions they have been given regarding their treatment. Now largely replaced with the term 'adherence'

Concordant   In health care this refers to a two-way relationship based on mutually understanding

Convenience sample   A group of research participants selected because they are available

Cost-effective   Value for money

Comorbidities   More than one health conditions that exist in the same person

Comparative study   A research study where one thing is compared to another

Content analysis   A means of analysing the written word by counting the number of times words or phrases appear

Correlation   A mutual relationship or connection between two or more things

Covertly   In secret; without being seen

Cultural anthropology   Cultural anthropology is a branch of anthropology focused on the study of cultural variation among humans

Dependent variables   A variable that is the event that is expected to change when the independent variable is manipulated

Descriptive statistics   A quantitative method for describing or summarising the key features of a collected set of data or information

Dichotomous   Able to be divided into two distinct parts or categories

Discrete   Individual, separate and distinct

Disease progression   Generally described as the worsening of a condition or disease over time, and used as a way of determining therapy options and prognosis

Dispersion   A measurement of how values of a variable differ from a fixed point such as the mean

Double-barrelled   Having two parts

Dyad   Consisting of two elements or parts

Efficacy   The ability to produce an intended or desired outcome or result

Empiricism   The belief that all knowledge is initially derived from sensory input and experiences; the basis for experimental science

English language literacy   The ability to read, write and understand English

Ethnography   A systematic and scientific description of the customs, behaviours and traditions of individual peoples or cultures

Exemplars   Serving as a typical positive or excellent example or model

Exclusion criteria   Individual characteristics that would disqualify a potential subject from being included in a study

Face validity   The extent to which a test is subjectively viewed (especially by test-takers) as actually covering the concepts it claims to be measuring; a way of describing the relevance and transparency of a test

Field notes   A method of recording thoughts, observations and anecdotes about a specific phenomenon during or after scientific research

Field research   Collection of data outside a controlled setting (such as a laboratory or library) in the "real world"

Format   The ways in which elements of a set are arranged

Frequency   A mathematical ratio expressing the number of actual to possible occurrences of an event

Grounded theory   A research methodology that uses the analysis of data to construct theory, rather than using theory to guide analysis of data

Group cohesion   The tendency for members or units within a collection to remain united and work towards a common objective or goal

HbA1c   Glycated hemoglobin, a form that is measured to identify average plasma glucose concentration over a period of time

Heisenberg Uncertainty Principle   A way of describing the fundamental limit to of precision with which variables can be simultaneously known; initially described in the context of subatomic particles, stating it is not possible to precisely know both the position and the momentum of a particle

Heterogeneity   Being diverse in description, character and content

Heterogeneous   Diverse in description, character and content

'H' factor   A regulatory protein that inhibits alternative pathway for complement activation

Homogeneity   Being the same or substantially similar, or all of the same kind

Hypothesis   A proposed explanation based on limited available data or evidence, used as a starting point for further subsequent investigation

Impact factor   A measure used by academic journals to describe the average number of citations to articles published in that journal; used to indirectly describe the extent of influence and impact a journal has on the scientific community

Inclusion criteria   Characteristics that prospective study participants must have to be included in a study

Independent variables   A variable (usually denoted by "x") that does not depend on another

Indicativeness   A description of the extent to which a data sample represents or is illustrative of the population as a whole

Inferential statistics   The use of mathematical analysis to deduce properties and underlying probabilities within a data set

Informed consent   Permission granted with full knowledge of possible consequences

Intention to treat (ITT) analysis   A form of data analysis that is based on the initial treatment assignment, not on the treatment which may have been eventually received. Designed to avoid issues related to non-random drop-out of participants from the study or crossover groups

Inter-   Between different but related groups

Interpretative phenomenological analysis   A form of qualitative research which aims to provide understanding into how a given person, in a specific situation, makes sense of a phenomenon of interest

Interval   Space between two points

Intervention   The act of intervening or interfering with a naturally occurring system or process

Interview schedule   A pre-established guiding list of questions used in qualitative research to enhance reliability of interviews

Intra-   Within a group

Knowledge translation   An umbrella term used to describe a variety of activities all aimed at moving research into the hands of individuals and organizations who can put it to actual, practical use

Latent variables   Variables that are not directly observed but instead must be inferred from other variables that can be directly measured

Level of probability   The p-value is used to describe the smallest level of significance at which the null hypothesis would be rejected

Linear regression model   A statistical tool most frequently used for prediction or forecasting, involving modeling of a relationship between a dependent variable (y) and an independent variable (x)

Logistics   Coordination of a complex operation involving many different elements

Longitudinal   Measurements over a period of time

Macro   At the largest scale or level

Matched sampling   Two different samples which are similar – or match – based on specific characteristics

Mean   The arithmetic average of a data set

Measurement tools   Description of a variety of different instruments used to count quantitative data

Median   The middle point in a data set

Meso   At the middle scale or level

Method   A systematic process for accomplishing an objective

Methodology   A system or set of processes (or methods), or a body or practices that informs the work within a discipline

Micro   At the smallest scale or level

Mixed-method   A methodology for research that involves integration of qualitative and quantitative research methods within a single study

Mode   The most frequently occurring element within a data set

Multimethod   The use of more than one method within a study or a group of related studies

Multivariate   Involving two or more variables

Nominal data   Discrete data that belongs to a definable category, differentiated by simple name without reference to qualities or preferences

Non-directional hypothesis   An alternative hypothesis which states that the null hypothesis is wrong; it does not predict whether the parameter of interest is smaller or larger than the reference value specified in the null hypothesis

Non-linear regression model   A form of regression model in which the dependent variables are modeled as a non-linear function; data are fitted by a method of successive approximations

Non-parametric   Not involving any assumptions as to the form of a frequency distribution

Normal distribution   A statistical depiction of the distribution of variables as a symmetrical, bell-shaped graph

Normal theory   A theory predicting that at the population level normal distribution will occur

Observer bias   Influence of researcher's cognitive biases in a way that subconsciously influences participants in research

Observer-expectancy effect   See *Observer bias*

Observer participant   A model of research in which the researcher is also simultaneously an active part of the group being studied

One-tailed t-test   A statistical test in which the critical area of distribution is one sided; that is it is either greater than or less than a certain value, but not both

Open-ended question   A type of question that allows the respondent great scope in providing information and that cannot be answered with a simple yes or no response

Ordinal Numerical scores that exist on an arbitrary numerical scale where specific number values have no significance beyond simply establishing a ranking over a set of data points

Outlier Any data point that is very much bigger, smaller or in some other way anomalous than the next nearest data point

Parametric A type of statistic that assumes sample data derives from a population that follows a probability distribution based on a fixed set of parameters

Participant observer See *Observer participant*

Pearson's chi-square test A statistical test applied to categorical data to evaluate likelihood that observed differences arose by chance

Pharmacokinetics The study of movement of drugs within the body – "What the body does to a drug"

Phenomenology A philosophy that concentrates on the study of consciousness and the objects of direct experience

PICO An acronym within evidence-based medicine that reminds clinicians to consider Patients, Interventions, Comparisons and Outcomes in evaluating quality and clinical applicability of published studies

Pilot study A small-scale, preliminary investigation that allows research to better understand how to design and implement a larger scale study

Pilot testing A method for preliminary evaluation of the quality and applicability of a measurement instrument and suitability for inclusion in a larger study

Population A finite collection of items or individuals that is under consideration and the interest of the researcher

Positivist A theory that knowledge is based on sensory experience interpreted through reason and logic

Power The probability that a statistical test will reject a false null hypothesis; it is inversely related to the probability of making a Type II error (beta)

Predictive validity In psychometrics, the extent to which a score on a test is correlated with a measurement on some other related criterion

Probability sampling A sampling method that uses some form of random selection that assures that different individuals within a population all have equal probability of being selected

Programme evaluation research Use of systematic research methods to assess the value, impact, outcomes, and responses to education or social programs or interventions

Proxy A substitute or alternative

Purposive sampling A non-probability/non-random sample selected based on desired characteristics of a population aligned with the objective of a study

Quantitative results Numerical data

Quasi-experimental design An empirical study without random selection; it shares similarities with randomized controlled trials but lacks the element of random assignment to treatment or control groups

Quota sampling A sampling technique that requires individual participants to be chosen from specifically defined population subgroups

Random error Measurement errors caused by factors that vary from one time or measurement to another time or measurement

Random sampling A sampling method in which each participant has an equal chance or probability of being selected to participate in the study

Randomisation A method used to generate a random allocation sequence for assigning subjects to treatment or control groups within a study

Range The difference between the largest and smallest value in a quantitative data set

Ratio data Interval data with a natural zero point; for example "time" since 0 in time has meaning.

Ratio scale Measuring data in a manner that allows for comparison of different values and to state differences between these values in the form of a ratio

Research output The results, findings, synthesis, and conclusions associated with a research project

Research protocol A detailed description of a study's methods and methodologies

Recruitment strategy The approach that the researcher will take to involving participants in the study

Red flag Warning indicator for potential danger or threat

Reflexivity The process of continuously examining oneself as a researcher and the researcher-participant relationship during qualitative research work

Reliability The consistency or reproducibility of measurement

Repeated measures design Use of the same subjects in all stages of research, including as part of the control group

Replicability Ability of other researchers to follow a research protocol and arrive at substantially similar outcomes and findings

Representative sampling A small subset of a population that accurately reflects characteristics of the larger group

Reproducibility Ability to copy or replicate

Respondents An individual who supplies information for a survey or questionnaire

Retrospective Looking back or examining past events and situations

Retrospective chart audit Research method involving analysis of completed clinical/medical records using structured criteria in a systematic manner to address research objectives

Riffing Improvising or building upon improvisation of others

Sampling bias Sampling in a way where some members of a target population are less likely to be included than others

Sampling error When a sample does not include all members of a population, statistical characteristics of that population may be mistaken or mis-estimated

Scientific Based on, using or characterized by the methods and principles of science; systematic, methodical, reproducible, defensible

Snowballing technique Also known as chain sampling or referral sampling, a non-probability sampling technique in which current study subjects are used to recruit future study subjects amongst their networks of friends and acquaintances

Social psychology   Branch of psychology interested in social interactions and their effects on individuals

Sociology   The study of the development, structure and function of human society

Sphygmomanometer   An instrument used to measure blood pressure

Spread   Also called dispersion, a measure of the extent to which items in a data set are scattered; common measures include standard deviation and variance

Standard deviation   A measurement of spread, used to indicate extent of deviation from the group as a whol

Statistical significance   Occurs when the observed p-value of a test statistic is less than the significance level defined for the study

Stratification   See *Stratified sampling*

Stratified sampling   Division of the population into separate groups (called strata) followed by a simple random sample drawn from each sub-group

Surrogate outcome   Also known as surrogate marker, aims to predict a clinical outcome or prognosis

Symbolic interactionist   A view of social behaviour emphasizing language and gestures as forms of communication and their subjective meanings and understanding, especially their role in the formation of children as social beings

Synthesis   Combining ideas and data to form a theory, hypothesis or explanation

Systematic error   Any error in which the mean is not zero, indicating that its effect will not be reduced when results of measurements or observations are averaged

t-test   A statistical test of whether a sample comes from a larger sample with a standard or normal distribution of statistical properties

Target population   The entire group of individuals to which researchers are interested in generalizing or applying conclusions

The Hawthorne Effect   Alteration of behaviour by subjects in a study due to their awareness of being observed by a researcher

Training   Teaching a person a particular skill or type of behaviour

Treatments   Medical, health or social care given to an individual

Triangulation   Use of two or more methods within a study in sequence to check and verify results

Trustworthiness   The ability to be relied upon as honest, accurate and truthful

Two-tailed t-test   A statistical test used to examine both sides of a data range to determine whether the null hypothesis is accepted or fails

Univariate   Involving one variable

Validity   Psychometric description of the extent to which a concept or measurement accurately corresponds to real-world experience

Vancomycin   Antibiotic used most frequently against resistant strains of streptococcus and staphylococcus

Variables   An attribute of a study object/person of interest that is capable of changing or varying within a group of objects/persons

Page numbers followed by "*f*" indicate figures, "*t*" indicate tables, and "*b*" indicate boxes.